The Fit and
Healthy Dancer

The Fit and Healthy Dancer

YIANNIS KOUTEDAKIS
School of Health Sciences, Wolverhampton University, UK

and

N. C. CRAIG SHARP
Department of Sport Sciences, Brunel University, Middlesex, UK

With contributions from

Colin Boreham, *Sport and Leisure Studies, University of Ulster, UK*
Ray Carson, *School of Health Sciences, Wolverhampton University, UK*
Paul Pacy, *Royal Free Hospital, London, UK*
Roger Wolman, *Royal National Orthopaedic Hospital, Stanmore, UK*
Susie Dinan, *Royal Free Hospital, London, UK*

JOHN WILEY & SONS
Chichester · New York · Weinheim · Brisbane · Singapore · Toronto

Other Wiley Editorial Offices

John Wiley & Sons. Inc., 605 Third Avenue,
New York, NY 10158-0012, USA

WILEY-VCH Verlag GmbH, Pappelallee 3,
D-69469 Weinheim, Germany

Jacaranda Wiley Ltd, 33 Park Road, Milton
Queensland 4064, Australia

John Wiley & Sons (Asia) Pte Ltd, Clementi Loop #02-01,
Jin Xing Distripark, Singapore 129809

John Wiley & Sons (Canada) Ltd, 22 Worcester Road,
Rexdale, Ontario M9W 1L1, Canada

Library of Congress Cataloging-in-Publication Data

Koutedakis, Yiannis.
    The fit and healthy dancer/Yiannis Koutedakis and N. C. Craig
Sharp, with contributions from Colin Boreham ... [et al.].
        p. cm.
    Includes bibliographical references and index.
    ISBN 0-471-97528-1 (alk. paper)
    1. Dancers–Health and hygiene.   I. Sharp, N. C. Craig.
II. Boreham, Colin.   III. Title.
RC1220.D35K68   1999
613.7′088′7928–dc21   98-30336
                                                            CIP

British Library Cataloguing in Publication Data

A catalogue record for this book is available from the British Library

ISBN 0 471 97528 1

Typeset in 10/12pt Palatino by Keytec Typesetting Ltd, Bridport, Dorset.
Printed and bound by Antony Rowe Ltd, Eastbourne
This book is printed on acid-free paper responsibly manufactured from sustainable forestry,
in which at least two trees are planted for each one used for paper production.

Dedications

Y. Koutedakis: To My Wife Fani and To My Sons
Romanos and Minos.

Craig Sharp: To the memory of My Mother Sheila;
A Swing Dancer of the 20's. And to the Creative
and Inspirational Students of Drama and Dance of
the University of Birmingham (Including Jean Butler
of Riverdance) to Whom I have been Privileged to
Teach Physiology over the Past 27 Years.

'There are two kinds of truth: the truth that lights the way, and the
truth that warms the heart. The first of these is science, and the second
is art. Neither is independent of the other or more important than the
other. Without art, science would be as useless as a pair of high
forceps in the hands of a plumber. Without science, art would become
a crude mess of folklore and emotional quackery. The truth of art
keeps science from becoming inhuman, and the truth of science keeps
art from becoming ridiculous.'

From: *The Notebooks of Raymond Chandler*, Ecco Press, NY, 1938, p. 7.

Quoted in 'Nature', Ficher E.P., 390: p. 330, 1997.

Contents

Bibliographies of Editors and Authors

Dr Yiannis (John) Koutedakis is Senior Lecturer at Wolverhampton University, UK, and Thessaly University, Greece. He has attended many Dance Festivals, World Sport Championships and Olympic Games as dancer, competitor, national coach, and scientific advisor. He is one of the founders of the British Olympic Medical Centre, and has worked with many Olympic squads, dance companies and dance schools. His research interests focus on the effects of fitness upon physical performance. He has published widely in English, Greek, Italian, and French.

Dr N. C. Craig Sharp graduated in Veterinary Medicine from Glasgow University, and worked in practice before joining the physiology department of the Glasgow Vet School, under Dr (later Sir) James Black, Nobel Laureate, later transferring to the Department of Experimental Medicine there. In 1971 he joined the Birmingham University Department of Physical Education and Sports Science, and was founder co-director of their human motor performance laboratory. He has been selected for four Olympic Games as coach or physiologist, and has been variously an international competitor, trainer, coach, team manager and team selector. He was co-founder of, and director of physiological services at the British Olympic Medical Centre, and is currently Professor of Sports Science at Brunel University, adjunct Professor of Sports Science at the University of Limerick, Ireland, and Honorary Professor of Sports Science at the University of Stirling.

Contributors

Dr Colin Boreham is Professor of Sport and Exercise Sciences at the University of Ulster in Northern Ireland. He has research interests in the effects of exercise upon the health of young people, and has published widely in the field. He is also interested in performance sport, having represented Great Britain and Northern Ireland in the Decathlon alongside Daley Thompson at the 1984 Los Angeles Olympics. He is married with three children and lives near Belfast.

Dr Ray Carson is currently Senior Lecturer in the Division of Biomedical Sciences at the University of Wolverhampton and teaches exercise physiology, human physiology and pharmacology. Previously he carried out research on lung physiology at the Royal Postgraduate Medical School and the London School of Hygiene and Tropical Medicine. His research interests include asthma and physiological responses to exercise, and he has published extensively in the field.

Susie Dinan is a Clinical Exercise Practitioner at the University Department of Geriatric Medicine, Royal Free Hospital Medical School, London, and the Wandsworth Community Team. She developed and delivers the RSA YMCA Exercise to Music and YMCA Fitness Training for the Older Person Modules, is co-author with Prof. Craig Sharp of Age Concern's 'Fitness for Life' book, and in 1994 was winner of the Exercise Association of England's Special Achievement Award. Susie was a former professional dancer and founder of the first Healthier Dance Medical Panel.

Dr Paul Pacy is a Consultant of Diabetes and Endocrinology at the Royal Free Hospital in London. Paul Pacy qualified from St George's Hospital Medical School in 1976 and after a conventional career in medicine in the UK and Canada began nutritional research for his MD in 1981. He worked for the Medical Research Council for 6 years during which time he obtained a PhD for work on insulin and protein metabolism. He also worked as a Senior Lecturer in Clinical Nutrition at the London School of Hygiene and Tropical Medicine. His research interests include energy expenditure, body composition, and regulation of protein metabolism.

Dr Roger Wolman is a Consultant in Sports Medicine and Rheumatology at the Royal National Orthopaedic Hospital in London. He is also the medical officer to several dance companies including Ballet Rambert and Riverdance and to the British Olympic Medical Centre. His main research interest is on Amenorrhoea and Osteoporosis in dancers and female athletes. He is the author of numerous scientific reports.

Foreword by Sir Peter Wright

In recent years a considerable amount of research has been carried out regarding the health of dancers and this has led to the conclusion that many of them are not as fit and healthy as they could be. Following on from that research this extraordinarily comprehensive reference book has now emerged that deals with the many problems, both physical and psychological, that face dancers from their early training days right through their performing years to the difficult times that come later when they retire from performing, usually at the relatively early age of about forty. It also looks at ways in which dancers can make better use of their bodies and how they can acquire more strength, power, stamina and resistance to injury and thus cope far better with the rigours of this very demanding and arduos profession.

This collaboration between Yiannis Koutedakis, with his great knowledge of both Dance and Fitness, and N.C. Craig Sharp, so highly respected as one of the foremost authorities on Sport, has resulted in an enlightening book which, for the first time looks at dancers not only as performing artists but also as performing athletes. This opens up whole new possible approaches to their training and healthcare, whereby they can benefit greatly from the training methods employed so successfully by athletes, and all the medical research that has gone into that training.

Every human being is of course different, both physically and mentally, and although some dancers can sail through their careers with very little adverse effect caused by the often unnatural and sometimes dangerous demands made on them, many are faced with chronic injuries, weight problems, stress fractures, nervous disorders, breathing problems, athritis and countless other problems that plague and hamper their short careers. This book points to ways of avoiding and preventing these setbacks and gives a very clear insight into the complexities of the human body and its miraculous functions. Added to this the excellent glossary, this ensures that all the terminology can be easily understood.

The demands made on dancers have increased enormously in recent years but training methods are slow to keep up with these developments and there is much in this book to spark off some new ideas, especially regarding increased power and stamina and the reduction in wear and tear of certain parts of the body. After all, the work of dancers today embraces not only the art of communicating the joy and aesthetics of movement executed in perfect harmony and style, the power to express ideas and emotions through movement and musicality and the effortless display of technical virtuosity, but also these days a far more athletic and often acrobatic approach to movement is required which choreographers are insisting on more and more as a result of the increased cross fertilisation between classical ballet and contemporary dance.

This book will be invaluable to teachers whose responsibility it is to make sure that the dancers of the future are properly prepared to meet these demands. Good dancers are the result of inspired and enlightened teaching which should maximise their students potential, but it is vital that this training goes hand in hand with the knowledge of how to look after their God-given instruments—the Human Body. Talent, good proportions, musicality, strength and many other gifts also go to making a good dancer, but without good health these will be wasted. The time has come to put the record straight and take advantage of all the knowledge contained in this book to ensure that our dancers are fitter and healthier in the future.

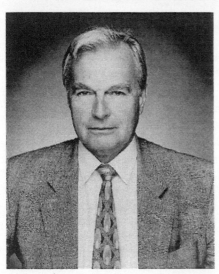

Sir Peter Wright, CBE.
Director Laureate,
Birmingham Royal Ballet.

Sir Peter Wright
(Photo by © Bill Cooper)

Foreword by Cynthia Harvey

American Ballet Theatre in the late 1970's was an exciting place to be. Guest artists flocked to dance with the company, and for me, a young dancer in her late teens, the roster and repertoire proved heady and awe inspiring. You can appreciate the surprise moreover, the sense of incredulity when one afternoon as I was warming up for a rehearsal, Rudolph Nureyev came up to me and said in a wistful tone, 'I wish I knew as much about dance and the body as you do when I was your age'. I understood what he meant. It was by no means simply a compliment and I felt it my duty to continue the process of education so that I would have no regrets during my career. That was over 20 years ago, and I was fortunate to have had a long career. It was not however, injury free. Most of my injuries were stress related with a couple of exceptions. It would be nice if I could say that I was virtuous because I knew about body conditioning excercises and practised them with my trainer diligently. As productive as that is, I can say to a young dancer today, that I too wish I knew what they now know, due to their good fortune in having access to intelligence such as that available in this book. Because of the reports made by Dance UK, it has been established that dancers are not always as healthy as they could be. The Fit and Healthy Dancer is not a 'how to' book filled with technical prose that is difficult and uninteresting to read. Yiannis Koutedakis and Craig Sharp have written a very comprehensive and informative book that delves into some of the reasons behind dance injuries and also provides the student reader or dance professional with an understanding of methods to improve the standard of fitness and eliminate some unnecessary dance injuries.

Dr Koutedakis and Professor Sharp have done extensive research into the topics that are of interest to the dancer; anorexia, performance anxiety and how nerves affect the body, optimum nutrition to achieve optimum performance levels, and information on the ageing dancer in society today. We learn that there are reasons why some physiques are more suitable to dance due to the muscle fibre content/type. We are informed of the voluntary control on the Autonomic System and the explanations provided give us the evidence to be able to answer so many of the questions that plague us during our performing career. There are also factors for which we do not have control, and these too are explained. No longer is it a mystery as to why there appears to be soreness following a performance, when the same activity during a rehearsal may seem to have little or no effect. There is also a formal study extoling the virtues of rest!

There are so many topics in this book that arouse my interest. No matter how informed you perceive yourself to be, The Fit and Healthy Dancer will clarify issues that you may have struggled with, but now, armed with knowledge and understanding, you are empowered.

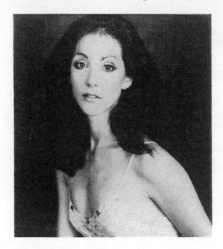

Cynthia Harvey

Cynthia Harvey
(Photo by Paul B. Goade)

Preface

We have been professionally involved with dance for many years. Yiannis was a dancer and a dance-teacher in the 70s and 80s, while Craig, the son of a swing dancer on the London stage in the 20s, was brought up on the legends of Pavlova and Nijinsky, although his later idols were Ulanova, Fonteyn and Nureyev. He first worked with dancers the Blue-bell Girls at the Glasgow Alhambra in the early 60s by measuring the astonishingly high pulse rates, immediately following their on-stage routines, and he discussed the physical side of training with members of the Bolshoi and Kirov Ballet Companies in the early 80s during a sports science visit to Moscow and (then) Leningrad. However, until recent years it did not seriously cross our minds that dance would also generate academic, research and scientific interests. In line with most others, we thought that dance was about technique, style and (especially) tradition. Meanwhile, sports science—together with sports medicine—were working hard to accumulate practical knowledge on performance-related issues such as *muscle function, cardiovascular* and *respiratory efficiency, diet, 'burnout'* or *overtraining, overuse injuries* and *osteoporosis.*

The outcome of this knowledge explosion is well known. Sports with history and tradition deeply rooted in classical Greece and beyond, eventually dismissed rhetoric such as 'this is how it has always been done', 'it worked for me; so, it will work for you' and 'no pain, no gain' by infusing preparation and training regimens with more objective methods. Scientific screening from physiology, biomechanics and psychology became the 'independent advisor' for the elite athlete and effective injury-prevention strategies were employed. All these resulted in increased performances, increased audiences, and better financial rewards. Indeed, most authorities agree that the last 25 years have been the *golden age* of sports, even though the appearance of illegal performance-enhancement substances have increasingly contaminated the spirit of sport. It was as part of these changes, that we were employed by the British Olympic Association to set-up and run the first ever dedicated service for the elite athlete in the UK. The result was the birth of the British Olympic Medical Centre, London.

The Centre was not only a place for sport-excellence. It was also the venue where an advanced contact with the science of dance was made, thanks to our then colleague Dr Roger Wolman (now Consultant at the Stanmore Royal National Orthopaedic Hospital and contributor in this book). Roger conducted a novel research project on osteoporosis using rowers, runners and dancers as volunteers. Although we were only involved in the assessment of a few of those volunteers, we realised that the dancers' impressive physicality was perhaps more the product of specialised selection procedures (via auditions) than the result of well designed fitness programmes. This was later partly confirmed by Dr Wolman's research findings, that the less fit dancers demonstrated the least bone density—thus being more likely to develop osteoporosis— compared to runners or rowers.

We also realised that many dancers seem not wholly to treat their body as the main instrument for their art. And if they did, they had relatively little idea of how it worked before, during, and after practice. They were happy discussing aspects related to history of dance and the usefulness of various teaching methods and techniques—with some of these developing a cult following!—but they had little scientifically based answers as to why one method is superior to another. In addition, (some) dancers and their teachers had the impression that they were quite different to athletes, yet both dancers and athletes have the same anatomy and physiological functions. Skeletal muscle and the heart, for instance, have no idea whether you dance, run or row!

The prospect of the application of physiology and movement science to dance promises to enhance not only performance, but also safety. This has been at least the case in sport. The scientific analysis of nutrition, strength, and cardiovascular demands of elite athletes has increased our understanding of the stresses placed upon the body in a great variety of sports, and in so doing has improved training techniques, enhanced performance, and helped to decrease the incidence of injuries. The application of these scientific analysis techniques to dance may reap similar benefits. The principle aim of this book therefore, is to contribute to the relevant body of knowledge, by attempting to answer the question '*how is the science of exercise of practical importance to the dance profession*?'

To achieve the set aims, it was important for us as editors to invite specialists with appropriate experience in dance and exercise science to contribute to the making of this book. By doing so, a great deal of knowledge was obtained directly from sports science, thus avioding a 'reinvention of the wheel'. The book has been written with the dancer and dance-teacher as the primary target audience, and it assumes that the reader is without an extensive scientific training, although we have not condescendingly watered-down the science so much that the work collapses under its own weight.

One of the problems we faced in producing this book, was the lack of scientifically generated data that is directly relevant to dance and dancers, with a major exception being the subject of injuries. We tried to rectify this problem by 'borrowing' information from sport activities that— from the physiological viewpoint—are close to dance.

The book is divided into three different parts. In the first, we start with the most important aspect of exercise, which is energy and its production, and finish with an introduction to nutrition. The second part consists of four chapters; the first on the various non-artistic components which contribute to dance and dance performance; the second chapter is on the principle tissue involved in dance, i.e., muscle and its function; the third chapter is devoted to the main fitness components, while the fourth chapter is on the principles of physical training. Finally, the third part of the book examines aspects relating to the young, mature, and retired dancer.

We hope that the reader will appreciate that increased physical fitness levels render dancers less vulnerable to injuries and possibly illness, and may even assist in better stage performances. We also hope that the reader will learn here that physical fitness training will not, for example, produce undesirable muscle bulk, or make dancers slower and reduce their flexibility levels. Last, but not least, we expect that the reader will understand that the physicality of dance concerns not only fitness, exercise and classes, but that a number of important health issues—such as 'burnout' and body weight-control, should also be considered.

Yiannis Koutedakis, BSc, MA, PhD
N.C. Craig Sharp, BVMS, MRCVS, PhD, FIBiol, FBASES, FPEA

Birmingham, 8-7-1998

Acknowledgements

The editors of this book wish to thank Dance UK, Birmingham Royal Ballet, Northern School of Contemporary Dance, English National Ballet School, London Contemporary Dance School, Northern Theatre Dance Company, the Bolshoi and the Kirov Ballet Companies, and the British Olympic Medical Centre for talks, advice, and help over the years; Mr Bev Parker and Dr Andrea Hass for illustrative help.

Part I

ENERGY AND FOOD FOR EXERCISE AND FITNESS

Yiannis Koutedakis

Chapter 1

Energy for Exercise and Fitness

1 SUMMARY

Energy is the essence of life. Mechanical, chemical, thermal (i.e. heat), electrical, solar and nuclear are the six main forms of energy in nature. The body's ability to convert chemical energy from food into muscular work is directly related to physical performance. This accounts for about 25% of the converted chemical energy; the vast majority (about 75%) appears as heat. All body cells obtain energy with the help of the specialized energy-carrier molecules of adenosine triphosphate (ATP), and the kilocalorie (kcal) is the main expression of energy. There are four components in food and drink with the potential to produce energy: carbohydrates, proteins, fats and alcohol. This energy is then used to build and repair body tissues and to power all forms of human movement, including dance. The framework for all this is known as *metabolism*, the basis for all physiological phenomena that one can observe or measure. There are three energy-releasing mechanisms (or systems) for ATP resynthesis: two *anaerobic* and one *aerobic*, operating without and with the presence of oxygen respectively. The two anaerobic mechanisms are better equipped to produce relatively large amounts of energy for short periods, whereas the aerobic mechanism can generate lesser amounts of energy for very long periods. Finally, optimal levels of physical fitness generally enhance the function of these energy-releasing mechanisms.

2   INTRODUCTION

The instrument used by dancers is their own body. But for the body to function, an optimal amount of energy is needed. Indeed, a successful stage performance depends—*inter alia*—upon the ability of the dancer to generate the right amount of energy and to control its application to the specific demands of his/her role. This 'specificity' stems from the fact that not all dance movements have the same energy requirements. Successful jumps and pirouettes depend upon the ability to produce energy very rapidly, whereas repeated 'glissade' is associated with the dancers' potential to produce energy at varying lesser rates. Therefore understanding the basics of energy and energy production allows clearer analysis of the demands imposed by different dance routines and assists in better preparation.

What is energy? It is definitely not something that can be described in terms of size, shape or mass. Yet we all use the term and expressions such as 'I have no energy to dance' and 'you look very energetic' are in constant use. The main objectives of this chapter are to help the reader to understand various aspects associated with energy, its production, storage and use.

3   DEFINITION OF ENERGY

Energy is the essence of life, as life itself implies the continuous supply and use of energy. Mechanical, chemical, thermal (i.e. heat), electrical, solar and nuclear are the six main forms of energy in nature, and they are all interchangeable according to laws of *thermodynamics*. However, the cells of the body are able to use energy from one source only: the *chemical energy* that was originally captured under the direct or indirect influence of sunlight. The sun is the ultimate source of energy, as solar energy is harnessed by plants, through *photosynthesis*, to produce plant or animal-based foods, all of which store chemical energy. This is then used to build and repair body tissues, and to power all forms of human movement including dance.

Fig. 1.1 shows the steps involved for the conversion of food into cellular chemical energy and subsequently into chemical, mechanical, electrical and muscular work. Chemical work refers to the supplying of the energy necessary to synthesize complex body components from simple ones, while mechanical work occurs when cellular chemical energy is converted into movement (e.g. to lift a weight, muscle must shorten). The partial conversion of cellular chemical energy into electrical work has been associated with the electrical charges across nerves and

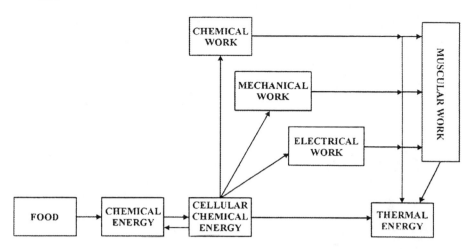

Fig. 1.1 Biological transformations of energy. Note that for muscular work the body uses energy from one source only: the chemical energy which is liberated by chemical reactions inside the cells

muscle cell membranes. According to Fig. 1.1, muscular work is related to chemical, mechanical and electrical equivalents. For our purposes, *energy represents the ability to perform physical/muscular work.*

The muscle's ability to convert chemical energy from food into muscular work is directly related to performance in sport and dance alike. However, the efficiency of the body to convert chemical energy to energy for muscular work is only about 25%. The majority of the cellular chemical energy— about 75%—appears as heat. Ironically, heat energy cannot be used for muscular work, simply because cells have no mechanism for this purpose. However, the heat is used to maintain a constant body temperature that provides the platform for the enzymes to regulate the chemical reactions. Indeed, most of the *enzymes* are highly active when body temperatures are between 36 to 40 °C.

The cell obtains energy with the help of specialized energy-carrier molecules. From bacteria to humans, the major energy-carrier is *adenosine triphosphate (ATP).* This is often referred to as the body's 'energy currency' and consists of a ring structure known as *adenine*, and three *phosphate* groups. In a procedure known as *hydrolysis*, energy is released when one phosphate is removed from the structure of ATP to form one molecule of *adenosine diphosphate (ADP):*

$$ATP \rightarrow ADP + P + Energy$$

Although some energy for muscular work is stored in ATP, its main function is not to store energy but to *transfer* energy from one part of the body to another for immediate use. So, are there any energy stores as a backup system? If so, what are they and where do we find them?

The body stores of carbohydrates, proteins and fats (or lipids) are also energy stores, which can provide ample amounts of ATP. Under normal conditions, well-fed individuals have substantial amounts of energy stored in their bodies, enabling them theoretically to work (e.g. running at a pace equivalent to 100 kcal per 1.6 km [= 1 mile]) for days, or even weeks (Table 1.1). However, this cannot happen in real life, as things tend to be slightly more complicated than they appear to be. For instance, large amounts of fats are involved in the construction of all body cell membranes, and proteins constitute most of the organs and muscles. Therefore, use of these fats and proteins as energy sources is not feasible.

4   MEASUREMENT OF ENERGY

Energy is ultimately given off from the body as heat. Although there are a number of different ways to express energy, the most common term used is *calorie*. One *small calorie* (cal) represents the amount of heat needed to raise the temperature of 1 gram of water by 1 °C. However, because the gram calorie is very small, the *kilocalorie* (kcal, i.e. 1000 cal) is the main expression of energy.

The *calorific value* of a nutrient may be defined as *the amount of energy produced in the body when this nutrient is consumed*. Again, the energy yield may be determined by measuring the heat that is liberated during the combustion of food materials. As can be seen from Table 1.2, there are four components in food and drink with the potential to produce energy: carbohydrates, proteins, fats and alcohol. However, only the first three

Table 1.1   The major energy stores in the body, and how far they would take us

Energy source	Storage form	Body calories[a]	Distance covered (km)
Carbohydrate	Liver glycogen	400	6.5
	Muscle glycogen	1500	24
Protein	Muscle protein	30 000	480
Fat	Muscle triglycerides	2500	40
	Adipose tissue triglycerides	80 000	1280

[a]Depending on gender, age, fitness levels, etc., values may show extreme variations
Source: Modified from Williams (1995)

Table 1.2 Calorific value of energy-yielding nutrients

Nutrient	Energy (kcal per gram)
Carbohydrate	4.1
Protein	4.3
Fat	9.3
Alcohol	7.0

components will be discussed in the present book, as alcohol is not a muscle fuel and it is only used by the liver.

It is interesting to note that one gram of fat provides more than double the energy of the equivalent amount of carbohydrate or protein. It is also worth mentioning that unlike carbohydrates and fats, proteins are not completely oxidized (i.e. utilized) in our body and end products of protein metabolism appear in the urine as urea. Urea therefore contains energy that is obviously lost. Thus, although the actual calorific value of protein is 5.6 kcal per gram—taking into account the lost urea energy— the true calorific value of protein is only 4.3 kcal per gram.

5 METABOLISM

It was mentioned earlier that energy is necessary to build and repair body tissues and to power all forms of human movement, including dance. The framework for all this is known as *metabolism*, the basis for all physiological phenomena that one can observe or measure. The term itself comes from the Greek word 'metabolismos' meaning 'change of matter'.

Metabolism may be defined as *the sum of all transformations of both matter and energy which occur within the body*, or *the total of all physical and chemical changes in the body* (Williams 1995). It involves two fundamental processes, *anabolism* and *catabolism*. Anabolism is a building-up process where complex body components—such as muscle and bone—are synthesized from basic nutrients. For a successful completion of this procedure, substantial amounts of energy are required. Conversely, catabolism is a tearing-down process where body compounds—such as liver glycogen, muscle glycogen and lipids (fats)—are disintegrating into their simpler components. During this procedure, energy becomes available for anabolic activities and, of course, muscular work (Fig. 1.2).

Basal metabolism is the *energy used by the body at complete rest*, or the *minimum amount of energy required for sustaining life at rest*. The beating of the heart, the inhaling and exhaling of air, and the transportation of nerve and hormonal messages to direct these activities are examples of basal

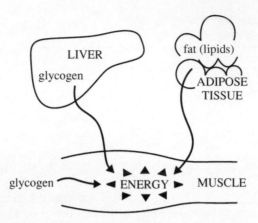

Fig. 1.2   Energy sources for muscular work
Source: Modified from Newsholme *et al*. (1994). Reproduced with permission of
John Wiley & Sons Limited

processes that sustain life at rest. Basal metabolism normally accounts for
the largest part of a person's daily energy expenditure. Lastly, *basal
metabolic rate* (or *resting energy expenditure—REE*) is the *rate at which the
body spends energy for the basal biological processes which are necessary to
maintain life*. This is the expression of basal metabolism in terms either of
kcal per square metre of body surface or kcal per kilogram of body
weight, per hour, and reflects how rapidly the body is using its energy
stores during periods of rest that exclude sleep.

The basal metabolic rate (BMR) varies from person to person and may
vary for a single individual with a change in circumstance or physical
condition. A BMR 10% below or above the expected average is not uncommon and is clinically classified as normal. However, a BMR that is 10%
lower or higher than average will mean lower or higher energy expenditure
per day respectively. In a year, such BMR fluctuations may easily make the
difference of an increased or decreased weight by about 10 kg of body fat.
Table 1.3 shows selected factors that affect basal metabolic rate.

6   ENERGY REQUIREMENTS

Energy requirements (or energy expenditure) may be defined *as the
amount of energy needed to maintain basic biological function and for physical
activity*. From this definition it is clear that two separate pieces of information are required to give satisfactory advice on the question of daily
energy needs: (1) the individual's basal metabolism (or basal metabolic
rate), and (2) the energy cost of physical activities.

Table 1.3 Factors that affect basal metabolic rate (BMR)

Factor	Effects on BMR	Examples
Age	↓	Adults have lower levels of BMR than children. In general, BMR continuously decreases with increase in age (the BMR of a 6 year old is about 70% higher than that of a 60-year-old man).
Diet	↑↓	Vegetarian meals require less energy for digestion than non-vegetarian meals.
Fasting	↓	Lower-calorie diets suppress energy needs at rest compared to high-calorie diets.
Fever	↑	Body temperature increases as the body fights against disease. Fever raises BMR by about 10% for each degree Centigrade.
Gender (pregnancy)	↑↓	Women have a 6–10% lower BMR than that of men of the same size and age. The BMR of the female increases markedly during pregnancy as the result of the additional metabolic activity of the foetus.
Hormonal status	↑↓	The thyroid hormone thyroxine is a key BMR regulator; it can speed up or slow down BMR by as much as 50%.
Muscle	↑↓	Muscle, due to its size, accounts for the largest part of BMR. The more muscle (relative to body weight) the higher the BMR.
Previous physical activity	↑	BMR may increase by up to 16%, for at least 4–5 hours, after the end of properly designed exercise programmes.

As already mentioned, basal metabolism represents the greatest proportion of energy use. In fact, maintenance of the bodily functions at rest requires—on average—two thirds of the daily energy needs. Therefore some knowledge of this energy expenditure is useful to dancers in a bid to regulate their energy intakes. This can be broadly achieved with the help of two specially devised formulae, one for men and one for women (Noble 1986). In the following example, application of the formulae gives us the daily energy requirements for basal metabolism in a man and a woman weighing 65 and 55 kg respectively:

	Energy/kg BW (kcal)		Hours		Body weight (kg)	Basal metabolism
Men	1.0	×	24	×	65	= 1560 kcal
Women	0.9	×	24	×	55	= 1188 kcal

As can be seen from this example, body weight (BW) together with the amount of energy (kcal) per kilogram (kg) body weight are needed to estimate basal metabolism. However, the individual's age and—especially—levels of physical fitness affect both of these factors. Relatively young and fit dancers may command up to 1.6 kcal per kg body weight, whereas the equivalent value in older and unfit individuals may be reduced by up to 50%. In general, women require about 15% less energy to fuel their basal metabolism than men, mainly due to differences in their body weight.

The second component necessary to estimate total daily energy requirements is the *energy cost* of bodily activities. Also called *exercise metabolic rate*, this energy cost represents the increase in metabolism—over and above resting levels—brought about by moderate or strenuous physical movement or exercise.

Kilocalories (kcal) per minute based upon body weight, kilojoules (kj) and METS (a unit based on multiples of the basal metabolic rate) are among the ways used to record the energy cost of different forms of activity. The energy cost of different forms of dance has been found to be similar to that of badminton, basketball and light (level) bicycling, with the actual values ranging from 0.083 to 0.181 kcal per kg body weight per minute (Table 1.4). For instance, if a 55 kg female is involved in aerobic dance for 60 minutes, she will burn 472 kcal ($55 \times 0.143 \times 60 = 472$ kcal), which includes the energy required for basal metabolism. To calculate the net cost of this 60 minute activity, we have to deduct 49.5 kcal (i.e. $1188 \div 24 = 49.5$) which the 55 kg female needs to maintain biological functions for the duration of the activity (i.e. 60 minutes). Therefore, the net cost is now reduced from 472 to 422.5 kcal.

Table 1.4 Approximate energy cost of different types of dance. The listed values are referred to both males and females

Reference (Type of dance)	Energy cost (kcal/kg body weight/min)
Jette and Inglis (1975) (Square dance)	0.083
Cohen, Segal, Witriol and McArdie (1982) (Ballet)	0.085
Léger (1982) (Disco dance)	0.143
Foster (1975) (Aerobic dance)	0.143
Wigaeus and Kihlbom (1980) (Swedish folkdance)	0.181

As in the case of basal metabolism, the calculated energy costs of human activities do not take into account important aspects such as technique of movement, age, climatological conditions and, again, fitness levels. These aspects have the capacity to slightly increase or decrease the energy cost levels of given activities. Nevertheless, people generally overestimate the energy cost of exercise. It may be disappointing to note that if one jogs on a summer's day for 25–30 min, covering a distance of about 5 km, he/she will use the equivalent of only 3 slices of bread as fuel, and lose half a litre of body fluid in the form of sweat. If the activity were a marathon run of 26 miles, the energy equivalent would amount to about a kilogram of bread and 3–4 litres of fluid.

7 ENERGY INTAKES

During the last two decades, scientists have calculated the daily energy-intake needs for healthy trained or untrained individuals (Table 1.5). In the dance world, however, not only fitness and health, but also the ability to conform to specific standards of body shape are of equal importance. Professional advancement may depend upon conformity to reigning standards of body proportion. Consequently, eliminating calories from energy intakes has increasingly become a built-in part of dancers' lives. It has to be stressed though that these practices have been based on an aesthetic ideal and not on scientific advice.

The tendency for lower energy intakes has been confirmed by the findings of several scientific studies. For example, female professional (ballet) dancers normally consume 70–80% of the recommended daily allowance of energy intake (Benson, Gillien, Bourdet and Loosli 1985; Bonbright 1989, 1990). Even dance students are not excluded from these patterns of reduced energy intake. Dahlström, Jansson, Nordevang and

Table 1.5 Reference daily energy intakes for non-active males (average body weight: 70 kg) and females (average body weight: 58 kg)

Age (years)	Males (kcal)	Females (kcal)
11–14	2700	2200
15–18	2800	2100
19–22	2900	2100
23–50	2700	2000
51–75	2400	1800

Kaijser (1990) reported that the energy intake of young dance students was only 66% of their estimated energy requirement. Yet, in most cases, body weight remains low but constant. It is not as yet clear which are the mechanisms involved in preventing dramatic body weight losses in active individuals with reduced energy intakes (Dahlström, Jansson, Ekman and Kaijser 1995). Nevertheless, reduced daily energy intakes often result in suboptimal overall nutrition. Studies have shown a relationship between reduced daily energy intakes on one hand, and low body weight, low body fat, amenorrhoea (or absence of periods) and anorexia nervosa on the other (Frisch, Wyshak and Vincent 1980; Warren 1983). As we will see later in this book (Chapter 10), bone calcium losses and the condition known as *osteoporosis* usually follow *amenorrhoea* and *anorexia nervosa*. Osteoporosis in turn increases the likelihood of stress fractures and other injuries in female dancers.

8   CALCULATION OF ENERGY INTAKES

Carbohydrates, fats and proteins are the three main energy-providing nutrients. However, carbohydrate is the preferred energy source for dance and other activities of high intensity and brief duration, while at the same time securing the function of important organs such as the liver and brain. To meet these demands, carbohydrate consumption should account for more than 55% of total daily energy intake in healthy and active individuals. The relative contribution of lipids and proteins to the total energy intake should be in the region of 30 and 15% respectively (Table 1.6).

The relative contribution of the three energy-providing nutrients to daily energy intake may be estimated by using the information in Table 1.7. Firstly, the total energy intake (or total calorie intake) is calculated from the weight of each of the three nutrients, and the amount of energy that is liberated from every gram of each nutrient. The relative contribu-

Table 1.6   The contribution of the three main nutrients to the total energy intake in a average (Western) diet and in a recommended diet for dancers

	Western diets	Dancers
Carbohydrates (%)	40–45	50–55+
Fats (%)	40–45	30–35
Proteins (%)	15–20	15

Table 1.7 Estimation of energy intake when the amount (in grams) of carbohydrates, proteins and fats consumed is known

	Total grams		Kcal/gram		Kcal
Carbohydrates	–	×	4.1	=	–
Protein	–	×	4.3	=	–
Fat	–	×	9.3	=	–

Total Energy Intake (kcal)

Energy from carbohydrates (%) = (energy from carbohydrates ÷ total energy) × 100
Energy from proteins (%) = (energy from protein ÷ total energy) × 100
Energy from fats (%) = (energy from fat ÷ total energy) × 100

tion can be obtained by dividing the energy (calories) from each individual nutrient by the total energy intake and multiplying by 100.

9 ENERGY BALANCE

According to the first law of *thermodynamics* (or law of the conservation of energy), *energy cannot be created or destroyed*. Therefore the total amount of energy taken in by a dancer must be accounted for by the energy output of his/her body. This balance between energy intake and output is given as follows:

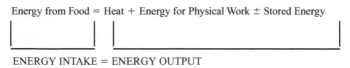

Energy from Food = Heat + Energy for Physical Work ± Stored Energy

ENERGY INTAKE = ENERGY OUTPUT

As seen in the previous section, most of the energy output by the body is in the form of heat. However, its rate of production depends on prevailing circumstances. When a dancer is exercising, for example, the rate of heat production is greater than when at rest.

If energy output (i.e. heat production, plus the energy for physical work) is balanced by the energy intake, then the stored energy in the body remains unchanged. In this case, individuals have a *neutral energy balance* and there are no changes in body weight (Fig. 1.3). Conversely, if there is no balance between energy intake and energy output, the stored energy by the body changes accordingly. In adults, increases in energy intake almost certainly result in energy store increases. Given that the body has only one way to store excess energy—by converting it to fat—energy store increases actually mean body fat increases. In this case, a *positive energy balance* occurs leading to a steady increase in weight due,

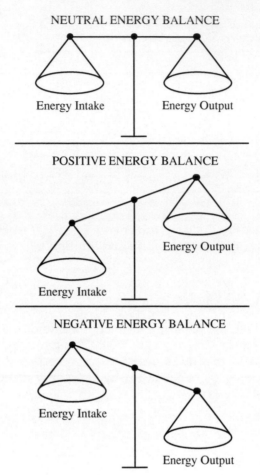

Fig. 1.3 Energy balance in humans

mainly, to an excess deposition of body fat. On the other hand, if energy needs exceed those provided by the consumed food, a *negative energy balance* occurs accompanied by body weight reductions (Fig. 1.3). The greater the negative energy balance, the faster the body loses weight. However, dancers should always remember that rapid weight loss may adversely affect *cardiac output*, plasma and blood volumes, kidney function, and may alter the individual's basal metabolic rate. Dancers should avoid diets of less than 1500 kcal per day, while diets of less than 800 kcal per day are dangerous.

10 PRODUCTION OF ENERGY: THE HUMAN ENERGY SYSTEMS

As previously discussed, the specific energy required for muscular work is provided by ATP. However, the ATP body stores would only last for a few muscle contractions if ATP could not be resynthesized at a rate equal to that of its use. ATP reductions of 25–30% are enough to prevent muscle from continuing to function.

A typical ATP molecule may exist for only 1–2 seconds before its energy is transferred to another molecule in the body. During this procedure ATP is reduced to ADP. The newly formed ADP is then rapidly reconverted into ATP through coupling to energy-releasing mechanisms involving *muscle fuels* such as phosphocreatine, carbohydrates, lipids and, to a lesser extent, proteins. These fuels are transported and transformed by various biochemical processes into the same end product—ATP:

$$ADP + P + \text{Energy from Muscle Fuel} \rightarrow ATP$$

There are three energy-releasing mechanisms (or systems) for ATP resynthesis: two *anaerobic* and one *aerobic*, operating without and with the presence of oxygen respectively. The two anaerobic mechanisms however, are better equipped to produce relatively large amounts of energy for short periods, whereas the aerobic mechanism can generate lesser amounts of energy for very long periods.

10.1 Anaerobic Breakdown of Phosphocreatine

When dance begins, rapidly produced energy is required. This need must be quickly fulfilled in a relatively easy and efficient way. Indeed, the anaerobic breakdown of *phosphocreatine* (PC) is the least complicated energy production mechanism. It does not involve the use of oxygen (hence the term 'anaerobic'), depends on rather short chemical reactions, makes use of the energy-rich PC stored directly in muscle cells, and leaves no fatigue-inducing products. However, this mechanism lasts only for about 10 seconds of intensive effort, such as repeated jumping.

PC is similar to ATP in that when its phosphate group is removed energy is liberated. This energy is then immediately used to generate ATP:

$$PC \rightarrow P + C + \text{Energy}$$

$$\text{Energy} + P + ADP \rightarrow ATP$$

The powerful start and execution of certain dance sequences (e.g. petite batterie, grand allegro) exemplify the importance of this anaerobic system, where especially rapid supplies of ATP are demanded. Re-formation of PC from inorganic phosphate (P) and creatine (C) occurs during recovery from exercise, in line with the replacement/resynthesis of most other muscle fuels.

10.2   Anaerobic Glycolysis

As exercise (dance) continues at relatively high intensities, levels of ATP decline to some extent. This reduction in ATP stimulates a rapid breakdown of the carbohydrate glucose (which is stored in the body as glycogen) to resynthesize ATP and, thus, maintain an adequate energy supply. This is the basis of the second anaerobic mechanism, which from the chemical viewpoint is more complicated than the first one. It involves ATP being formed within muscle cells from the energy derived by the incomplete breakdown of glucose to lactic acid:

$$\text{Glucose (Glycogen)} \rightarrow \text{Lactic acid} + \text{Energy}$$

$$\text{Energy} + \text{P} + \text{ADP} \rightarrow \text{ATP}$$

More specifically, the incomplete breakdown of one molecule of glucose leads to the formation of two molecules of pyruvic acid followed by two molecules of lactic acid, and in the process a *net* of two ATP molecules are produced (in fact, four ATP molecules are produced in total, but two are used up). These take place in the absence of oxygen, in a biochemical procedure known as anaerobic *glycolysis* (Fig. 1.4). It should be stressed that the proceeding equations and the associated descriptions are much simplified. In reality, they are far more complex as the release of the ATP molecules requires the presence of several enzymes, selectively involved in the various stages of the anaerobic glycolysis.

Lactic acid is unfairly perceived among dancers and their teachers as the demon of their art. This stems from the fact that increased amounts of lactic acid in the body cause muscular fatigue, which in the end affects dance performance. However, dancers often forget that lactic acid is, in essence, a protection mechanism against severe energy depletion, and against injury due to intensive muscular work. Nevertheless, the body has more than one way of maintaining a balance between lactic acid production and its removal from the muscle and blood. This balance depends upon the dancers' levels of fitness and the relative intensity of muscular work, and it can be partly achieved by converting some lactic acid back to pyruvic acid (Fig. 1.4). However, when either the fitness levels are low or the intensity of dance is high, or both, lactic acid production is greater than its removal. The substance begins then to accumulate, causing muscle hyperacidity, and eventually brings physical effort to an end (Houston 1995). Aspects related to *cardiovascular* proficiency—such as an increased number of muscle capillaries—may contribute to faster rates of lactic acid removal.

Anaerobically generated energy could be the main limiting factor during intensive dance lasting from 10 seconds to about 2 minutes, where a continuous supply of ATP at very high rates is required. However, the contribution of anaerobic metabolic pathways to the overall energy production of a given dance is considerably reduced during routines of several minutes. For dance lasting for more than 2 minutes, aerobic glycolysis is the main energy provider.

Glycolysis is common to both aerobic and anaerobic energy production systems. If sufficient oxygen is available, the pyruvic acid enters into another biochemical procedure—the *Krebs cycle*—where a further 36 molecules of ATP may be produced (Fig. 1.4). If, on the other hand, the demand for energy is too great, pyruvic acid is transformed to lactic acid to allow the process to go on longer. Nevertheless, the two pathways for ATP formation are not alternatives. Rather, they are intimately connected procedures that run in parallel and are utilized to extents depending on the exertion level. Indeed, depending on the type, intensity and duration of the activity, the road divides and one or the other route is primarily used. During a highly intensive 100 m run, about 95% of the required energy is produced anaerobically, whereas the same energy-releasing procedures will provide less than 5% of the energy needed to complete a

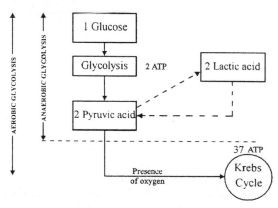

Fig. 1.4 Energy (ATP) production: a simplified diagram of anaerobic (without oxygen) and aerobic (with oxygen) glycolysis
Source: Modified from The Runner's Guide, Koutedakis (1994). Reproduced with permission

successful marathon run (Fig. 1.5). In dance, the energy required for 'travelling' work during contemporary classes mainly comes from anaerobic sources; these sources will only contribute a fraction of the energy needed for a slow sequence centre-work.

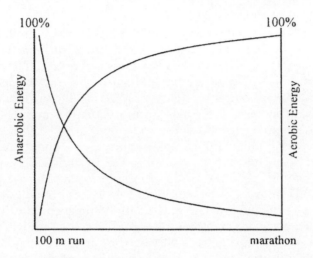

Fig. 1.5   The contribution of the anaerobic and aerobic energy-releasing mechanisms depends on the *type, intensity* and *duration* of the physical activity

10.3   Aerobic Energy Production

In the presence of oxygen, carbohydrates, fats and proteins are broken down (Fig 1.6). During this biochemical procedure (also known as *Krebs cycle*) energy is liberated for ATP resynthesis. The total of 36 molecules of ATP may be produced if the fuel is glycogen. If the fuel is fat, more than double this amount of energy may be produced. Such energy yield, however, involves hundreds of reactions and specialized enzymes, which inevitably make the Krebs cycle much more complex than the two anaerobic energy-production mechanisms.

Apart from the apparent complex nature of the Krebs cycle, the involvement of such a large number of reactions and enzymes makes this process of ATP formation relatively slow. If we now add on top of this the time needed for the atmospheric oxygen to reach the energy production sites, it becomes clear why the aerobic pathway release is best suited for relatively slow physical activities requiring lower rates of energy supply.

For the purpose of aerobic energy production in muscle cells—as indeed in all body cells—oxygen meets carbohydrates, fats and proteins

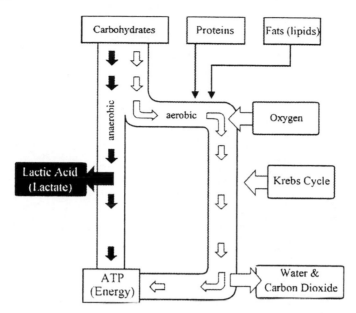

Fig. 1.6 Energy (ATP) production: a simplified diagram of anaerobic (without oxygen) and aerobic (with oxygen) mechanisms

in specific aerobic energy-production sites. These sites are specialized cell organelles known as *mitochondria*.

The term comes from the combination of two Greek words (*mitos* = thread and *chondros* = granule) which characterize the general appearance of these organelles. Most mitochondria are cylindrical in shape, and can be found in varying numbers in all body cells except red blood cells. In particular, mitochondria populations vary with the size and the energy expenditure of the cell in question. Thus, given that levels of energy expenditure are generally proportional to fitness levels, fitter dancers tend to have greater numbers of mitochondria in their muscles than their untrained counterparts.

The primary function of the mitochondria is to couple the energy liberated during the breakdown of food molecules to the resynthesis of ATP. In fact, 95% and 100% of the ATP molecules synthesized from glycogen and fat breakdown respectively take place within this organelle. No wonder that energy production via the aerobic route makes it the body's preferred source from which to power most energy-demanding biological functions at rest, and to fuel long spells of dance.

In well-fed and healthy dancers, glycogen and fat win over protein in the contest for ATP generation. However, while glycogen contribution to energy production remains relatively unchanged, the roles of fat and protein may change under special circumstances. In cases of strict diets with very low daily energy intakes (i.e. 800 kcal or less), a significantly higher percentage of the required energy is supplied by protein rather than fat (Fig. 1.7), at the expense of lean tissue, that is muscle, and with deleterious effects on both health and physical performance. It should be added here that protein metabolism is more complex than fat or carbohydrate metabolism, with the reason being placed squarely on the chemical structure of proteins.

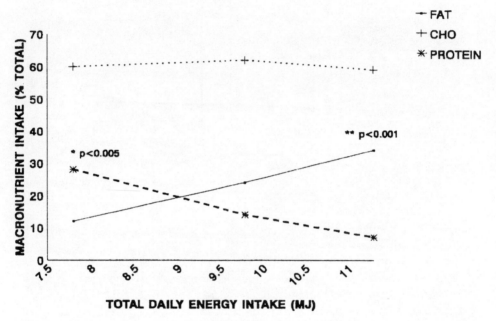

TOTAL DAILY ENERGY INTAKE (MJ)

Fig. 1.7 Relationships between total daily energy intake, and energy supplied by carbohydrates and fats. At lower daily energy intakes, a significantly (p <0.005) higher percentage of the required energy is supplied by protein rather than fat. However, protein contribution to energy production is significantly less (p <0.001) at higher levels of energy intake
Source: From Koutedakis, Hitchcock, Pacy and Sharp in 13(1): 36 Journal of Sports Sciences (1995). Reproduced with permission of E. & F. N. Spon

11 THE EFFECTS OF FITNESS ON THE HUMAN ENERGY SYSTEMS

Physical fitness and its components will be discussed in detail in Part III. However, for the purpose of this section it could be said that—compared to untrained conditions—optimal levels of physical fitness generally enhance the function of the energy pathways involved in the execution of different exercises and dance routines. For instance, appropriate levels of fitness are associated with a slight increase in resting muscle ATP and PC stores. This enhanced capacity for fast and 'explosive' dance movements is further matched by a greater and specialized muscle mobilization that is also the result of optimal fitness.

Appropriate physical preparation or physical 'tuning'—and therefore fitness—can elevate the individual's capacity for anaerobic glycolysis too. This may be accomplished partly due to increases in the muscle glycogen stores and partly because of a more efficient removal of metabolic by-products (i.e. lactic acid) from the working muscle. Such adaptations permit greater energy release through anaerobic mechanisms, for relatively longer periods of time before the onset of fatigue.

Aerobic fitness is primarily accompanied by improved delivery of oxygen to the muscle cells and their capacity to use it. However, better oxygen supply and use means that, potentially, more ATP may be resynthesized through the aerobic energy system. This is further supported by the fact that good aerobic fitness implies increases in intramuscular storage of substrates, particularly glycogen and *fatty acids*. However, the main point concerning dancers lies with the fact that aerobically trained muscles become better at using fat and sparing glycogen. This means that dancers are able to exercise for longer before the limited glycogen stores are depleted and fatigue sets in. In general, the fitter the dancer, the lower the proportion of glycogen and the higher the proportion of fat the muscles will use at any given exercise intensity (Fig. 1.8).

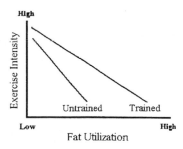

Fig. 1.8 Fat utilization during exercise. For the same exercise intensity, fit (trained) individuals utilize proportionally more fat than their untrained counterparts

12 CONCLUSIONS

All body cells obtain energy with the help of the specialized energy-carrier molecules of adenosine triphosphate (ATP). This energy is then used to build and repair body tissues and to power all forms of human movement, including dance. The framework for all this is known as *metabolism*. There are three energy-releasing mechanisms (or systems) for ATP resynthesis: two *anaerobic* and one *aerobic* operating without and with the presence of oxygen respectively. The two anaerobic mechanisms are better equipped to fuel intensive dance for short periods only, whereas the aerobic mechanism can generate energy for much longer periods. Optimal levels of physical fitness generally enhance the function of the energy-releasing mechanisms. More scientific work is needed on aspects related to energy production and supply during different forms of dance.

13   FURTHER READING

Åstrand PO, Rodahl K (1986) *Textbook of work physiology: physiological bases of exercise* (3rd edition). New York: McGraw-Hill

Bean A and Wellington P (1995) *Sports nutrition for women*. London, A and C Black

Bloomfield J, Fricker PA, Fitch KD (1995) *Science and medicine in sport* (2nd edition). Victoria, Australia: Blackwell Science

Montoye HJ, Kemper HCG, Saris WHM, Washburn RA (1996) *Measuring activity and energy expenditure*. Champaign, IL: Human Kinetics

Newsholme E, Leech T, Duester G (1994) *Keep on running. The science of training and performance*. Chichester, UK: Wiley

Williams MH (1995) *Nutrition for fitness and sport* (4th edition). Madison, WI: Wm C Brown & Benchmark

Chapter 2

Food for Exercise and Fitness

1 SUMMARY

Energy is produced in the watery medium of the cell from carbohydrates, proteins and fats, with the help of vitamins and minerals. *Carbohydrates* are the preferred energy source for dance and other activities of high intensity and brief duration. Given that the available stores in the body will last for about 90 minutes of strenuous physical activity, regular carbohydrate replacement should be amongst the dancer's priorities. The importance of *fat* as an exercise energy source depends on the intensity of activity as well as on the availability of carbohydrates. Fats are primarily used when the body performs low intensity muscular work, thus sparing the store of carbohydrate. The fitter the individual the greater the carbohydrate sparing. Fats should not form more than 35% of the total daily energy intake. *Protein* is one of the most essential and multipurpose nutrients. Animal sources such as meat, fish, eggs and/or dairy products are often referred to as 'complete' protein foods, whereas vegetable sources are described as being 'incomplete' as far as protein content is concerned. *Vitamins* contribute to chemical processes that regulate metabolism, energy release, and tissue repair. No vitamins can be synthesized by the human body. Lack of certain vitamins is associated with a number of undesirable conditions, including fatigue and underperformance in physical tasks. *Minerals* make up 4% of our body weight. They are involved in many biological functions including energy production, bone structure and oxygen carrying. Although *water* is essential for energy production, health and, of course, exercise it is seldom thought of as a nutrient because it has no calorific value. Although increased sweating rates translate into better regulation of body temperature, a 2% body weight loss as fluid may affect the ability to dance. Ingestion of extra water prior to exercise allows dancers to work with lower heart rates and provides for increased sweating rates. Finally, while some *nutritional aids*, such as glutamine and creatine, have been recommended for performance enhancements, their long-term effects are as yet unknown.

2   INTRODUCTION

Citizens of (Western) industrialized countries tend to regard the intake of food in a rather passive manner. This seems to be the result of a general lack of understanding of what constitutes optimal nutrition, and how the latter regulates our bodily functions. What is surprising, however, is the fact that this general attitude towards food can also be found in apparently 'active' individuals, for whom appropriate nutrition is as important as fuel for a car or aeroplane. An alarmingly large number of these individuals fail to recognize that unvaried diets with limited food choices may lead to suboptimal nutrition with devastating results for both health and physical performance.

Regarding dance and dancers, only a small percentage of dancers receive dietary advice from qualified specialists (Fig. 2.1). This was among the findings of a recent study (Koutedakis, Pacy, Carson and Dick 1997) leading to the assumption that, for the majority of dancers, profes-

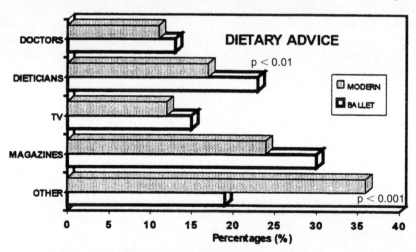

Fig. 2.1 Sources of dietary advice (expressed in %) in a sample of 324 professional ballet and modern dancers. The majority of the dancers failed to approach qualified specialists for dietary advice
Source: From Koutedakis, Pacy, Carson and Dick Vol. 12, Medical Problems of Performing Artists (1997). Reproduced by permission of Hanley & Belfus, Inc.

sional dietary advice is not a priority. Furthermore, it is also often forgotten by many of us that, as over 96% of the molecules of the human body are completely replaced every 12 months, at the end of the day we are what we eat.

It was noted in the previous chapter that some of the food we eat is used to build, maintain or repair the body cells, while the majority is processed (i.e. metabolized) for energy (ATP) production. Most of this energy appears as heat and is used to keep the body warm, some is used for the work of the cells, and some for muscular contraction (e.g. dance). Body-building requirements determine the *quality of diet*, whereas the energy needs of the individual determine the *quantity of diet*. Therefore, optimal nutrition is a *dietary balance* of different nutrients to keep the bodily functions at the required levels. In the watery medium of the cell, delicate blending of carbohydrates, proteins and fats, along with vitamins and minerals, makes this possible. In this chapter, aspects related to these nutrients will be briefly discussed.

3 CARBOHYDRATES

As discussed earlier, carbohydrate is the preferred energy source for dance and other activities of high intensity and brief duration. At rest, optimal levels of carbohydrates secure the function of important organs such as the liver and brain. To meet these demands, their consumption should account for more than 55% of total daily energy intake in healthy and active individuals (Williams 1995). However, published data suggested that the daily carbohydrate consumption in dancers is too low for optimal energy yield (Cohen, Potosnak, Frank and Baker 1985).

Carbohydrates are organic compounds that contain carbon, hydrogen and oxygen in various combinations. These combinations then form different carbohydrates that may be categorized as *simple* carbohydrates, *complex* carbohydrates and *dietary fibre* (Fig 2.2). Simple carbohydrates can be either *monosaccharides* or *disaccharides*. The monosaccharides—glucose, fructose, and galactose—are the smallest carbohydrate molecules with 6-carbon atoms; the disaccharides—sucrose, lactose, and maltose—are formed by linking two monosaccharides together to make a 12-carbon structure. Link three or more monosaccharides together and a *polysaccharide* (i.e. complex carbohydrate) is formed, such as starch and glycogen. Some polysaccharides contain up to 3000 monosaccharides (i.e. glucose molecules).

Simple carbohydrates are sugary and sweet in taste, whereas complex carbohydrates are starchy and not very sweet. However, in simple carbohydrates and refined polysaccharides (e.g. white flour), vitamins, mineral

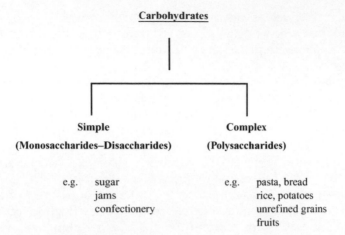

Fig. 2.2   Carbohydrate classification

salts and trace elements are often reduced or missing. In this case carbohydrates have limited health value and are usually referred to as 'empty
calories'. It should also be stressed that the brain is only fuelled by the
monosaccharide glucose.

The type of carbohydrate consumed—and whether it is consumed
before, during, or after the end of a class and/or rehearsal—may play a
significant role in maintaining optimal levels of this nutrient. In particular, the type of carbohydrate can indicate how rapidly its digestion
product moves from the small intestine into the blood. To better describe
the degree to which various foods affect carbohydrate concentrations in
the body, the term *glycaemic index* (GI) has been introduced. It simply
means the extent to which a particular food item causes the key monosaccharide glucose to increase in the blood after the food has been
consumed.

Consumption of foods with high GI is associated with *insulin* release,
and dancers should avoid these foods at least one hour prior to intensive
exercise. For example, eating a rapidly digested chocolate bar—with high
GI—would cause a rapid and high blood glucose rise and a corresponding high insulin response. The latter may then lead to *hypoglycaemia* (i.e.
reduced blood sugar levels) and the associated fatigue during exercise. In
addition elevated insulin encourages the conversion of carbohydrate to
fat. In contrast, a pear with its low GI would result in a gradual rise in
blood glucose involving a relatively small amount of insulin. It is safe,
however, to eat foods with high GI after exercise where a speedy return
to pre-exercise carbohydrate levels is required. Aspects such as the
degree of ripeness of fruits may also affect the rate of glucose release—
and therefore their GI—given that the fruits' composition changes as they

ripen. The starch content of a banana is about 37% when unripe, falling to 3% during ripening when starch converts to sugar.

Carbohydrates are stored in limited amounts as *glycogen* in the liver (80–110 g) and in the muscle (300–450 g). Both muscle and liver glycogen can be exhausted by hard exercise; the available stores in the body will last for about 90 minutes of strenuous cycling, running, dancing, and so on.

Increased stores of *muscle glycogen*—through appropriate diet as well as exercise—can positively affect dance in terms of its intensity and duration. According to the original (or classical) method known as *carbohydrate loading*, if muscles are first depleted of glycogen and then replenished by consumption of a high-carbohydrate diet, the glycogen content is about twice that achieved with a low-carbohydrate diet. Nevertheless, muscle glycogen is utilized rapidly during exercise, and fatigue occurs when it is depleted to low levels. Such fatigue may then be related to poor dance technique and to the increased incidence of injury often seen in the latter parts of dance sessions.

The *liver glycogen* can be made available to muscle when it is broken down to *glucose* and then released into the blood. Other tissues or organs (e.g. the brain) also take up blood glucose. This leads to rapid falls of total glycogen, especially when it is not promptly replaced. Reduced levels of the body's glycogen may then contribute to the feelings of 'lack of energy' which dancers often experience after a long day in the studio.

Glycogen is restored in the muscles at a rate of about 5% per hour. With a normal diet, it takes at least 20 hours to fully replenish stocks (Fallowfield and Williams 1993). However, in the first 1–2 hours after exercise, glycogen restoration is faster and—with a high-carbohydrate diet—muscle glycogen can be restored by almost 50% during this time. Failure to do so may lead to situations where dance sessions the next day may be fuelled by lower glycogen reserves than the previous day, with obvious implications for both technique and injuries. However, the question always asked is '*how much carbohydrate do dancers and other active individuals need per day?*'

The Colgan Institute in the US has developed a system where body weight and hours of exercise are taken into account for the estimation of an individual's daily carbohydrate requirements (Table 2.1). If a dancer weighs 50 kg and spends 6 hours at classes in a day, he/she will need to consume about 700 g of carbohydrates by the end of that day. This strategy would enable the dancer to maintain a balance between carbohydrate intake and its use as exercise fuel. However, during periods of reduced physical effort (e.g. holidays), the dancer's carbohydrate intake should also decrease. Thus, for the same 50 kg dancer, intakes should not be more than 250 g, or the equivalent of five cups of baked beans. The

Table 2.1 How much carbohydrate? Estimates of daily carbohydrate needs (in grams) for different body weights and duration of physical activity

Body weight (kg)	Exercise per day (hours)						
	1	2	3	4	5	6	7
40	100	200	300	400	500	600	700
45	150	250	350	450	550	650	750
50	200	300	400	500	600	700	800
55	250	350	450	550	650	750	850
60	300	400	500	600	700	800	900
65	350	450	550	650	750	850	950
70	400	500	600	700	800	900	1000
75	450	550	650	750	850	950	1050
80	500	600	700	800	900	1000	1100

carbohydrate content of certain foods appears in Table 2.2. It should also be remembered that:

- Greater amounts of carbohydrate intakes will *not* further increase availability and use
- Excess carbohydrate is converted into *body fat*
- Large carbohydrate portions are *not* better than frequent smaller ones

4   DIETARY FIBRE

Dietary fibre, a carbohydrate polysaccharide, represents the most resistant parts of the skeletal framework of the plant. Dietary fibre is resistant to

Table 2.2 Examples of the carbohydrate content of foods measured in grams

Food	Amount	Carbohydrate (g)
Apple	1 medium	20
Apple juice	8 fl oz	30
Baked beans	1 cup	50
Baked potato	1 large	55
Banana	1 medium	20
Fruit Yoghurt	1 cup	35
Lentils	1 cup (cooked)	40
Muesli	$\frac{1}{2}$ cup	36
Orange	1 medium	20
Orange juice	8 fl oz	25
Rice	1 cup (cooked)	35
Spaghetti	1 portion (cooked)	40

digestion and absorption by the intestine, and hence leaves some residue in the digestive tract. This property has led to the formation of a theory whereby fibre is an unnecessary part of the human diet. However, this theory overlooks the fact that the majority of the indigestible fibre continues to be broken down in the colon via the fermentation process, and that fibre is essential for the health of the whole digestive system.

Dietary fibre exists in two basic forms: water-soluble and water-insoluble. The latter type of dietary fibre passes through the entire gastrointestinal tract showing little or no effects on metabolism. In contrast, soluble fibres may be metabolized mainly in the large intestine. There are a number of reasons supporting the use of dietary fibre:

1. *Protect teeth.* Less chewing may lead to a lack of abrasion on the teeth, which dietary fibre would have created. Hence, the cleansing action doesn't occur, resulting in forms of dental decay.
2. *Protect the stomach.* Foods containing dietary fibre empty out of the stomach faster than processed foods, thereby preventing gastric ulcers, as no excessive acid is released.
3. *Protect the large intestine.* Fibre enters the colon where much of it will be fermented, thereby providing protection for the cell lining. This is thought to protect against cancer. Also, fibre provides a 'grip' for the colon.
4. *Control energy intakes.* Chewing fibre-rich foods stimulates the secretions of saliva and gastric juice that are directly involved in the stomach distension, which, in turn, evokes the sensation of satiety. With fibre-reduced/depleted foods, overconsumption (and thus increased energy intakes) may result in order to achieve satiety.
5. *Contribute to blood glucose control.* Ingestion of fibre-depleted carbohydrates may cause blood glucose to rise suddenly with a correspondingly high insulin response. For example 38 g of sugar can be swallowed in a single can of cola drink within one to two minutes. For the same 38 g of sugar to be ingested in unrefined form (containing a lot of fibre), 330 g of, say, apples have to be chewed for several minutes, therefore preventing a sudden blood glucose rise.

Since it is unlikely that refined carbohydrate foods will be totally avoided, dancers are advised that fibre, preferably in the form of fresh fruits and vegetables, should be added in sufficient quantities to their meals.

5 FATS

Fats (or *lipids*) are organic substances with limited water solubility. Despite the negative publicity, they serve a variety of functions, including:

The importance of fat as an exercise energy source depends on the

- Organ support (e.g. eyes)
- Absorption of the fat-soluble vitamins A, D, E and K from the gut
- Forming an essential part of cell membranes and nerve fibres
- Providing up to 70% of the energy requirements at rest
- Preservation of body heat, especially fat under skin
- Body shape
- Production of steroid hormones
- Together with carbohydrates they constitute the main sources of energy for exercise; fat may provide about 50% of the energy requirements in dance, but up to 90% in marathon running

intensity of activity as well as on the availability of carbohydrates. Fats are primarily used when the body performs low intensity muscular work, thus sparing the store of carbohydrate (i.e. glycogen). The fitter the individual the greater the carbohydrate sparing. However, if the body starts to run low on carbohydrate (e.g. during chronic food deprivation or prolonged exercise) it will increase its use of fat. Fig. 2.3 shows that as the glycogen stores decrease over time, the use of fat for energy production increases. From this it becomes clear that dancers may do themselves no favours when, in an attempt to lose weight, they ingest little or no fat, and that such practices should be discouraged.

The body stores most of its fat in the adipose tissue as *triglycerides* that are composed of three molecules of *fatty acids* and one molecule of *glycerol*. Stored triglycerides are mobilized by *lipolysis* to provide *free fatty acids*, which are then released into the blood and transported to the active

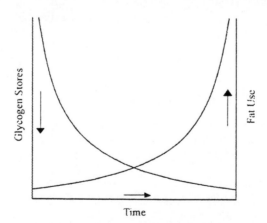

Fig. 2.3   The contribution of fat to energy production during exercise in relation to glycogen stores

muscle for the purpose of energy production. Under normal conditions, the body's stored fat could provide energy for continuous exercise lasting for several days, unlike the carbohydrate stores that would last less than 90 minutes. This is partly related to the fact that fats generate more than twice as much energy per gram than carbohydrates (i.e. 9.3 vs 4.1 kcal). If fat was the only substrate, this would theoretically enable individuals to run continuously at marathon speeds for more than 70 hours (Newsholme and Leech 1983).

For both health and fitness, it is advisable to reduce fat intakes to about 30–35% of the daily energy needs (Coyle 1991), with a simultaneous increase of carbohydrate intake. A low-fat diet will be easier to achieve if dietary fat is replaced with a mixture of energy from sugar and starch (Drummond, Kirk and de Looy 1996). Dancers should also include in their fat intake an 'omega-3' family of unsaturated fatty acids found mainly in the oils of seafish, such as mackerel, salmon, sardines, and herring. Research has indicated the potential health and fitness benefits of these fatty acids as they upgrade blood flow to the muscles, prevent blood clotting, contribute to lower blood pressures, result in better red blood cell plasticity, and reduce symptoms of some inflammatory conditions.

Increased dietary fat intake, especially *triglycerides* and *cholesterol*, has well-established implications in the development of cardiovascular disease, and diseases such as cancer. However, moving towards lower-cholesterol diets is not without potential problems. Cholesterol—despite its reputation as the 'black sheep' of human nutrition—actually plays some key roles inside the body, such as in sex hormone formation and maintenance of the integrity of brain-cell membranes. Cholesterol is also found in the nerves, liver and blood.

5.1 Saturated and Unsaturated Fats

According to their chemical structure, fatty acids occur in two forms: *saturated and unsaturated*. In food, the proportions of each form determine whether the fat is hard or liquid, how the body handles it and how it affects health. Saturated fatty acids are solid in room temperatures and found primarily in animal food products. The major exceptions to this rule are the tropical fats. Coconut and palm oils are unusually high in saturated fats even though they are treated as vegetable oils. Only 5–10% of the daily consumed calories should come from saturated fats. To achieve this, avoid products that provide details of high saturated fat content on their labels. Beware of foods claiming to be 'low' or 'no cholesterol'—they may be high in saturated fat. Also avoid products which list the above mentioned tropical oils as major ingredients, as well as those vegetable oils which have been artificially saturated with hydrogen—known as *hydrogenated oils* and *fats*.

Found primarily in plant foods, there are two varieties of unsaturated fatty acids: monounsaturated and polyunsaturated. Both are liquid at room temperature. However, monounsaturated fatty acids may solidify at cold temperatures, while polyunsaturated are liquid. The main source of monounsaturated fat is olive oil, while polyunsaturated fats may be obtained from different vegetable oils including corn oil and sunflower oil. The omega-3 fatty acids—already mentioned in this section—are highly polyunsaturated fats. Monounsaturated fatty acids are thought to have the greatest health benefits. They can reduce the harmful low-density lipoprotein (LDL) without affecting the beneficial high-density lipoprotein (HDL). Intakes of polyunsaturated fatty acids can reduce LDL, but also lessen the good HDL.

6 PROTEINS

Protein is one of the most essential and multipurpose nutrients. It has a wide variety of physiological functions associated with both health and fitness (Lemon 1991; Koutedakis 1994). These functions may include:

- Formation of the structural basis of muscle tissue (which is the largest protein pool within the body)
- Growth and repair of damaged tissue
- Involvement in the metabolic processes, by forming enzymes which facilitate (catalyse) chemical reactions for energy production
- Formation of antibodies (the key elements of the body's defence system)
- Synthesis of many hormones
- If carbohydrate and fat fail to provide enough energy—as in cases of starvation or exhaustive and prolonged exercise—protein can be used as fuel. To do this, protein has to be converted into glucose

Unlike carbohydrates and fats, protein contains nitrogen that enables it to form *amino acids*, the building blocks of proteins. Twenty amino acids have been identified as necessary in adults, which can further be divided into *essential* and *non-essential* amino acids (see Table 2.3). The essential amino acids cannot be manufactured in the body and have to be found in our food.

Animal sources such as meat, fish, eggs and/or dairy products are often referred to as 'complete' protein foods as they contain all nine

Table 2.3 The essential and non-essential amino acids

Essential	Non-essential
Isoleucine	Alanine
Leucine	Arginine
Lysine	Asparagine
Methionine	Aspartic acid
Phenylalanine	Cysteine
Threonine	Glutamic acid
Tryptophan	Glutamine
Valine	Glycine
Histidine	Proline
	Serine
	Tyrosine

essential amino acids and therefore have higher biological value (Table 2.4). Vegetable sources are described as being 'incomplete' as far as protein content is concerned, as they lack at least one of the essential amino acids, and therefore show lower biological value. However, mixing single proteins from either animal or vegetable sources may result in meals with higher biological value than any single protein can provide (Table 2.4). *Vegans, lactovegeterians* and *ovovegetarians* should be careful in the selection of the foods they eat, if dance performance is not to suffer from insufficient protein intake.

The human body has no protein reserve/store comparable to its large energy stores of fat and moderate stores of glycogen. The average person needs 0.8 g of protein per kg of his/her healthy (non-obese) body weight per day (Trichopoulou and Vassilakos 1990), which provides 10–15% of total daily energy intakes. For health purposes, the recommended daily allowance (RDA) for protein for the average Briton is 45–56 grams per day. However, males and females who engage in repeated, high-intensity physical activities lasting up to several hours, would probably benefit from an increased protein intake of 1–2 g of their body-weight (Phillips, Atkinson, Tarnopolsky and MacDougal 1993; Lemon 1994). Any excess protein intake is converted to fat and stored, or excreted.

It is generally agreed that most conventional, but well designed, diets meet the protein needs of the average dancer, and that protein supplements are not required. However, this may not be the case with individuals who consume low calorific diets, or with those who have relatively low daily protein intakes in their diets (e.g. some vegetarians). Even if protein sources are appropriately mixed, vegetarian dancers should consume approximately 10–20% more food than meat-eaters, mainly

Table 2.4 Commonly used single and mixed proteins. Appropriately mixed proteins give higher biological values than single proteins alone

BIOLOGICAL VALUE		
		MIXED PROTEINS
		Egg & potato
		Egg & milk
		Egg & wheat
	SINGLE PROTEINS	Milk & wheat
	Egg	Beans & maize
	Beef	Red beans & rice
	Fish	Green peas & rice
	Milk	Green beans & almonds
	Soya	
	Rye	
	Beans	

Foods

because of the differences in protein quality between vegetable and animal protein sources. In such cases, protein (or amino acid) supplementation may be necessary for maintaining an optimal nitrogen balance and for reducing impairment in exercise status. Supplementation of certain amino acids, such as glutamine, may also be advisable as it has been suggested that this amino acid is essential for the optimal function of the immune system, and that it is known to be decreased in overtrained athletes (Parry-Billings, Budgett, Koutedakis *et al.* 1992). However, it should be stressed that most of the available data are negative regarding the benefits of amino acid supplementation.

7   VITAMINS

Vitamins are a group of 13 unrelated organic compounds that are involved in important functions related to growth, health and physical fitness. They contribute to chemical processes that regulate metabolism, energy release, and tissue repair. Most cannot be synthesized by the human body. Lack of certain vitamins is, *inter alia*, associated with fatigue and underperformance in individuals with increased levels of physical activity. Vitamins are either *water-soluble* or *fat-soluble* in nature.

The four fat-soluble vitamins are A, D, E, and K (Table 2.5). Apart from their role in energy release, these vitamins play an important role in the treatment of various medical conditions such as gastric ulcers (A), osteoporosis (D), sunburn, joint and muscular pain (E). Daily ingestion of fat-soluble vitamins is not necessary, given that they are normally stored in small quantities in the liver and in the fat cells of the adipose tissue. However, these vitamins are sensitive and can be destroyed during cooking (Table 2.6).

The nine water-soluble vitamins are: B1, B2, B6, B12, biotin, folic acid, niacin, pantothenic acid, and C (Table 2.7). They are absorbed from the

Table 2.5 Fat-soluble vitamins

Vitamin	Major sources	Major functions	Daily reference values (for adults)
A	Not widely present in plants. Pro-vitamins for the formation of A in egg yolk, carrots, fruits, oils, milk products.	Needed for synthesis of mucopolysaccharides, maintenance of normal epithelial structure. Formation of visual pigments	1000 μg (males) 800 μg (females)
D	Fish oils, liver, milk, egg yolk. Action of sunlight on the skin.	Increases calcium and phosphorus absorption. Helps calcium deposition in bones and teeth.	10 μg
E	Leafy green vegetables, wheat germ oil, liver, peanuts, eggs.	Helps red blood cells resist haemolysis. Aids in muscle and nerve maintenance. Acts as antioxidant.	10 mg (males) 8 mg (females)
K	Yoghurt, molasses, sunflower oil, liver, leafy green vegetables.	Aids in prothrombin synthesis (clotting factors VII, IX, X) in liver.	80 mg (males) 65 mg (females)

Table 2.6 Vitamin losses in cooking

C	100%	B6	40%
B1	80%	D	40%
B2	75%	A	40%
Biotin	60%	Niacin	25%
E	55%	B12	10%

Table 2.7 Water-soluble vitamins

Vitamin	Major sources	Major functions	Daily reference values (for adults)
B1 (Thiamine)	Organ meats, whole grains, oysters, yeast, molasses, yoghurt, nuts.	Helps regulate carbohydrate metabolism.	1.5 mg (males) 1.1 mg (females)
B2 (Riboflavin)	Milk, eggs, beef and veal, liver, whole grains and cereals, spinach, nuts, yeast, molasses, beets.	Forms enzymes (FAD, FMN) involved in oxidative phosphorylation. Aids cellular respiration. Energy release.	2.0 mg (males) 1.5 mg (females)
B6 (Pyridoxine)	Whole grains, liver, milk, molasses, leafy vegetables, bananas, yeast, tomatoes, corn, yoghurt, fish.	Helps amino acid metabolism; transport of amino acids across plasma membranes.	2.0 mg (males) 1.6 mg (females)
B12 (Cyanocobalamin)	Organ meats, milk, cheese, eggs, yeast, fish, oysters.	Nucleic acid and amino acid metabolism. Erythrocyte formation to prevent anaemia.	3.0 μg (males) 2.0 μg (females)
H (Biotin)	Liver, yeast, vegetables, eggs, and intestinal bacteria.	Assists CO_2 fixation, transamination and nitrogen metabolism. Aids cell growth.	300 mg (males) 150 mg (females)
Folic Acid	Organ meats, leafy green vegetables, eggs, milk, salmon, intestinal bacteria.	Nucleic acid synthesis and DNA formation. Aids growth, reproduction, digestion.	200 μg (males) 180 μg (females)
Niacin	Whole grains, liver, chicken, seafood, yeast, nuts, dried beans.	Aids carbohydrate metabolism. Aids production of sex hormones. Reduces cholesterol.	20 mg (males) 15 mg (females)
Pantothenic acid	Yeast, liver, eggs, nuts, salmon, green vegetables, cereals.	Forms part of coenzyme A. Glucose production from lipids and amino acids.	8.0 mg (males) 5.0 mg (females)
C (Ascorbic acid)	Citrus fruits, butter, tomatoes, green peppers, broccoli, potatoes.	Necessary for oxidation reactions, synthesis and maintenance of collagen, bone and tooth formation, healing.	75 mg (males) 60 mg (females)

digestive tract along with water and are not stored in the body tissues to any appreciable extent. They are used for therapy of many painful conditions such as sciatica, lumbago (B1), mouth and gastric ulcers (B2), and muscle fatigue (B6). Vitamin C is used to increase the rate of healing after accidental and surgical injury, while biotin is used to treat skin problems. Water-soluble vitamins are thought to be depleted with strenuous exercise, and—as in the case of fat-soluble vitamins—they are easily destroyed in processing and cooking (Table 2.6).

Many dancers believe that vitamin supplements will help them feel stronger, have better health and even elevate their performance levels. However, there are no data supporting that intakes above the *daily* (or dietary) *reference values* (Tables 2.5, 2.7) are indeed beneficial. Furthermore, most studies have shown that active individuals can actually receive the necessary vitamins through their diets. A varied diet, with plenty of fruit and vegetables, can provide all dancers need. However, individuals who are on weight-reduction schemes or on low body weight maintenance programmes may require some vitamin supplementation (Williams 1995). So do vegetarians who often become deficient in vitamin B12.

It should be remembered that excess supplementation of certain vitamins—apart from the obvious expense—can be associated with toxicity symptoms. For example, excess levels of vitamin D can cause vomiting, constant thirst and head pains, while excess vitamin E can cause muscle weakness and proneness to fatigue. Therefore, only a multi-vitamin supplement with 100% or less of the daily reference amounts is recommended if it is needed.

Foods that are rich in vitamins C and E may provide some protection against cancer and heart diseases. They also serve as *antioxidants*. These are compounds that protect other compounds (such as lipids in cell membranes) from attack by oxygen. Oxygen triggers the formation of the highly reactive chemicals known as *free radicals*, which, if left uncontrolled by the body, can damage cell structures, disrupt metabolic processes and cause fatigue.

8 MINERALS

The body is composed of at least 31 known chemical elements. The most abundant chemical element is oxygen that amounts to 65% of a person's body weight. Three other elements constitute 31% of the body mass; these are carbon (18%), hydrogen (10%), and nitrogen (3%). The remaining 4% of our body weight is composed of a group of 21 metallic elements called *minerals*.

Minerals can be classified into 7 *macrominerals* and 14 *trace elements* (or *microminerals*) based upon the extent of their occurrence in the body (Tables 2.8 and Table 2.9). Macrominerals each make up at least 0.01% of the total body weight. Optimal levels of calcium, magnesium and phosphorus have been related to increased and demanding physical efforts. The four remaining macrominerals are not thought to directly affect physical performance.

Trace elements each comprise less than 0.001% of total body weight. Apart from those appearing in Table 2.9, the trace mineral list includes molybdenum, nickel, silicon, vanadium and arsenic. Although five trace elements (i.e. chromium, copper, iron, selenium and zinc) have been suggested to act as physical performance stimulators (Clarkson 1995), more data are needed to confirm this.

Minerals are essential for numerous biological functions, as they are found in enzymes, hormones, and vitamins. They are essential substances for the musculoskeletal system, play an important role in the efficient extraction and utilization of energy from carbohydrates, fats and proteins, and activate energy transfer throughout the body.

Minerals are found in the soil and are incorporated in growing plants, and subsequently in grazing animals. Humans obtain their mineral nutrition from both plants and animals, while drinking water is an excellent source of many minerals. As with vitamins, healthy and physically active people who eat well-balanced meals obtain enough of the essential mineral elements to maintain proper physiological functioning. Mineral supplements may be necessary, however, in some geographic regions where mineral elements (such as iodine) in the soil or water supply are relatively scarce.

Because many of the minerals are only required in small amounts, minor changes in their intake can make a critical difference to both health status and performance capabilities. For instance, undersupply of calcium, phosphorus and magnesium has been found to be associated with impaired skeletal development, muscle weakness, muscle cramps and increased incidents of bone and muscle injuries. Together with reduced physical activity levels, inadequate supply of these minerals—calcium in particular—also contributes to increased cases of *osteoporosis* in both pre- and post-menopausal women (Alekel, Clasey, Fehling *et al.* 1995; Santora 1987). Heavy sweating, heavy menstrual flow, increased destruction of red blood cells and passing blood may be associated with iron deficiency (more commonly found in women). Last but not least, low levels of zinc may bring about appetite loss, poor wound healing and possibly impair growth in children.

The minerals sodium, potassium, chloride, calcium and magnesium have quite similar functions and they are collectively called *electrolytes*.

Table 2.8 Food sources, functions and daily requirements for the *macrominerals*

Mineral	Major sources	Major functions	Daily reference values (adults)
Calcium	Dairy products, eggs, fish, soya/tofu.	Bone/teeth formation, heart action, blood clotting, muscle contraction, excitability, nerve synapses, mental activity, buffer systems.	1.2 g (males) 1.0 g (females)
Chloride	All foods, table salt.	Principal anion of extracellular fluid. Necessary for acid-base balance, osmotic equilibrium.	Unknown
Magnesium	Green vegetables, milk, meats, nuts.	Bone structure, regulation of nerve and muscle action. Catalyst for intracellular enzymatic reactions, especially carbohydrate metabolism.	350 mg (males) 280 mg (female)
Phosphorus	Dairy products, meats, fish, poultry, beans, grains, eggs.	Necessary for proper bone structure, intermediary metabolism, buffers, membranes. Phosphate bonds essential for energy production (ATP), nucleic acids.	About 1.5 g
Potassium	All foods, especially meats, vegetables, milk.	Major component of intracellular fluid. Needed for muscle contraction, nerve impulse transmission.	Unknown
Sodium	Most foods, table salt.	Major component of extracellular fluid. Necessary for ionic equilibrium, nerve impulse conduction, buffer systems.	3.0 g (males) 2.0 g (females)
Sulphur	All protein-containing foods.	Component of hormones, several vitamins and proteins.	Unknown

Table 2.9 Food sources, functions and daily requirements for selected *trace elements*

Mineral	Major sources	Major functions	Daily reference values (adults)
Chromium	Meats, vegetables, yeast, beer, unrefined wheat flour, corn oil, shellfish.	Necessary for glucose metabolism, formation of insulin for proper blood-sugar level.	50–200 μg
Cobalt	Meats	Involved in red blood cell formation.	Not known
Copper	Liver, meats, oysters, margarine, eggs, wheat products.	Necessary for haemoglobin formation, maintenance of certain copper-containing enzymes, proper intestinal absorption of iron.	1.5–3.0 mg
Fluorine	Fluorinated water, toothpaste, milk, tea.	Hardens bones and teeth. Suppresses bacterial action in mouth.	1.5–4.0 mg
Iodine	Iodized table salt, fish, seaweed.	Necessary for synthesis of thyroxin, which is essential for maintenance of normal cellular respiration.	150 μg
Iron	Liver, eggs, red meat, shellfish, beans, nuts, raisins.	Component of haemoglobin, myoglobin. Necessary for transport of oxygen, cellular oxidation.	15 mg (males) 10 mg (females)
Manganese	Meats, bananas, bran, beans, leafy vegetables, whole grains, nuts.	Necessary for formation of haemoglobin, activation of enzymes.	350 mg (males) 280 mg (females)
Selenium	Most foods, especially liver, other meats and seafood.	Enzymes, lipid metabolism, antioxidant (protects plasma membrane from breaking down).	70 μg (males) 55 μg (females)
Zinc	Meats, milk, seafood, eggs, legumes, green vegetables.	Component part of many enzymes.	15 mg (males) 12 mg (females)

Their major functions are to enable neural impulses to control muscle activity and to manage and maintain the proper rate of fluid exchange within the body. They can also activate enzymes to guide a variety of metabolic activities in the cell.

Sodium, potassium and chloride are the three major electrolytes. Sodium and chloride are primarily found in the fluid outside the body's cells and blood plasma, but potassium is located inside the cells. When sweating excessively, the body loses the electrolytes present in sweat, leading to impairment in exercise performance. One litre of sweat loss is accompanied by a loss of about 1.5 g of electrolytes. It is common, therefore, for active individuals to increase electrolyte intake to offset the effects of dehydration. However, megadosing of these minerals is never advisable. Excess potassium can cause heart failure, and high levels of sodium have been associated with high blood pressure.

9 WATER AND FLUID REPLACEMENT

Although *water* is essential for energy production, health and, of course, exercise, it is seldom thought of as a nutrient because it has no calorific value. *Inter alia*, water is needed for the body's cooling system, for transportation of nutrients throughout the tissues, for optimal functioning of the heart, and for the maintenance of adequate blood volume.

Approximately 60% of the body's weight is water. About 60 to 65% of this water is contained inside the cells and is referred to as *intracellular fluid*. The remainder is outside the cells and is known as the *extracellular fluid*. With respect to dance and exercise in general, water makes up about 72% of the weight of muscle tissue and only 20–25% of the weight of fat. Thus differences between individuals in terms of total body water are determined largely by differences in body composition; in individuals with the same body weight, the total body water will be larger in those with the greater muscle mass.

The total amount of water in the body is kept constant by delicate balancing mechanisms (Table 2.10). On a daily basis water losses must be matched by water intakes, and it is the body itself which controls both water excretion and water intake. In sedentary persons most of the water losses are associated with kidney function and evaporation through the lungs and skin. In fact, the body must excrete a minimum of about 500 millilitres each day as urine, in order to carry away the waste products of metabolic activities. During exercise, however, sweating accounts for a greater proportion of the fluid losses. Sweat rates in the order of 1.5 litres/hour are commonly encountered in strenuous exercise. In hot and humid conditions, well-acclimatized athletes may sweat at rates greater

Table 2.10 Example of water balance per 24 hours in a sedentary person at rest

Gains		Losses	
Liquids	1200 ml	Evaporation (lungs/skin)	800 ml
Foods	900 ml	Sweat loss	50 ml
Metabolic water	350 ml	Faeces	100 ml
		Urine loss	1500 ml
Total	2450 ml	Total	2450 ml

than 2 litres/hour. In general, the harder and longer the exercise, and the hotter and more humid the environment, the more body fluid will be lost. Let us now consider the basic physiology behind sweating.

During exercise muscles produce extra heat. In fact, about 75% of the energy we put into dance—and other forms of exercise—is converted into heat. This extra heat has to be dissipated to keep body temperature within safe limits (around 37 °C). This is mainly accomplished by sweating. Water from inside the body is carried from the hot muscles to the skin surface in the blood capillaries, and as it evaporates heat is lost. For every litre of sweat that evaporates, the body loses about 600 calories of heat. Dancers cannot prevent their body from losing water. However, they can estimate the sweat loss and, thus, the quantity of water they should take by simply weighing themselves before and after a class.

The effects of dehydration on the ability to perform physical tasks and on health have been known since the era of classical Greece and the ancient Olympic Games. Even small unreplaced fluid losses can impair maximal physical performance, mainly due to decreases in plasma volume which in turn affect carbohydrate utilization (Armstrong, Costill and Fink 1985; Buskirk, Lampietro and Bass 1985). Apart from the element of performance, large unreplaced losses can further bring about alterations in numerous biological functions and cause muscular cramps, nausea, vomiting, weakness, reduced mental concentration, confusion and even death. For example, a 2% body weight loss as fluid may affect the ability to dance, given that under these circumstances the capacity for maximal exercise is reduced by about 15%. At 5% body weight loss as water the capacity for maximal physical work will decrease by 30%, while water loss of 9–12% of body weight can be fatal. It should be noticed that it requires about 24–36 hours to voluntarily rehydrate oneself, after a body fluid loss equivalent to 4.0–6.0% of body weight (Costill 1972).

The water needs of the body are mainly met from liquids. However, solid foods also serve as water sources. One kilogram of fat, protein or, especially, carbohydrate produces about 350 ml of water when broken down for energy. The adult water intake directly from liquids ranges from 800–1600 ml each day. This amount will vary considerably under certain conditions, especially during exercise and thermal stresses, where fluid intake may increase 5–8 times above normal. A common mistake is that we rely on feeling thirsty as the signal to drink. But feeling thirsty is only a fail-safe device that prevents us from becoming severely dehydrated. Pale and plentiful urine indicates that you are well hydrated.

Ingestion of extra water prior to exercise allows dancers to work with lower heart rates and provides for increased sweating rates—and a comfortable decrease in body temperature as a result—during exercise. It is therefore advisable to drink about 300 ml of plain water (cold at 5 °C) 30–45 minutes before exercise. During exercise a volume of 150–250 ml of plain water ingested at 10–20-minute intervals is a realistic goal, as larger volumes at one time tend to produce feelings of uncomfortable fullness.

9.1 Sport Drinks

In the last 5–10 years, a number of commercially available sport drinks have appeared. Based on their content, these products can be generally categorized as fluid replacement or energy drinks, although most of them can be safely treated as both.

Fluid replacement drinks principally contain electrolytes (mainly sodium) and carbohydrates. Their aim is to replace fluid faster than plain water. Energy drinks carry more carbohydrates than fluid replacement drinks and their aim is fast and effective replacement of energy losses. The composition of energy drinks is not crucial as glucose, sucrose and *glucose polymers* are all suitable, although fructose is best avoided on account of the risk of gastrointestinal upset.

Sport drinks can also be classified as *hypotonic* (or *low osmolality*), *isotonic* (or *normal osmolality*) and *hypertonic* (or *high osmolality*) drinks. A hypotonic drink contains fewer particles (i.e. electrolytes and carbohydrates) per 100 ml than the body's own fluids, thus it is absorbed faster than plain water. Isotonic drinks normally contain the same electrolytes and carbohydrates per 100 ml as the body's fluids and are therefore absorbed as fast as plain water. By contrast, hypertonic drinks have more particles (i.e. electrolytes and carbohydrates) per 100 ml than the body's own fluids, which means that they are absorbed more slowly than plain water.

When dancers exercise in hot environments, drinks with up to 5% solution (i.e. hypotonic) permit quick supply of water, electrolyte and carbohydrate. For exercise in normal temperatures, isotonic drinks may be more appropriate. Recent research shows that drinks with 6–10%

solutions provide optimal absorption rates. These may be commercially available as isotonic drinks. Products with higher than 10% solutions should be avoided during exercise, as gastric emptying is inhibited, thus providing less water and carbohydrates per given time. However, such drinks can be safely consumed after exercise. Dancers can always make their own cheap and very effective sport drink simply by combining five tablespoons of table sugar (sucrose) and one third of a teaspoon of salt with two pints of water.

10   GENERAL DIETARY RECOMMENDATIONS

- Choose a diet from a variety of foods
- Try to eat fresh fruit, dried fruit, nuts
- Eat more cereals, vegetables and salads of all kinds
- Cook green vegetables for shorter periods of time in less water
- Use natural vegetable cooking oils and try grilled foods in preference to fried
- If you cook chips have thick-cut varieties to keep the fat content down
- Eat no more than 4–5 eggs per week
- Eat about 6 bread slices per day and preferably wholemeal rather than white
- Buy foods as close as possible to their natural state (e.g. honey instead of sugar)
- A light meal should be eaten 1–3 hours prior to exercise
- Avoid big late-evening meals

- Carbohydrate consumption should account for 55+% of total energy intake
- Following exercise, the amount of stored glycogen in the working muscles falls, so glycogen stores must be refuelled after every session, and soon!
- Large carbohydrate meals are not more effective than frequent smaller meals
- Eating 50–100 g of carbohydrate every 2 hours is advisable
- Sugar consumption should only be one quarter of total carbohydrate intake

- Fat intake should not be more than 30–35% total energy consumption
- Avoid commercially available minced-meat products, as they are normally high in fat

- Cut down on beef, lamb, and pork, and eat more poultry and fish
- When choosing dairy products, select those marked *low fat*
- Buy cooking oils marked *high in polyunsaturated fat*

- No vitamin or mineral supplementation is needed if dancers are eating well and wisely
- Drink plenty of water
- When losing a lot of sweat, drinks need to be low in carbohydrate ($<6\%$)
- If you are not losing much sweat but are at risk of developing fatigue due to low glycogen stores, drinks need a relatively high carbohydrate content ($>10\%$)

11 ERGOGENIC AIDS

Up to date, scientific research continues to support the proven way for fitness/performance maintenance or enhancement: optimal training and practice in the studios and gymnasiums and, of course, proper diet. However, given the emphasis placed on better performances, many dancers—along with an ever-increasing number of sport competitors—are prepared to pay a high price for an 'aid' which will secure these much-desired performances. That has led to the development of an entirely new industry specializing in the production of substances and/or design of techniques that can be employed beyond the normal training and preparation regimens. A brand-new word, *ergogenic aids*, had also to be found to categorize these diverse methods. The term is derived from the Greek noun *ergo* (= work) and verb *geno* (= to produce, create) and is usually defined as *to increase potential for physical work (performance)*. Ergogenic aids in sports and exercise are grouped into five main categories (Williams 1995):

- Pharmacological ergogenic aids (e.g. amphetamines, anabolic steroids)
- Physiological ergogenic aids (e.g. blood doping, oxygen)
- Psychological ergogenic aids (e.g. hypnosis, stress management)
- Mechanical ergogenic aids (e.g. equipment such as better dance shoes)
- Nutritional ergogenic aids (e.g. proteins, carbohydrates, caffeine, water)

Although no scientific research has yet supported claims that 'ginseng will make you faster' and 'bee pollen has special energy-enhancing effects', recent research does suggest that certain food substances may indeed have an ergogenic effect. For example, adequate carbohydrate consumption may reduce mental fatigue during prolonged exercise, while supplements of the amino acid glutamine may be required for a strong immune system in active individuals (Brouns 1993). Also, taking about 0.3 of a gram per kg body weight of bicarbonate (as in baking soda) one to two hours before an intensive physical activity may buffer the produced lactic acid and consequent deleterious effects of muscular fatigue (Clark 1997), but may be associated with nausea.

11.1   Creatine Supplementation

Creatine has been among the commercially available substances that have hit the world of sport and exercise in the last 5–10 years, aiming at improved performances through better and more efficient energy supplies. However, dancers should remember that this chemical is still expensive, and it results in weight increase, also the long-term effects of such practices are as yet unknown.

Creatine is a naturally occurring compound found in meat and fish, and plays a significant role in energy production during highly anaerobic efforts as part of the energy-rich compound *phosphocreatine* (PC). The latter is normally present in the muscle at a concentration of about 3–4 times that of *adenosine triphosphate* (ATP).

To allow the muscle to do very intensive work and to change quickly from rest to work the assistance of PC is always necessary. In fact, PC backs up ATP in providing energy for fast and powerful muscular contractions. More specifically, the enzyme creatine kinase catalyses the transfer of the phosphate group (P) from PC to the always present ADP, resulting in the formation of new ATP and the release of free *creatine* (C):

$$ATP \rightarrow ADP + P$$

$$PC + ADP \rightarrow ATP + C$$

The theory behind creatine supplementation is that the PC muscle content will also increase, making it more effective during brief and very intensive exercise bouts (Greenhaff 1995). Creatine supplementation may also accelerate the recovery process (i.e. PC restoration) following intensive muscular efforts. Indeed, PC is restored from the available creatine and by transfer of a phosphate group (P) from ATP:

$$P + ADP + \text{energy from oxidative metabolism} \rightarrow ATP$$

$$C + ATP \rightarrow PC + ADP$$

Apart from high-intensity (anaerobic) exercise, elevated creatine levels—and therefore PC—can also be of benefit in the following two ways:

- It increases the muscle's buffering capacity against lactic acid (cell acidity is buffered by a number of processes, including the breakdown of PC)
- Facilitates transfer of energy within the muscle cells (PC is involved in energy 'crossing' from the mitochondria membrane to the muscle contractile machinery)

In 1995, The British Olympic Association produced a Position Statement regarding creatine supplementation. The four main points are as follows:

- 20 g/d for five days of creatine can increase the substance's content in the muscle
- Such doses may result in better performances in short but 'explosive' events
- There is no evidence for improvements resulting from low-dose supplementation
- Vegetarians may experience the biggest benefits

12 CONCLUSIONS

Carbohydrates are the preferred energy source for dance, and should constitute more than 55% of the total energy intake. The amount of carbohydrate required per day by dancers depends on their body weight and hours of exercise. *Fats* are primarily used when the body performs low-intensity muscular work, thus sparing the store of carbohydrate. The fitter the individual the greater the carbohydrate sparing. Fats should not form more than 35% of the total daily energy intake. *Protein* is one of the most essential and multipurpose nutrients. One to two grams of protein per kg body weight per day should be an optimal intake for most dancers. *Vitamins* contribute to energy release, tissue repair, and physical fitness. Variable diets with plenty of fruit and vegetables will meet most vitamin requirements in dancers. *Minerals* are involved in many biological functions including energy production. Again, variable diets with plenty of fruit and vegetables will satisfy most mineral needs. Ingestion of extra *water* prior to exercise allows dancers to work with lower heart rates and provides for increased sweating rates. During exercise a volume of 150–250 ml of plain water ingested at 10–20-minute intervals is advisable. Finally, the long-term effects of certain *nutritional aids*, such as creatine, are as yet unknown.

13   FURTHER READING

Clark N (1997) *Sports nutrition guidebook*. Champaign, IL: Human Kinetics
Colgan M (1993) *Optimum sports nutrition*. New York: Advanced Research Press
Katch FI, McArdle WD (1993) *Introduction to nutrition, exercise, and health*. Phila-
    delphia: Lea & Febiger
Whitney EN, Cataldo CB, DeBruyne LK, Rolfes SR (1996) *Nutrition for health and
    health care*. Minneapolis: West Publishing
Williams MH (1997) *Ergogenics edge*. Champaign, IL: Human Kinetics

References to Part I

Alekel L, Clasey JL, Fehling PC *et al*. (1995) Contribution of exercise, body composition, and age to bone mineral density in pre-menopausal women. *Medicine and Science in Sports and Exercise*, **27**: 1477–85

Armstrong LE, Costill DL, Fink WJ (1985) Influence of diuretic-induced dehydration on running performance. *Medicine and Science in Sports and Exercise*, **17**: 456–61

Benson J, Gillien DM, Bourdet K, Loosli AR (1985) Inadequate nutrition and chronic calorie restriction in adolescent ballerinas. *Physician and Sportsmedicine*, **13**: 79–90

Bonbright JM (1989) The nutritional status of female ballet dancers 15–18 years of age. *Dance Research Journal*, **21**: 9–14

Bonbright JM (1990) Physiological and nutritional concerns in dance. *Journal of Physical Education, Recreation and Dance*, **61**: 35–7

Brouns F (1993) *Nutritional needs of athletes*. Chichester, UK: Wiley

Buskirk T, Lampietro PF, Bass DE (1985) Work performance after dehydration; effects of physical conditioning and heat acclimatisation. *Journal of Applied Physiology*, **12**: 189–94

Clark N (1997) *Sports nutrition guidebook*. Champaign, IL: Human Kinetics

Clarkson PM (1995) Minerals: exercise performance and supplementation in athletes. In: Williams C, Delvin JT (eds), *Foods, nutrition and sports performance*. London: E & FN Spon, pp. 113–46

Cohen JL, Potosnak L, Frank O, Baker H (1985) A nutritional and haematological assessment of elite ballet dancers. *Physician and Sportsmedicine*, **13**: 43–54

Cohen JL, Segal KR, Witriol I, McArdle WA (1982) Cardiorespiratory responses to ballet exercise and the VO2 max of elite ballet dancers. *Medicine & Science in Sports and Exercise*, **14**: 212–17

Costill DL (1972) Water and electrolytes. In: Morgan WP (ed.), *Ergogenic aids and muscular performance*. New York: Academic Press: pp. 293–320

Coyle EF (1991) Timing and method of increased carbohydrate intake to cope with heavy training, competition and recovery. *Journal of Sports Science*, **9** (Special Issue): 29–52

Dahlström M, Jansson E, Ekman M, Kaijser L (1995) Do highly physically active females have a lowered basal metabolic rate? *Scandinavian Journal of Medicine Science in Sports*, **5**: 81–7

Dahlström M, Jansson E, Nordevang E, Kaijser L (1990) Discrepancy between estimated energy intake and requirement in female dancers. *Clinical Physiology*, **10**: 11–25

Drummond S, Kirk T, de Looy A (1996) Are dietary recommendations for dietary fat reduction achievable? *International Journal of Food Science & Nutrition*, **47**(3): 221–6

Fallowfield JL, Williams C (1993) Carbohydrate intake and recovery from prolonged exercise. *International Journal of Sport Nutrition*, **3**: 150–64

Foster C (1975) Physiological requirements of aerobic dancing. *Research Quarterly for Exercise and Sport*, **46**: 120–2

Frisch RE, Wyshak G, Vincent L (1980) Delayed menarche and amenorrhoea in ballet dancers. *New England Journal of Medicine*, **303**: 17–9

Greenhaff P (1995) Creatine and its application as an ergogenic aid. *International Journal of Sport Nutrition*, **3**(Suppl): S100–S110

Houston ME (1995) *Biochemistry primer for exercise science*. Champaign, IL: Human Kinetics

Jette M, Inglis H (1975) Energy cost of square dancing. *Journal of Applied Physiology*, **38**: 44–5

Koutedakis Y (1994) The physiology of fitness. In: *The runner's guide*. London: Collins Willow: pp. 115–30

Koutedakis Y, Hitchcock A, Pacy PJ, Sharp NCC (1995) The effect of reducing energy diet on resting energy expenditure and nutrient intake in elite lightweight oarswomen. *Journal of Sports Science*, **13**(1): 36

Koutedakis Y, Pacy PJ, Carson RJ, Dick F (1997) Health and fitness in professional dancers. *Medical Problems of Performing Artists*, **12**: 23–7

Léger LA (1982) The energy cost of disco dancing. *Research Quarterly for Exercise and Sport*, **53**: 46–9

Lemon PWR (1991) Effect of exercise on protein requirements. *Journal of Sports Science*, **9**(Special Issue): 53–70

Lemon PWR (1994) Are dietary protein needs affected by regular exercise? *Insider*, **2**(3): 1–4

Newsholme EA, Leech AR (1983) Integration of carbohydrate and lipid metabolism. In: *Biochemistry for the medical sciences*. Chichester, UK: Wiley: pp. 336–56

Noble BJ (1986) *Physiology of exercise and sport*. St. Louis, MO: Times Mirror/ Mosby College Publishing

Parry-Billings M, Budgett R, Koutedakis Y *et al.* (1992) Plasma amino acid concentrations in the overtraining syndrome: possible effects on the immune system. *Medicine and Science in Sports and Exercise*, **24**: 1353–8

Phillips SM, Atkinson SA, Tarnopolsky MA, MacDougal JD (1995) Gender differences in leucine kinetics and nitrogen balance in endurance athletes. *Journal of Applied Physiology*, **75**(5): 2134–41

Santora AC (1987) Role of nutrition and exercise in osteoporosis. *American Journal of Medicine*, **82**(suppl 1B): 73–9

Trichopoulou A, Vassilakos T (1990) Recommended dietary intakes in the European Community member states. *European Journal of Clinical Nutrition*, **2** (Suppl.): 51–101

Warren MP (1983) Effects of under-nutrition on reproductive function in the human. *Endocrine Review*, **4**: 363–77

Wigaeus E, Kihlbom Å (1980) Physical demands during folk dancing. *European Journal of Applied Physiology*, **45**: 177–83

Williams MH (1995) *Nutrition for fitness and sport* (4th edition). Madison, WI: Wm C Brown & Benchmark

Part II

FIT TO DANCE

**Yiannis Koutedakis and
N. C. Craig Sharp**

Chapter 3

Non-artistic Components of Dance Performance

1 INTRODUCTION

Dance performance is not a single act. It is a continuum of different but interrelated constituents which derive from such unlikely and diverse areas as material science, body science and medicine and, even, space science. More specifically, dance performance is a very complex phenomenon depending, *inter alia*, on a large number of technical, medical, psychological, nutritional, physiological, economic and environmental elements (Table 3.1). At professional level, these elements may be divided into those that directly affect dancers' performance and those with an indirect role. It is conceivable, however, that two similar performances may be achieved by various combinations of participating factors.

In the present text it is not possible to examine everything that may potentially affect dance. However, after a brief introduction of aspects that may directly affect dancers and their performance, we will concentrate on the *physiological* elements of dance. A knowledge of these is mainly useful to assess *physical fitness*, to detect areas of weakness that require special attention, and to prescribe the most suitable form of supplementary training for the needs of the individual dancer.

2 BIOMECHANICAL

Biomechanics is the scientific discipline that studies the mechanical principles of human movement, and is an integral part of a larger scientific area known as *kinesiology*. It mainly involves two- or three-dimensional high-speed filming of a particular movement and subsequent video analyses.

Table 3.1 Selected consistuents of professional dance performance with direct and indirect effects

Constituents	Elements
Direct effects	
* Biomechanical (Kinesiology)	Skill, style, technique
* Hereditary	Genetic predisposition, talent identification
* Medical	General health, injury treatment, postural defects, osteoporosis and the problems of the asthmatic and diabetic dancer
* Nutritional	Muscle fuel and body fluid replacement, healthy eating
* Psychological	Stress control, motivation, goal settings
* Technological	Material science (e.g. shoes, dance surfaces)
* Physiological (Physical fitness)	Aerobic (cardiovascular) capabilities
	Anaerobic capabilities
	Muscular strength & power
	Joint mobility/Muscle flexibility
	Body composition (proportionality)
Stage-fright	Pre-performance nervousness
Indirect Effects	
* Artistic	Choreography, music, costumes
* Environmental	Temperature, facilities, working environment
* Individual	Financial state, personal–family relationships
* Managerial	Selection, administration, finances
* Methodological	Teaching methods
* Sociological	Type of dance, ethnic background
* Travelling	Living conditions, dance practice facilities
* Paediatric	Limits and requirements of exercise in children

Angular, linear and peak velocities of the limbs during the execution of a movement, and sequence and length of muscle recruitment are items contained in the long list of information obtained from such analyses.

As a body of knowledge, biomechanics was primarily developed during the 1970s when there was a widespread tendency for sport coaches to slavishly copy the training methods and technique of the current champion and present him or her as a model to the young hopefuls. It has now been established that—based on body dimensions and muscular function—every individual is mechanically different, and what we understand as superior technique is normally reserved for a specific individual. Attempts to copy him/her will most probably fail.

Although the classical ballet teacher may, at first glance, be horrified by a computer analogue analysis of a grand jeté, the information gained from such studies may help him or her to decide when a young dancer is ready for such a technique, or to demonstrate a technical deficiency in its performance. In general, biomechanics may help dance teachers to:

- Enhance their ability to detect the root causes of faults (e.g. anatomical imbalances) that may arise during particular movements
- Secure the best possible use of the natural abilities (talent) that their dancers have
- Avoid movements that may potentially cause injury

3   HEREDITARY

Human genetics is the study of how people develop according to the characteristics passed on from the parents. Given that no training/teaching methods and techniques can completely alter these characteristics, the right heredity is necessary for individuals to achieve elite sport or dance performances, hence the expression 'the champion is born'. Optimal muscle fibre profile and skeletal dimensions are two examples of hereditary factors that may directly affect dancers and their performance.

Assessing the young hopefuls' parents for established dance-related genetic characteristics may become a common practice in the future, as it is already in gymnastics. It is known, for example, that children have body types (or *somatotypes*) more similar to their mothers than their fathers. It has also been confirmed that the ability to respond to different forms of physical training and exercise is genetically determined (Klissouras 1971; Simoneau, Lortie, Boulay *et al.* 1986). However, only about 40% of fitness has been linked to genetic factors, leaving an estimated 60% within our control through regular exercise and appropriate diet (Paffenbarger and Olsen 1996). Nevertheless, to reach the highest performance levels, one definitely needs this 40% of genetic contribution, which is why correct identification and selection of young talents is becoming increasingly important. Fig. 3.1 shows how heredity and other external factors can, through general health and physical activity, affect both fitness and physical performance. Racehorses and, to some extent, the racing greyhound provide living examples of how heredity can influence performance, and how winners are often mated to provide the genetic characteristics of successful racing.

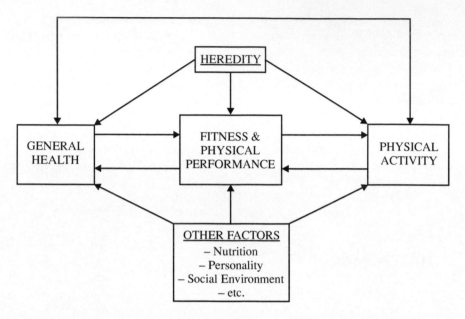

Fig. 3.1 Heredity and physical performance

4 MEDICAL

A good state of general health is a significant element in the route to professional dance. Anomalies in the skeletal system (e.g. kyphosis, scoliosis, deformity of the chest), hypertension, chronic infections and sight disorders are among the medical conditions that elite dancers should be free from. Conditions such as asthma and diabetes are no longer regarded as unsurpassable obstacles in achieving high levels of physical performances. On the other hand, there are a number of medical conditions (e.g. osteoporosis) which, although they do not affect performance directly, may impair one's long-term health.

   Injury is perhaps the single most frequent cause forcing dancers to stay away from action. Indeed, in a period of 12 months, almost 50% of a large sample of professional dancers reported one to six days off action due to a musculoskeletal injury (Fig. 3.2). The lower back seems to be the most frequently injured site, which together with pelvis, legs, knees and feet, accounts for more than 90% of the injuries (Koutedakis, Pacy, Carson and Dick 1997a). Both *external* (e.g. type of movement, velocity of limbs, number of repetitions, etc.) and *internal* (e.g. muscular activity) factors have been held responsible for developing such injuries. A poor posture

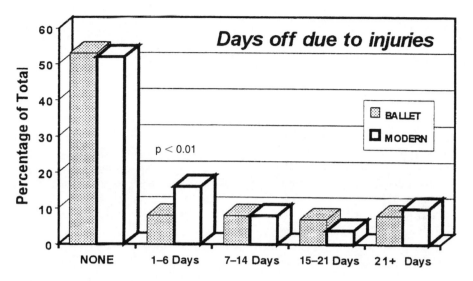

Fig. 3.2 Days off due to injuries in professional ballet and modern dancers (Data expressed in % of the total [$n = 324$] sample)
Source: From Koutedakis, Pacy, Carson and Dick Vol. 12, Medical Problems of Performing Artists (1997). Reproduced by permission of Hanley & Belfus, Inc.

increases the stress on supporting structures (e.g. bones and ligaments) and therefore the chances of developing an injury. As we shall discuss in the next chapter, low levels of physical fitness may also contribute to injuries in dancers.

5 NUTRITIONAL

It was stressed in Part I that diet and dietary habits can affect physical performance (Cohen, Potosnak, Frank and Baker 1985; Coyle 1991; Peterson 1986). This is mainly because the foods dancers—and all other humans!—eat contain the chemically bonded energy needed to sustain life, and to permit general bodily movement and dance. Adenosine triphosphate (or ATP) is the energy currency that the body is using at any given time. An uninterrupted supply of this energy compound must, therefore, always be available.

The raw fuel for ATP synthesis takes the form of carbohydrates, fats and proteins, while the efficient extraction of energy from these foods requires the delicate blending of other nutrients (e.g. vitamins, minerals) in the finely regulated watery medium of the cell. Thus, optimal food and fluid intakes before, during and after dance should be a key component of every dancer's education and lifestyle.

6   PSYCHOLOGICAL

What makes an individual behave in a certain way is an extremely complex issue. We are born with a behavioural blueprint but we are also products of our environment and our past experiences. Added to this, we also have the power of self-determination, which means that we are outcomes of our thoughts, hopes, dreams and visions of the future. However, for successful careers, dancers must also be able to provide a constructive answer to a number of performance-related questions such as: Can you concentrate efficiently and quickly on the main movement you have to do during a performance? Can you keep your excitement and nervousness under control? Can you set realistic goals for your dance development? Are the set goals matched by adequate motivation?

In the last 20 years, scientists in the field of exercise (or applied) psychology have developed a number of techniques for coping with the mental part of physical activity. These were initially geared for sportsmen and women, but in the hands of qualified specialists these techniques can now be applied to dancers too. In fact, the recent report of the national inquiry into dancers' health and injury (Brinson and Dick 1996) recommended that dancers should incorporate some mental techniques (e.g. mental focusing) in their daily practices.

7   TECHNOLOGICAL

Technology and art are among those attributes that separate humans from other species. They make our lives both easier and more colourful, and they are happily passed on and built upon by successive generations. As can be seen from Fig. 3.3, there are well-established links within the three-component 'system' (i.e. technology, art and man) which inevitably affect outcomes and may lift physical (dance) performance to dazzling heights. This is better understood in sport where technology—through aerodynamic javelins, high-performance tennis rackets and rowing blades with improved 'water-grip'—has made significant contributions towards the succession of the world-record-breaking performances experienced in the last two decades. In dance, technology and science have, among other factors, helped in the design and construction of dance shoes, studio floors and trampolines. These developments are crucial in the prevention and control of injuries, while at the same time they allow performance levels to increase. Technology has also provided great support in the more accurate diagnoses of injuries, faster rehabilitation, and in technique and movement modifications, through to better and

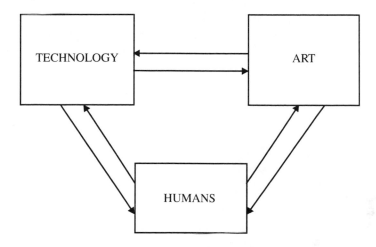

Fig. 3.3 Links between technology, art and humans

more reliable equipment such as scanners, ultrasound machines and video cameras.

8 PHYSIOLOGICAL

Physiology consists of all the normal workings of the body. In the context of dance, the branch of physiology concerned is that designated 'exercise physiology'. This is the description and explanation of all the short- and long-term physical changes which occur when the body undergoes movement, whether slow or fast, or whether for very short or very long periods of time. Here, the physiology of dance is no different from the physiology of many vigorous sports, and the main organs and tissues concerned are the lungs, the heart, the blood, the blood vessels and tendon, ligament, bone and muscle. Muscle produces energy which it changes into force. And these systems are backed up by the skin, as a heat exchange unit, the liver as a supplier of blood glucose, the fat depots as suppliers of fatty acid fuels, various endocrine glands to secrete hormones to help regulate body functions, the kidney to help with fluid balance, and the brain, spinal cord and autonomic nervous system to co-ordinate it all.

As discussed earlier, there are five main physiological elements that can affect dance performance: (1) aerobic capabilities; (2) anaerobic qualities; (3) muscle strength and power; (4) joint mobility and muscle flexibility; and (5) body composition. All these five elements are also the basic components of *physical fitness*, which will be separately discussed in the following chapter. However, before this, the physiological aspect of 'stage-fright', or nervousness, will be considered, the effects of which have been felt by most dancers, regardless of their experience, gender or status.

8.1   Pre-Performance Nervousness

'Stage-fright', nervousness or anxiety, is felt or seen as a cluster of effects. These include: widening of the pupil; dry mouth; yawning (there is a 'nervous' yawn and a hunger yawn, as well as a sleepy yawn); production of sweat initially on the palms, under the arms and in the pubic area; gooseflesh and/or erection of body hair; an increase in heart and respiration rate; 'butterflies' in the abdomen; tremor of the hands and sometimes of the legs ('the shakes', or knocking of the knees); and finally the feeling of needing to go to the toilet, when you have only just been.

Although such nervousness is not pleasant, it is nevertheless an indication that the body is preparing itself well for a physical ordeal, such as a performance. To understand the mechanism of stage-fright, it is first necessary to have a brief look at the nervous system. As a whole this consists of: (1) the brain, the spinal cord and all the associated nerves which come and go from the brain or the cord, and either receive sensations or issue instructions; and (2) what is known as the autonomic nervous system, which is, *inter alia*, responsible for the physical side of nervousness, and will be described below.

NERVOUS SYSTEM—SOMATIC AND AUTONOMIC

The whole responsive nervous system is organized into two main divisions—the *somatic* and the *autonomic*. The somatic division deals primarily with conscious sensations, such as touch, taste, hearing and sight, which can be treated as 'information coming into' the body. The somatic division is also responsible for instructions 'going out of' the body, such as all the muscle actions which we perform voluntarily, together with reflex actions (as when we right ourselves following a near-fall).

The autonomic system plays the major part in keeping constant the internal environment of the body, for example body temperature. If you get too cold, your skin goes pale as the blood vessels constrict to minimize blood flow and reduce heat loss. Shivering may also start. In general, the autonomic system unconsciously deals with the vital functions which are too important to be left to the forgetful conscious mind when awake, and which simply cannot be left to it when you are asleep.

But the autonomic system integrates with the spinal cord and brain in a hierarchy of levels of operation. For example simple autonomic reflexes, such as operating the bladder, arise in the spinal cord. More complex responses such as breathing, blood pressure, and vomiting are integrated in the *medulla* or lower part of the brain. Even more complex responses such as the pupil reflex and accommodation or focusing of the eye, are integrated in the midbrain. At the most complex level, body temperature and blood chemistry are organized higher up the brain still, in the region known as the *hypothalamus*.

The autonomic nervous system is also divided into two parts, known as the *sympathetic* and the *parasympathetic*, and they tend to have completely opposite actions.

The Sympathetic Division: the Basis of Pre-performance Nervousness

The sympathetic division acts to meet minor or major emotional or physical crises—from blushing with embarrassment, to nervousness before a performance, to total evacuation of bowels and bladder in situations of sheer terror. In other words, it operates in situations of frolic, fright, flight or fight, by getting the body ready for some kind of action. Signs of this preparation are well seen in animals, a cat faced with a dog, for example.

The autonomic nervous system probably regards a dance performance as a cross between flight and fight, so it activates its sympathetic division to deal with it. Sympathetic nerves stimulate the iris to dilate, body-hair erector muscles to contract, the heart to beat faster and breathing to speed up, blood vessels in muscles to dilate, sweat glands to secrete, and vessels in skin to constrict at first then dilate as you get hot, the air passages to widen, and often yawning to occur to help fully aerate the lungs. Sphincters constrict between stomach and intestine, and between small and large intestine, and at the anus. Sympathetic nerves stimulate the liver to secrete more glucose and the adrenal gland to secrete adrenaline. All these effects are conducive to activity.

At the same time, the stomach and intestinal walls, and the bladder wall relax (partly producing 'butterflies'), while salivary glands are inhibited (hence the dry mouth, to stop you inhaling saliva), and blood vessels in the abdomen constrict (the vascular shunt, described above under aerobic fitness). The reason for this is that digestion and excretion are not required when the body is very active, so they are shut down. However, before bladder and rectum relax, they constrict quite strongly (hence the feeling of needing to go to the toilet, even when there is nothing left to void). The slight feeling of nausea is similarly due to the changes in the gastric muscle and sphincters. Performers may feel slightly nauseous, but they are very rarely actually sick.

Thus, more oxygen is potentially available (deeper breathing, greater cardiac output of blood), more blood is available for the muscles which are themselves tenser and ready for action. The eye is keener, the sweat mechanism ready to start—and 'vegetative' functions (digestion of food and excretion of waste) are held in abeyance. You are ready to dance.

All this so far without a mention of adrenaline. The point is that most of the body's sympathetic preparation for activity is carried out by actual nerves. Where these nerves end in organs or tissues, they secrete the substance noradrenaline, and it is this which causes the various effects just described. However, one of the organs innervated by such sympathetic (but not the parasympathetic) nerves is the pair of adrenal glands, or more accurately the inner part of the adrenal glands. In the adrenal medulla are two main types of cell, one which secretes *adrenaline* and the other secretes *noradrenaline*. These are then directed not onto any particular organ or tissue, as is the case with the nerves of course, but into the blood, so that the whole body benefits, wherever there are receptor sites for the chemicals to lock into. Their main job is to reinforce the general sympathetic response, with a full adrenal secretion being about 10% as effective as full sympathetic system stimulation.

THE PARASYMPATHETIC DIVISION: 'HOUSEKEEPING' WHEN THE PERFORMANCE IS OVER

The parasympathetic side of the autonomic nervous system tends to switch on when the performance is over, and it is related to what might be called the 'vegetative' or housekeeping functions of the body, such as eating, digesting and the elimination of waste. The best way to think of parasympathetic function is when you get home in the evening after performance or rehearsal or training, have eaten a meal, and are sitting in a soft chair in a warm, quiet, low-lit room. Then your pupils constrict, as does your bronchial muscle, while your salivary glands will have been secreting, as well as the digestive glands in stomach and small intestine. In addition, the sphincters of your stomach (top and bottom, or cardiac and pyloric) will have relaxed, as will those between small and large intestines, to allow the free passage of food. This will be helped on its way by active movements of the walls of the stomach, and of the small and large intestine.

The external genitalia are much affected by the autonomic system, as will be noticed by men in particular. During exercise, there is a strong sympathetic vasoconstriction which causes a marked shrinkage in size of the penis, which is totally dependent for its size changes on its content of blood. This is why it can be difficult for a man who is nervous, and sympathetically stimulated to achieve an erection. However, under a parasympathetic response, there is vasodilatation of genitalia and erection (of penis and clitoris) is much easier. Interestingly, the sexual act unifies the two sides of the autonomic nervous system in a unique way; the parasympathetic is responsible for getting the two sets of genitalia properly together, but the orgasm is mediated by the sympathetic—and this accounts for the breathing and sweating, which is out of proportion to the actual energy being expended.

POSSIBLE VOLUNTARY CONTROL ON THE AUTONOMIC SYSTEM

Normally, the autonomic system is not under voluntary control, indeed this is the main point of it. However, it is possible to gain a modest degree of control over some autonomic functions, at times with the aid of simple 'biofeedback' devices, such as heart-rate monitors. Some yoga practitioners are able to reduce their heart rate for example, seemingly by increasing the parasympathetic impulses, which act to slow the heart. And they can reduce blood pressure, by what appears to be autonomic control. Also, biofeedback-conditioned autonomic control techniques have shown promise in the modest control of conditions such as migraine and even epilepsy.

Interestingly from the viewpoint of stage performances, the mechanics of facial muscle movement are closely tied to the autonomic nervous system. Thus, producing facial expressions of fear or anger on the one hand, or happiness on the other, may induce a degree of sympathetic or parasympathetic activation. Given that, to some extent, members of an audience tend to mimic the expressions of actors, dancers or mime artists, the dancer in performance may affect the audience physically as well as intellectually. Finally, nervousness or stage-fright forms a manifestation of a set of physiological functions, which have strong psychological overtones. Therefore the way to deal with excessive nervousness is through psychological relaxation and stress-coping techniques.

9 CONCLUSIONS

Dance performance is a continuum of different but interrelated constituents that are able to satisfy the physical, mental, and artistic aspirations of both dancers and audiences. Dance performance depends on a large number of medical, psychological, nutritional, physiological, economic and environmental components, with direct and indirect effects. Heredity is also an important component that may account for about 40% of dance performance, while technology has an increasing share in the quality of dance. More multidisciplinary scientific research is needed on the different forms of dance, as the current relevant data are rather limited.

10 FURTHER READING

Bejjani FJ (ed.) (1993) Current research in arts medicine: a compendium of the MedArt international 1992 world congress on arts and medicine. Pennington, NJ: a cappella books/Chicago Review Press
Brinson P, Dick F, (eds) (1996) Fit to dance? The report of the national inquiry into dancers' health and injury. London: Galouste Gulbenkian Foundation
Fitt G (1996) Dance kinesiology (2nd edition). USA: Schirmer Books
Fox KR, (ed.) (1997) *The physical self: from motivation to well-being*. Champaign, IL: Human Kinetics
Taylor J, Taylor C (1995) *Psychology of dance*. Champaign, IL: Human Kinetics
Whiting WC, Zernicke RF, (eds) (1998) *Biomechanics of musculoskeletal injury*. Champaign, IL: Human Kinetics

Chapter 4

Muscle and its Physiology

1 INTRODUCTION

Most movements of the body and inside it are the result of the contraction or shortening of muscle cells. Laughing, talking, sneezing, swallowing, crying, blinking, goose-pimples, being sick, urinating, childbirth, constricting the pupil, the heartbeat—and, of course, walking, running, jumping, dancing, singing and playing music—are all carried out by muscle. Just about the only obvious body movement which is not directly due to muscle contraction is that of erectile tissue, as in nipple, clitoris and penis. Here the change in size is due to 'turgor movement', as in plants. However, even these fluid-based turgor movements start by the relaxation of tiny smooth muscle cells in the walls of appropriate blood vessels, thus dilating them, and greatly increasing the local blood flow. Blushing is due to a similar mechanism. If you think about it, you will see that virtually all human communication comes about from muscle action—the muscles of the diaphragm, thorax, larynx, tongue, cheeks and lips for speech, facial muscles for expression, and other skeletal muscles for gesture and general 'body language'.

Muscle is a wonderful tissue capable of causing very large variations in force, speed, power and range of movement, as it very elegantly converts chemical energy from food (originally from the sun) directly to mechanical energy. In contrast, most man-made engines (whether using oil, coal or nuclear fuel) need to convert the chemical energy into steam, or electricity or heat, before it can be converted to mechanical energy. Some muscle (e.g. limb muscle) is controlled by motor nerves, some (e.g. in blood vessels) by autonomic nerves and some (e.g. uterus) by hormones. Some only contract when stimulated by a nerve, and some have an inherent rhythm (stomach, intestine, the heart), which can be modified by other stimuli. These different contractile functions and methods of control are associated with the three main different muscle types as seen under the light microscope, namely *skeletal muscle, smooth muscle* and *cardiac muscle*.

In dancers, skeletal muscle accounts for somewhere between 38 to 45% of body weight, contains about half of the body water, and during exercise can raise their metabolic rate by over 20 times. For all its volume, it is a relatively low source of primary cancers, neither is it at all a fertile tissue in which secondary tumours might grow.

Muscle as a tissue is made of many hundreds, thousands or indeed millions of muscle cells. Because in skeletal muscle these are very long and thin, these cells are often referred to as muscle fibres. Either way, cells or fibres, they are the individual constituents of skeletal muscle tissue.

2   TYPES OF MUSCLE

The differences in function and control of muscle indicated above are associated with differences in the structure of the cells making up the muscle. This gives three main types of muscle.

First is *skeletal muscle*, which most people think of as 'muscle'. It forms the muscles of our trunk and limbs and is, to a greater or lesser extent, under voluntary control, although it can act on its own. For example, if you put your hand into water which is too hot, a 'reflex' contraction occurs whereby the biceps and brachialis flexors of the arm contract to pull the hand out. This is initiated by a reflex, which occurs via the spinal cord, and is not connected to voluntary control. Indeed, for a second or two after your hand is out, you are still waiting for the pain to hit you.

Skeletal muscle consists of long (up to 10 centimetres) thin (30–60 micrometres, or 30–60 thousandths of a millimetre wide) cells which appear striated or striped under the microscope, due to ordered arrays of the contractile protein rods, *actin* and *myosin*, as will be described below.

Second is *cardiac muscle*, forming the 'myocardium', the muscle wall of the four chambers of the heart. Its cells are also seen as striated under the microscope, but they are much shorter, being only 100 micrometres long, and are branched and joined together with neighbouring cells as a network. In the embryo, each individual cardiac cell contracts to its own rhythm, but as they join up the cell with the fastest rhythm drives the others. There is a group of these 'fastest cells' known as the *pacemaker*. This is located in the right atrium, and initiates the heartbeat. Its free-running rhythm would be about 140, but this rate is kept damped down to around 70 to 80 by the *parasympathetic nervous system*.

Third is *smooth muscle*. Here the cells are cylindrical and about 200 ×

Table 4.1 Selected anatomical and physiological characteristics of smooth, skeletal and cardiac muscle

	Smooth	Skeletal	Cardiac
Alternative names	Involuntary, non-striated, plain	Voluntary, striated	Heart
Fibre length	0.02–0.05 mm	1–100 mm	0.08 mm or less
Fibre diameter	8–10 μm	30–60 μm	15 μm
Fibre composition	Small single cell, no branching	Very large single cell (many nuclei at edge of each fibre), no branching	Branched single cells
Type of contraction	Slow, rhythmic, sustained	Variable sustained	Moderately rapid (with rests between contractions), no sustained
Distribution	Stomach and intestines, respiratory, urinogenital tracts; blood vessels; ducts of glands; hair; muscles of skin; ciliary muscle (eye)	Locomotor muscles; subcutaneous muscle; diaphragm	Heart only

10 micrometres in size. They do contain the contractile proteins actin and myosin, but not in parallel arrays, hence they are not striated. They can increase in size to a remarkable extent, as seen in the pregnant uterus. Smooth muscle is mainly under control of the *autonomic nervous system*, to a greater or lesser extent. Smooth muscle is located in the iris, blood vessels, and the bronchial tree, and in the hollow organs such as stomach, intestine, gall bladder, urinary bladder and uterus, and in the hair follicles in the skin. An important function of smooth muscle is its property of 'accommodation', whereby it can 'reset' itself to a new length, after a period of being stretched. In terms of the function of the urinary bladder, this is the main reason why the urge to urinate can 'wear off'. One needs a bit of patience, and perhaps endurance, but it will happen. A summary of selected anatomical and physiological characteristics of the three types of muscle appears in Table 4.1.

3   TYPES OF SKELETAL MUSCLE FIBRE

Above, three major types of muscle, skeletal, cardiac and smooth, have been described. But skeletal muscle itself consists of three main types of muscle fibre, graded on two main abilities: their speed of contraction and their major energy source (which also determines how quickly they fatigue). They tend to be called simply 'slow' or 'fast' muscle, with two types of fast. Many animals, such as cats, rabbits, birds and fish, have entire muscles which are fast and slow respectively. For example, the white meat in fish is fast muscle, the brown is slow. Fish use fast muscle to catch prey, or to escape, and slow muscle to remain at a particular depth in the water with slow movements. Chickens and many non-soaring birds have their flight muscles entirely fast, and their leg muscles slow, for perching. Indeed, chicken breast (fast muscle) is white due to lack of *myoglobin* and low blood supply, and sweet due to its rich store of glycogen, the predominant fuel of fast fibres. Chicken leg muscle is brown due to myoglobin and a richer blood supply, and less sweet as it uses fat as a major fuel.

Humans tend to have mixtures of fast and slow fibres, genetically determined. Most of us have around 50:50 fast to slow, although some of our muscles always contain a higher proportion of slow fibres than others. For example, the soleus muscle just above the Achilles tendon, being a muscle of posture, always contains more slow fibres than the gastrocnemius or calf muscle, a muscle of propulsion. Gifted individuals may have a muscle profile distinguishably different from that 50:50 mentioned above. The great sprinters have up to 90% of their muscle cells fast (Fig. 4.1) and conversely the great marathon runners may have over 90% of their muscle cells slow, while those who can jump well have a varying preponderance of fast fibres.

Although the slow–fast muscle fibre profile appears not to be altered in number (except possibly in ageing), with training, the area of both may be altered, but especially that of the fast fibres. Hence on similar training, 'muscular' individuals (who probably have a higher percentage of fast fibres to begin with), will hypertrophy their muscle more than 'slimmer' men or women. The types of muscle fibre are described below.

## 3.1	Slow (or Type I) Fibres

These operate mainly through *Krebs cycle*, using carbohydrate or fat as required, depending on the level of effort. The fibres have a relatively rich blood supply, with some five to eight capillaries per fibre. They are rich in *myoglobin*, which transports and stores the oxygen, and they are rich in *mitochondria*, wherein the oxygen is used to release the fat energy and most of the carbohydrate energy. Thus these fibres are mainly oxidative, and their waste products are primarily carbon dioxide (breathed out) and water. The limited data on dancers' muscle profiles

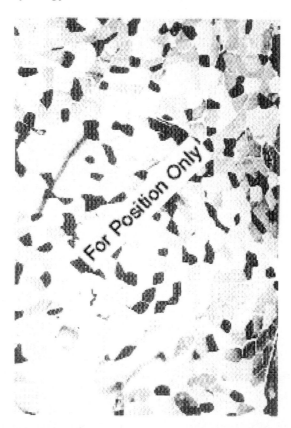

Fig. 4.1 Cross-sectional area of a muscle sample obtained from the vastus lateralis muscle of an elite international male sprinter. Slow muscle fibres have black colour, while fast have either grey or white, corresponding to fast oxidative and fast glycolytic fibres respectively. As expected, around 90% of the sample's area is covered by fast muscle fibres, hence the ability of this athlete to excel in events where speed of muscle contraction is important

have shown that (ballet) dancers have predominately slow fibres (Dahlström, Esbjörnsson, Gierup *et al.* 1997).

Slow fibres are organized into relatively small *motor units* (i.e. the number of muscle fibres controlled by a single nerve fibre, as described below). This gives the slow motor units a better measure of fine control. For example, darts players lob their darts slowly at the board, they do not throw them hard and fast. Similarly, squash players going for a very precise shot will play it as slowly as the tactical situation in the rally will allow. Therefore, if you want accuracy, make your movements as slow as reasonably possible.

In terms of speed, average mammal slow fibres contract in about 140 milliseconds. It is worth noting that slow mouse muscle fibres are faster than the fastest human fast fibres. And it may well be that within humans there is a range of 'fast' and 'slow' speeds even within the same fibre type grouping.

3.2   Oxidative Fast (or Type IIa) Fibres

These fibres form a halfway house between extremes. In terms of contraction speed, they contract nearly twice as fast as slow fibres, that is they take about 80 milliseconds to contract. In terms of metabolism, they derive their energy approximately equally from oxidative (aerobic) and anaerobic sources (phosphocreatine and glycolysis). They do not have as many mitochondria as slow fibres, or as much myoglobin or capillaries. Their motor units span a range of size and fatigability which on average is in between the two other fibre types.

Cell for cell, fast fibres are 30–40% or more larger than slow fibres. So dancers with more fast fibres will tend to look more 'muscular' than dancers with more slow fibres in their bodies.

3.3   Glycolytic Fast (or Type IIb) Fibres

These are called 'glycolytic' because they derive most of their energy from glycolysis, and much of the remainder from phosphocreatine. It will be remembered that glycolysis is the first phase of carbohydrate metabolism, whereby glucose-from-blood, or quantitatively far more glucose-from-glycogen, is metabolized down to pyruvate, which goes into Krebs cycle. If there is too much pyruvate for Krebs to handle, it is changed to lactic acid, a potent cause of fatigue. So, the type IIb fibres can produce a lot of energy quickly, but they fatigue quickly. 'A lot of energy quickly' translates into force at speed, or simply, power—as in leaps or jumps, and these fibres take only about 70 milliseconds to contract. However, their motor unit size is large, giving much force and power, but not the control of type I motor units.

4   MOTOR UNITS AND THEIR FUNCTION

As mentioned above, skeletal muscle fibres are organized into *motor units*, which are varying sizes of groups of muscle fibres all supplied with electrical impulses from one motor neurone or nerve cell (Fig. 4.2).

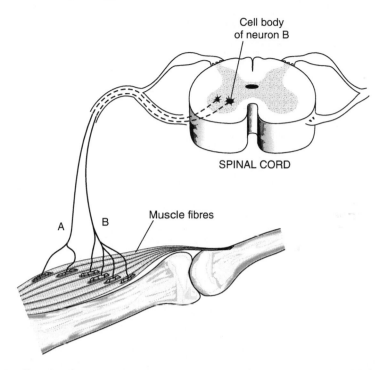

Fig. 4.2 Sketch of two motor units consisting of two (A) and four (B) muscle fibres

The number of muscle fibres in a motor unit may be as few as 10 in a small muscle in the finger, to several thousand in a large muscle such as the hamstrings. The number of fibres in a motor unit depends partly on the size of the muscle, partly on the power needed, and partly on the degree of control required. The bigger the motor unit, the greater the power (usually). The smaller the motor unit, the finer the control.

There appears to be a specific pattern of recruitment of motor units, whereby small (slow) motor units are recruited during low-force contractions, with small type IIa units coming in at higher force movements and larger type IIa higher still. The large type IIb motor units seem only to be recruited during high-force contractions. This recruitment by motor unit size makes for a very good modulation of force and control, as by progressive recruitment of motor units, the force generated in a muscle can be increased in a stepwise fashion. The small steps begin with smooth initial increases in force (so one doesn't crush a paper cup on lifting it), but at higher forces the increments are much larger, consequently control is less precise.

This motor unit recruitment pattern has implications for strength training in that if one is training for strength, the loading needs to be heavy in order, if for nothing else, to recruit right through the fibre bed to the recalcitrant type IIb fibres.

What makes one motor unit fast, and another slow is, oddly enough, not primarily the genetic coding of the muscle fibres themselves, but the expression of that coding as teased out by the nerves. This is done, not by any substance which the nerves secrete, but by their pattern of electrical impulses. Fast nerves tend to transmit their impulses at a rate of around 40/second (i.e. 40 Hertz). Slow nerves operate around 10 Hertz. Were one to cut the nerves supplying a whole slow and fast muscle respectively, and reconnect them the other way round, the slow muscle would gradually become fast, and vice versa.

Birmingham professor David Jones believes that, in effect, this is what happens to some motor units with ageing. Young and Dinan (1994) found that ageing muscle loses power quicker than force, at a rate of 3.5% compared to 1.8% per year respectively. Jones and Round (1990) have found areas in ageing muscle which are completely devoid of any fast fibres, and Jones believes that this might be due to the fast fibres losing their nerve connections (possibly due to disuse?), but being reinnervated with slow nerve sprouts from adjacent slow fibres. If a muscle replaces fast with slow motor units in this way, it would indeed lose power (the product of force and velocity) quicker than strength (force), exactly as Young and Dinan have described.

Speed in muscle movements is probably based on much more than simply having a fairly high proportion of fast fibres. Virtually all fibres must be recruited for a jump, for example. And they must all be recruited in the smallest window of time, in other words there must be the closest possible synchrony of contraction. If, in a jump, it takes 100 milliseconds to get off the ground, it is no use the type II motor unit recruitment time being spread over 130 milliseconds, that is with some of the units not coming into action until the dancer is already in the air. It may be that plyometric and rebound training helps such motor unit synchrony. Indeed, those dancers who do a lot of elevation work in class or rehearsal may be doing just the right type of training for improving synchrony. Elevation is also influenced by the force of the contraction, so that has to be worked on as well, in terms of strength training to increase the force.

Thus on the basis of size, speed and fatigability, motor units are found to lie within a spectrum of being large, fast and fatigable at one end, and small, slow and endurant at the other.

5   MUSCLE FORCE AND CROSS-SECTIONAL AREA

In addition to slow–fast fibre percentage, recruitment of motor units and synchrony of contraction, the force a muscle generates is proportional to its cross-sectional area, rather than to its length. But speed of shortening is also dependent on length. The longer the muscle, all else being equal, the quicker it shortens. Power, the rate of generating tension, is the product of force times velocity, and as force is proportional to area, and velocity to length, then power is proportional to length times area, which is volume. Thus, a short thick muscle will produce high force at low speed, and a long thin muscle will produce low force at higher speed. In both cases the power may be the same. Which is why dancers of different physiques can achieve the same elevation. One can draw a graph of muscle power, by plotting force against velocity, and for many skeletal muscles it is found that maximum power is usually achieved at about one third of maximum shortening speed.

In moderately trained men or women, about 3 kg (some 30 Newtons) of force are produced per square cm of muscle area. This implies that the calf muscle, the gastrocnemius, can exert a tension of over 250 kg. Gluteus maximus, on which you may be sitting as you read this, is the strongest body muscle and can develop up to 1200 kg. And all the skeletal muscles together could in theory produce a tension of around 20 000 kg, over 20 tons.

The relationship between muscle force levels and cross-sectional area has also been confirmed in dancers. Kuno, Fukunaga, Hirano and Myashita (1996) assessed female Japanese classical ballet dancers, who had done no exercise or training whatever other than long-term ballet classes and performances, and found that their cross-sectional muscle area was greater and their leg muscle strength was significantly higher than appropriate controls.

6   THE STRUCTURE OF THE MUSCLE

To understand how a muscle functions, one needs to know its structure, from the gross anatomy, down to the organization of the very molecules of contraction themselves, as all have a bearing on the understanding of movement, fatigue and injury. Such knowledge will further assist the understanding of strength, speed, local muscle endurance and muscle flexibility, together with their training and limitations.

6.1   The Whole Muscle

Anatomy has long been shared between medical science and art, with their greatest mutual glory in the anatomical studies of Leonardo da Vinci in the fifteenth century, and art students have long worked in human and veterinary anatomy dissecting rooms. There is no room in a text such as this to go into the details of musculoskeletal anatomy, with its 215 pairs of skeletal muscles, but the anatomy of one muscle, for example the sartorius, will illustrate how a muscle is constructed.

Sartorius comes from the Latin word for 'tailor', as the muscle helps in keeping the knees poised when you sit in the cross-legged tailor's position. Each skeletal muscle has an 'origin' and an 'insertion'. Sartorius originates from the anterior suprailiac spine, near the front of your hipbone (or ilium), and it inserts on the medial tibial condyle, that is on the inside of your knee on the tibia (main bone of the lower leg). Apart from helping to maintain a cross-legged position, sartorius helps in a dancer's turn-out, that is it rotates the thigh outwards (Fig. 4.3).

At its 'origin' a muscle usually ends in a short strong mass of fibrous tissue which is embedded into the bone. The 'insertion' is where the tendon of the muscle is equally firmly attached to bone. Tendon and fibrous tissue (and ligament) are all made from very strong fibrous collagen, which is a protein consisting of strong thin molecules like strands in a wire rope. At the muscle end, the collagen molecules of tendon attach to various parts of the muscle, including the fibrous sheaths around bundles of muscle fibres, sometimes penetrating into the end of the muscle cells themselves. At the bone end, the collagen molecules penetrate into the bone, and bond with the osseous material of the bone itself.

If we were to dissect a sartorius (or indeed any skeletal muscle), we would first cut through the *epimysium*, an outer fibrous (or connective tissue) covering of collagen sheets which holds the whole muscle together. Once through the *epimysium*, we would see small bundles of muscle fibres, wrapped in more collagen sheeting known as the *perimysium*; these bundles are called *fasciculi* (a word which has the same origin as fascist; from fascisti—the bundle of rods which was the Italian fascist movement's symbol). Cutting through the epimysium into a *fasciculus* under a low power dissecting microscope would reveal individual muscle cells, each invested with a final covering of collagenous sheeting, the *endomysium* (Fig. 4.4). All this collagen is manufactured by cells known as fibroblasts, and once synthesized, the collagen molecules are rolled out like long logs at a lumbar camp. The logs of collagen are then lined up according to the force lines, and embedded in a ground substance, in much the same way as fibreglass is made, with glue and glass-fibres.

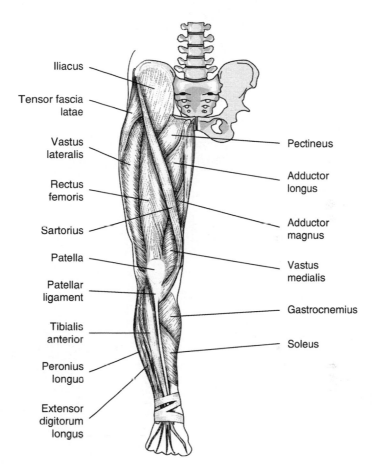

Iliacus

Tensor fascia
latae

Vastus
lateralis

Rectus
femoris

Sartorius

Patella

Patellar
ligament

Tibialis
anterior

Peronius
longuo

Extensor
digitorum
longus

Pectineus

Adductor
longus

Adductor
magnus

Vastus
medialis

Gastrocnemius

Soleus

Fig. 4.3 The main muscles of the front of the leg that move the leg and foot. Sartorius muscle also appears

Each muscle is innervated by a particular nerve, in this case a branch of the femoral nerve. On entering the sartorius, at its *motor point* the nerve begins to separate into its component motor nerve fibres, which separate into as many nerve fibres as there are motor units to innervate. Even then, each individual nerve has to split into as many strands as there are muscle fibres in the motor unit. There are also nerve fibres running the other way, from the muscle back to the spinal cord, and possibly up to the brain, carrying sensory information from a variety of receptors such as pain receptors, *muscle spindles* and *tendon organs*. For the brain to control muscle, it must have information on what the muscle is doing.

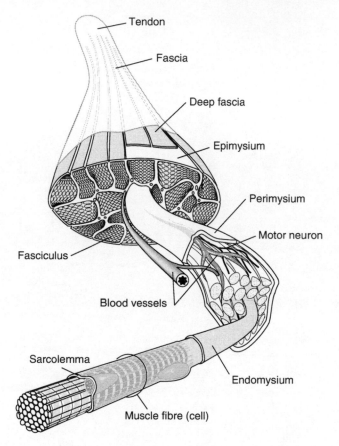

Fig. 4.4 Various stages of magnification of muscle, from the whole, to fasciculi—and on down to muscle fibres, blood vessels and motor neurons

6.2   The Muscle Fibre and its Structure

This term is synonymous with the single skeletal muscle cell. Each muscle fibre/cell has an anatomy, an 'ultrastructure', of its own—as do all cells. Whether fast or slow the deep structure of the muscle fibre is much the same. It consists of at least 9 elements which will be briefly considered:

1.   The muscle cell membrane or *sarcolemma*, helping transmit the contraction signal.
2.   The *myoneural junction*, where the nerve and its impulse meet the muscle cell.
3.   The *T-system* which further transmits the contraction signal.

4. The *sarcoplasmic reticulum*, which manufactures proteins and releases calcium.
5. The *sarcomere*, the unit of contraction, containing 'z-lines', actin and myosin.
6. *ATP molecules*, phosphocreatine molecules for instant (anaerobic) high-intensity energy and the enzyme clusters for anaerobic glycolysis.
7. The *mitochondria* which supply aerobic energy.
8. The muscle cell *nuclei*, which hold all the information and instructions for the cell.
9. The *'satellite cells'*, very small adjunct muscle cells, very closely invested with each muscle cell proper, which act as a repair system

THE SARCOLEMMA

Many aspects of muscle are preceded by the prefix 'sarco' (e.g. *sarcolemma*), which is from the Greek work for flesh. Indeed when people talk of 'flesh', it is muscle which is usually meant. The sarcolemma itself is the muscle cell membrane, holding the whole cell together. It is made from a strong flexible lipoprotein: the protein for strength, and the lipid or fat (plus incorporated water) for malleability. These qualities are particularly suited to dealing with the problem of all living cells, which is the 'water problem'.

Because all cells exist in a watery environment, and because they contain huge numbers of molecules inside a semi-permeable membrane, 'osmotic pressure' tends to strongly attract water from areas of low concentration (outside) to areas of high concentration (inside). This would burst the cells open, had they not devised a defence. Plant cells tend to deal with the problem by brute force. They encompass the cell membrane in a rigid wall of cellulose or lignin, too strong to burst. The advantage of this is it does not require much energy to maintain, but its penalty is that the whole structure is fairly immobile. Plant movement is very limited. Also, it deprives plants of the ability to think.

Animal cells have solved the water problem by means of the *sodium extrusion pump*, a sort of rotating molecular cage in the cell membrane, whereby sodium is pumped out of the cell, and with each sodium ion go two molecules of water. This permits a flexible membrane, with the disadvantage that it requires a constant energy supply, to keep the pump working. However, an advantageous spin-off is that the sodium ions are electrically positively charged, so the outside of the cell membrane is positive with reference to the inside. This sets the stage for the generation of nerve impulses, which are circles of altered electrical charge travelling along the nerve fibres, as in brain or motor nerve to muscle. It also sets the stage for the electrical impulses along the sarcolemma, which is the signal for muscle fibre contraction. Thus, by taking the easy way out of the water problem, plants forfeited the ability of thought and quick movement.

When a muscle fibre is at its resting length, as in a dancer lying on a couch, the sarcolemma is folded, with small corrugations, which straighten out as the muscle fibre is stretched, and exaggerate as it is contracted. In this way the sarcolemma can cope with the large changes in muscle fibre length without damage.

THE MYONEURAL JUNCTION

The *myoneural junction*, as the name suggests, is an enlargement at the end of a motor nerve fibre where it meets the muscle fibre. When the nerve impulse reaches it, it secretes the substance *acetylcholine* which, in turn, alters the electrical state of the adjacent sarcolemma, thus triggering a wave of altered electrical charge along the sarcolemma.

THE T-SYSTEM

The *T-system* (or Tubular system) is a set of invaginations at regular intervals all along the sarcolemma, and it serves to bring the sarcolemma's wave of electrical charge much deeper into the muscle cell, into very close contact with the sarcoplasmic reticulum.

THE SARCOPLASMIC RETICULUM

The *sarcoplasmic reticulum* is a netlike meshwork of membranes in the muscle cell, with two main functions. Firstly, on the arrival of the electric impulse down the T-system, it is stimulated to release calcium into the interior of the muscle cell, which paves the way for actin and myosin to make contact. The other function of the sarcoplasmic reticulum is to manufacture all the proteins which the muscle cell needs, whether functional proteins such as enzymes, or the contractile proteins such as actin and myosin.

THE SARCOMERE

The *sarcomere* is the unit of contraction of the muscle cell, the point of the entire muscle cellular operation, and where dance—and all other physical actions—originate. It is bounded at each end by a 'z-line', composed of a zigzag mesh of proteins, containing parallel arrays of the protein filaments *actin* and *myosin* (Fig. 4.5).

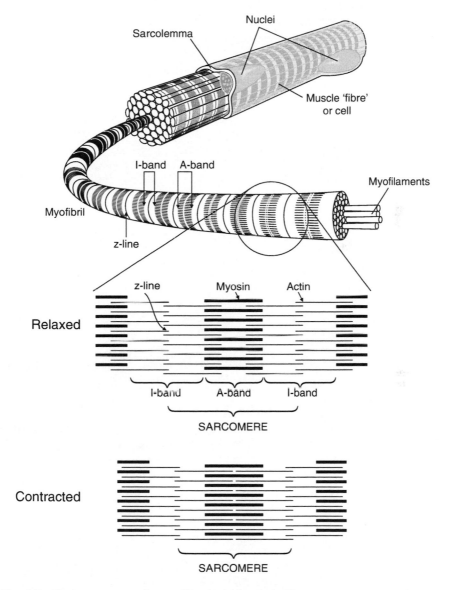

Fig. 4.5 Various stages of magnification of muscle fibre

They are joined end-to-end to form a chain up to about 10 000 to 15 000 units long. This long chain is called a *myofibril*, and there are about 2000 myofibils in a single muscle fibre. Each myofibril is surrounded by sarcoplasmic reticulum—more so in fast fibres, where the need is to get the calcium to the sarcomere as quickly as possible (and to remove it as quickly as possible; it is as important for a muscle to relax as to contract, to avoid injury for example).

Human sarcomeres are about 4 micrometres long in a fully extended muscle, and 1.6 micrometres long when the muscle is fully contracted. However, for maximal performance, the sarcomere has to be at about two thirds of its longest length. In terms of a whole muscle, that is often about two thirds of its fully extended length. This is why the sprinter starts from a crouch position, with all the muscles set to about two thirds of their resting length, to maximize the force at the start. And also why one crouches down before a jump, or bends one's arms before catching something heavy.

ENERGY MOLECULES

ATP, the energy currency of the cell, as described in Part I, provides the energy for muscle contraction, to shorten the sarcomere, and hence the muscle. Muscle may, of course, generate a force without shortening, and even while lengthening. In both these cases, the force is still developed by the same mechanisms, which will be briefly discussed later in this section.

Molecules of *ATP* are far too small to be seen with the electron microscope. The same applies for *phosphocreatine*. The enzyme clusters for *glycolysis* are not housed in an organelle as are those of Krebs cycle, and they too cannot be seen with the electron microscope. However, *glycogen* granules may be seen as small black dots, more plentifully in fast fibres, whereas small droplets of *fat* may be seen more in slow fibres.

MITOCHONDRIA

Mitochondria can also be seen with the electron microscope. These sausage-shaped organelles contain the enzymes for Krebs cycle, which together with the final phase of electron transport, provide the aerobic energy for the cell. All the oxygen used by the body is used in mitochondria, which respond to aerobic training by multiplying. They contain DNA of their own, so control themselves to a considerable extent. Moreover, all our mitochondria come from our mothers, via the ovum. No mitochondria are transmitted in the sperm, hence Adam could not have been good at aerobic endurance, but could have excelled at high-intensity dance routines. In anything aerobic, Eve would have beaten him out of sight. Somehow she obviously acquired more than just the genetic information from Adam's rib cells.

MUSCLE CELL NUCLEI

All cells except red blood cells contain a nucleus, which houses the cellular DNA, which is the information storehouse of the cell, its repository of genetic information and instructions. Muscle is unique in having from about 2000 to 30 000 nuclei per fibre, depending on size. This is really because in development muscle is formed by the fusion of thousands of myoblasts (embryonic muscle cells), to make the relatively enormous cells needed for muscular function in terms of high force development.

SATELLITE CELLS

These are also developed from embryonic myoblasts. They are very small, having one nucleus and only a small amount of surrounding *cytoplasm*. They exist closely attached to, but just outside, the sarcolemma. They form a real back-up repair system in that if muscle is damaged, they are stimulated to multiply, fuse, and form new muscle cells. Thus each muscle fibre carries its own genuine repair/replacement system with it, a quite extraordinary system. This is perhaps to compensate for the fact that individual muscle fibres do not appear to divide, although there is some debate over this.

7   THE MECHANISM OF MUSCLE CONTRACTION

Within each muscle fibre and at the level of the above mentioned contractile filaments, muscle contraction occurs when the *cross-bridges* of the thick (myosin) filaments bind to selected sites on the thin (actin) filaments (Fig. 4.6) with the assistance of calcium ions. More specifically, an impulse passes down a motor nerve to the motor end plate where it releases acetylcholine. This changes the permeability of the adjacent circle of sarcolemma, so that some of the positively charged sodium ions flow back in again, thus 'depolarizing' the sarcolemma. This electrical wave of depolarization spreads at about 7.5 m/sec over the sarcolemma and down all the T-tubules, virtually simultaneously. The wave triggers the release of calcium from those parts of the sarcoplasmic reticulum nearest the T-tubules. Calcium then floods the sarcomeres, initiating the displacement of *tropomyosin* from actin's cross-bridge binding sites, thus allowing the myosin cross-bridges to fix onto the sites, and contraction to begin.

As a result of this selective binding, the filaments actin and myosin slide past one another, maintaining their original lengths but reducing the overall length of the sarcomere (Fig. 4.7). The actual force to do this is

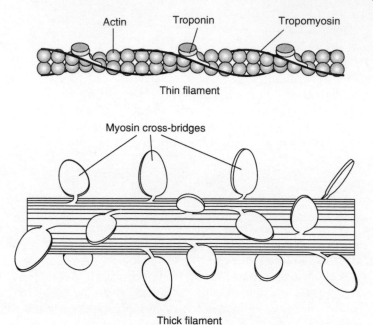

Actin   Troponin   Tropomyosin

Thin filament

Myosin cross-bridges

Thick filament

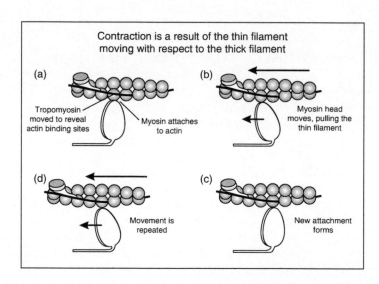

Contraction is a result of the thin filament
moving with respect to the thick filament

(a)
Tropomyosin
moved to reveal
actin binding sites
Myosin attaches
to actin

(b)
Myosin head
moves, pulling the
thin filament

(d)
Movement is
repeated

(c)
New attachment
forms

Fig. 4.6 The muscle contractile filaments. The thin filament contains three different proteins: Actin, Troponin, and Tropomyosin. In the absence of calcium, tropomyosin blocks the attachment sites for myosin. In the presence of calcium, troponin changes its shape and pulls tropomyosin away from the myosin attachment sites on actin. Thus contraction begins

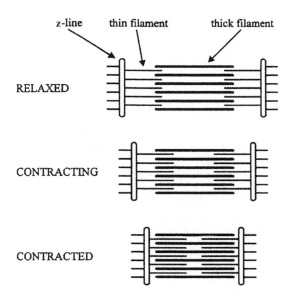

Fig. 4.7   Skeletal muscle contraction. The thin and thick filaments slide past one another, resulting in a shortening of the overall length of the sarcomere. The sarcomere is contained between two z-discs (or z-lines) and is the contractile unit within the muscle fibre

generated by *cross-bridges*, which extend from the thicker myosin fila-ments to corresponding attachment sites on the thin actin filaments (Fig. 4.6). These attachment sites at rest are blocked by a regulatory protein, tropomyosin and its partner troponin, but when the calcium comes flooding out of the sarcoplasmic reticulum, troponin nudges aside the tropomyosin, allowing the cross-bridges to make contact, and then to move, like the arms of a line of dancers passing a colleague overhead. When the cross-bridge has completed its movement it detaches, swings back, re-engages, and moves again. This goes on until the calcium is withdrawn (by being pumped back into the sarcoplasmic reticulum), or until the myosin molecules physically bump against the z-line.

When the electrical activation at the T-tubules stops, that is when you stop willing a muscle to contract, calcium release is halted, and the 'calcium pump' of the sarcoplasmic reticulum pumps the calcium back into its 'terminal cisterns', to be stored for reuse. Sometimes, when energy demands are very high, there is not quite enough ATP to fully activate the calcium pump, so calcium stays around the sarcomere, and relaxation is slowed up. Such 'relaxation fatigue' may lead to poor co-ordination at best, or injury at worst.

At longest and shortest sarcomere lengths, relatively few cross-bridges can be engaged, so the force developed is less. If you do a series of chin-ups to a bar, or press-ups on the floor, you fatigue at full arm extension on the chin-ups, and on the floor in full arm flexion in the press-ups. However, if you lift the chin-upper half way to the bar, he can easily pull himself all the way up; and if you lift the press-upper half way up, she can easily complete the movement. In both cases you have allowed the muscles involved to reset their sarcomeres to about the half-way point of optimal cross-bridge engagement.

8   TYPES OF MUSCLE CONTRACTION

A summary of the different types of muscle contraction appears in Table 4.2. Note that most muscle contraction, of the type known either as *isotonic* (= 'same tension') or *concentric* (ends move towards the centre) does indeed shorten the muscle fibre. However, *isometric* (= 'same length') contraction is the name given when you put the palms of your

Table 4.2   Types of muscle contraction

1. *Isotonic* contraction is defined as *the contraction that produces the same amount of tension—while muscle is shortening—as it overcomes a constant resistance.* The tension exerted by the contracting muscle may be affected by several factors including: the *speed* of muscle fibre shortening, the initial *fibre-length*, and the *angle* of pull in relation to the skeleton.

2. *Concentric muscle contraction is when a muscle shortens as it overcomes an external constant resistance.* Concentric is also the most common contraction used in strength training, e.g. 'bench-press'.

3. *Eccentric contraction refers to the lengthening of a muscle during contraction.* Walking down steps or downhill running would be two examples. This type of muscle contraction normally demonstrates higher maximal forces compared to the concentric equivalent.

4. *Isometric contractions refer to situations in which muscle tension is developed, but there is no change in the external length of the muscle.* Pushing against a wall may form an example where there are no changes in the muscle's length, but a substantial development of tension.

5. *Isokinetic contractions involve the development of maximal tension as the muscle shortens at a constant (iso) speed (kinetic) throughout the range of motion.* A good example is the arms' movement during swimming. Compared to isotonic, isokinetic contractions are potentially capable of generating maximal forces throughout the full range of motion. In strength training, isokinetic exercises provide the 'best of both worlds' in terms of isotonic and isometric contractions.

hands together in front of your chest and push hard—a lot of force is developed, but no movement. Just as in holding a partner aloft. And there is a third mode of 'contraction', which is where a muscle may exert a strong force while it is lengthening. This is termed an *eccentric* contraction (ends moving away from the middle). For example, when you walk downstairs, as your leading foot is feeling for the next stair, your uppermost leg is increasingly flexing, which implies that your quadriceps is getting longer. (Think of the quads stretching exercise where you stand on one leg and flex the other and pull your foot behind you up to your bottom). So your trailing leg is increasingly flexing, the quads are lengthening, yet they are developing an increasing force until your other foot takes the weight on the next step.

This also happens every time a dancer lands from a jump or leap; the landing leg(s) flexes, yet is generating forces much greater than body-weight to absorb the impact. Actually, muscle can generate up to the order of 30–40% greater force eccentrically than concentrically, and this forms part of the rationale behind the form of strength/power training known as plyometrics or depth jumping.

9   CONTROL AND REFLEX

The only active movement a muscle can make is to shorten, thus muscle can only pull. No matter how hard you push a set around a stage, the working muscles are all shortening and pulling; but the pull is converted to push by the body levers—the bones. When you push with your arms, the triceps at the back of the upper arm pulls on the olecranon, the elbow outgrowth of the ulna. The olecranon pivots over the end of the humerus as a fulcrum, and the rest of the ulna moves in the opposite direction, thus straightening the arm. Even in a rugby scrum, every muscle is pulling.

Muscle may twitch involuntarily when it is fatigued, or it may lock into the painful contraction of cramp, when it is fatigued, or cold—these are examples of muscle out of control. Normally muscle is under control. 'Ordinary' body skeletal muscle is under the voluntary control of motor nerves, from the spinal cord, which in turn is an extension from the brain. Other muscle, such as in the walls of blood vessels, or which attaches to hairs, giving goose-pimples, or that of the iris, is controlled by autonomic nerves, as described earlier. Still other muscle, such as that of the uterus, is controlled by hormones, as at menstruation and childbirth. Some muscle can only contract when stimulated by a nerve impulse; other muscle, such as heart or intestine, has its own internal rhythm—which can be altered by nerve impulses, or chemical or mechanical stimuli.

Much of the action of all muscle types occurs because of a reflex. A reflex of skeletal muscle may be defined as an *involuntary response to a stimulus*. It may be involuntary, but it is programmed, and reflexes may also be learned. The 'reflex saves' of hockey goalkeepers are not instinctive, they are acquired by much practice. The reflex whereby you whip your hand out of a basin of overhot water does not need to be learned, it is pre-programmed. An important reflex related to dance is the 'stretch reflex', whereby when a muscle is stretched suddenly, it contracts 'involuntarily'. When the doctor taps just below your kneecap with a small rubber hammer, and your knee jerks forwards, that is a stretch reflex. The sequence of events is that the hammer tap depresses the patellar ligament running from the bottom of the kneecap to the tibial tuberosity (the bony lump below your knee). This in turn pulls the patella a few millimetres downwards, thus fractionally stretching your quadriceps muscle, which inserts on the top of the kneecap. Muscle spindles scattered through the quads are highly sensitive to length changes, and send signals to the spinal cord, via their sensory nerves if suddenly stretched. These impulses then contact and activate motor nerves to the quadriceps, which then contracts, and your lower leg jerks forwards.

All the major skeletal muscles demonstrate such a contractile reflex on being suddenly stretched. Where it may be important to dancers concerns stretching, especially at the beginning of the day, in that stretching of any major muscle group should be done slowly, as is usually the case in a classical class, but not always in other dance forms. If one stretches too fast, especially in dynamic bouncy types of stretch, a danger is that a stretch reflex might be invoked, so that the lengthening muscle suddenly reflexly tries to shorten, which may lead to injury.

The elaborately named technique of 'proprioceptive neuromuscular facilitation' (or PNF) was developed in order to nullify some of the muscle spindle's contribution. It was found that if a muscle is held in a strong isometric contraction, this inactivates spindle function to some degree, and the muscle may be stretched further immediately thereafter (see more about PNF in Chapter 5 under muscle flexibility and joint mobility).

Going back to the doctor's surgery. If your leg does *not* jerk forward after two or three taps, then the doctor would ask you to clasp your hands in front of your chest and pull hard. Then your 'patellar reflex' should work. Activating any large muscle group, such as your arms and shoulders, causes all muscle spindles to reset to a higher level of sensitivity. Hence the fact that the patellar reflex will now be present. But a lesson from this is that if you inadvertently tense your shoulders before going on stage, you may alter spindle activity and make your movements a little less accurate in your first few steps, especially if they are delicate and precise. Hence the physiological importance of relaxation just before skilled movement. The warm-up also helps here, as large body movements also help to relax or desensitize muscle spindles. It is for that reason that pianists, classical and jazz, usually open a concert or set with an up-tempo and/or forte number, to 'shake the nerves out of my fingers', as they say.

On the other hand, if one has to make a grand entry, as in 'Spectre de la Rose', for example, then one may want a degree of muscle tension, just as the sprinter on the blocks does not want to be relaxed. The movement may not be quite as controlled, but it will be a bit more powerful, from a tense start.

10 CONCLUSIONS

As far as muscle as a whole is concerned, there are four ways in which it can act. It can exert a strong force, which is its *strength*; it can contract fast—and this is its *speed*; it can go on contracting and relaxing for a period of time, which is its *endurance*; the fourth aspect is *flexibility*, related to its extended length. Each of these attributes is important in different proportions for different dance activities. Each can be measured in the laboratory. And each of them can be improved by specific modes of exercise training. Dance, gymnastics, martial arts—and an increasing number of drama performances—require all the attributes of muscle, at an increasingly higher level of training. An understanding of their structure and function is essential to getting the best out of one's muscles.

11 FURTHER READING

Blakey P. (1992) *The muscle book*. Stafford, UK: Bibliotek Books
De Vries HA, Housh TJ. (1994) *Physiology of exercise for physical education, athletics and exercise science* (5th edition). Madison, WI: Brown and Benchmark
Jones D, Round J. (1990) *Muscle in health and disease*. Manchester, UK: Manchester University Press
Wilmore JH, Costill DL (1994) *Physiology of sport and exercise*. Champaign, Il: Human Kinetics
Wirhed R. (1984) *Athletic ability and the anatomy of motion*. London: Wolfe Medical Publications

Chapter 5
The Main Physical Fitness Components and Dance

1 INTRODUCTION

The last two decades have witnessed an unprecedented exercise and fitness boom, reflected in the large number of people engaged in some form of physical activity. It has been estimated that the industrialized countries have about 35% of their populations actively involved in a variety of physical activities ranging from gentle dance classes to aerobic sessions in gymnasiums, studios and swimming pools, through weekend sport, to national, international and world-class competition for men and women of all ages and socio-economic status. Never before has so much capital and effort been invested by so many nations in an attempt to maintain, regain or improve *fitness* and increase performance both in the exercise field and the working environment.

The World Health Organization defines fitness as *the ability to perform work satisfactorily* (Bouchard and Shephard 1994). However, the wording of this definition makes its interpretation somewhat dependent on personal inclinations and social context.

It has been suggested that fitness can be approached from objective and subjective viewpoints (Sharkey 1997). The former is more physical, can be measured, and is about bodily systems and functions, such as heart rates, volumes of oxygen consumption and levels of muscle strength. In contrast, approaching fitness from a subjective viewpoint is more related to individuals' emotions and psychology. For our purposes, the term fitness will be considered as synonymous to *physical fitness.*

Physical fitness may be defined as *the individual's ability to meet the demands of a specific physical task,* and primarily consists of aspects related to muscle and its function. It depends on the individual's ability to work under *aerobic* and *anaerobic* conditions, and on their capacity to develop high levels of muscle tension (i.e. *muscle strength*). *Muscle power, joint mobility, muscle flexibility* and *body composition* are also important parts of physical fitness, together with the less researched *body balance*.

Regardless of their performance level, sex and age, all dancers use one or more of these elements of fitness during their daily practice. However, no single fitness component or measurement can predict success in dance, as they vary markedly depending on the individual, the specific task (or role), and the level of performance. Hence, all components of physical fitness should be simultaneously considered, as they are parts of the complete fitness jigsaw (Fig. 5.1).

The investigation into physiological and fitness components of dance and dancers has mainly concentrated on classical ballet dance (Cohen, Segal, Witriol and McArdle 1982a; Cohen, Segal and McArdle 1982; Claessens, Beunen, Nuyts *et al.* 1987; Chmelar, Schultz, Ruhling *et al.* 1988; Hamilton, Hamilton, Marshall and Molnar 1992; Galanti, Holland, Shafranski *et al.* 1993). Relatively few reports on modern and contempor-

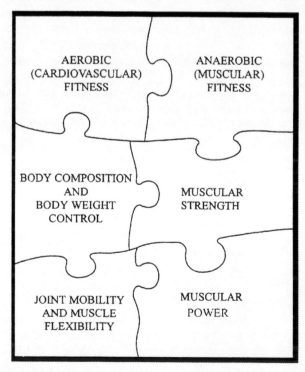

Fig. 5.1   Fitness jigsaw

ary dance have been published up to now (Chatfield, Byrnes and Foster 1992; Dahlström, Inasio, Jansson and Kaijser 1996).

In essence, one might view physical activity as being concerned with movement physiology below the level of the head. From the neck up are located all the skills and interpretations of dance, together with the ability of controlling anxiety, nervousness and stress, and kinetic memory of the dance itself. Of course all the motor patterns originate in the brain, but in this section the emphasis will be on the body, and not the mind. Before considering each individual fitness item in greater detail, a summary of the main functions of these fitness items would probably assist the reader to better appreciate their value and contribution to different forms of dance.

- *Aerobic fitness,* or stamina, more technically called cardiorespiratory fitness. It involves all aspects of the uptake, transport and utilization of oxygen to release moderate levels of energy (for many hours if necessary) from the muscle fuels, mainly carbohydrate and fat. This in turn involves the lungs, the blood, the heart, the blood vessels delivering the oxygen, and the muscles, with their capillaries, myoglobin and mitochondria, all receiving and utilizing the oxygen.
- *Anaerobic fitness,* or local muscle endurance. This operates without the need of oxygen, and involves two high-energy sources, creatine phosphate and glycolysis, producing up to ten times the rate of energy of the aerobic system. This energy is then used for fast and 'explosive' movements, such as jumping. However, it either completely exhausts itself in seconds (i.e. creatine phosphate) or inhibits itself with end products in less than a minute (i.e. glycolysis).
- *Muscle strength.* In its purest form, strength is demonstrated by weightlifters, and *inter alia* in dance it is shown in the lifts. It is the ability of muscle to generate force, measured (in Newtons) on various equipment. It responds well to optimal training, and plays an important role in injury prevention and rehabilitation.
- *Muscle power.* Strength is the ability to produce force, but power is the rate of development of the force. In other words, it is the ability to produce force fast, so power invokes the speed of muscle contraction. This attribute is trained by concentrating on moving loads at speed, either as free or fixed weights.
- *Muscle flexibility and Joint mobility.* This involves the range of movement of a limb or limb segment about a joint. It is measured as the angle through which the movement has occurred, in degrees of arc. It is the main fitness component that dancers have traditionally sought to improve. Its training involves plastic deformation of ligament, tendon, and muscle, and lengthening of muscle itself.

• *Body composition* relates to the percentage of body weight which is fat, and that which is 'fat-free'. The two main elements which can alter body weight are fat and muscle. Too much or too little body fat can markedly affect performance and injury rates, while body weight is influenced by the balance between calorie intake (i.e. diet) and calorie expenditure (i.e. physical activity).

2 AEROBIC (CARDIORESPIRATORY) FITNESS

2.1 Introduction and Definition

'*Aerobic*' literally means 'with air'. Because in life and dance the vital ingredient of air is its content of oxygen, aerobic is taken to mean 'with oxygen'. In opera terms, the singer utilizes all the expired air to vibrate the vocal chords, so singing is truly 'aerobic'.

We take oxygen for granted, but on Earth it was not always so. The early atmosphere was extruded from innumerable volcanic vents and fissures as the cooling Earth contracted, and it contained very little free oxygen. In other words, the early atmosphere was *anaerobic*—without oxygen. After about one billion years, life began to evolve—and it was anaerobic life. Towards the end of the next billion years, when life was well established on land, the early plants began gradually to increase the atmosphere's content of oxygen through photosynthesis. Indeed, they began to pollute the atmosphere with oxygen, because the gas is, surprisingly, toxic. Long ago, one of the present authors published an article which included work on the toxicity of oxygen, if breathed at pressures and concentrations very much higher than normal (Sharp 1966).

Simple life forms, partly because they replicate into so many generations in a short space of time, can evolve very rapidly. That is why bacteria so readily develop resistance to antibiotics, and why the pharmacologists have to strive to keep a step ahead of them. Faced with oxygen pollution, it is thought that the simple life forms developed a means of dealing with the oxygen and its associated toxic *free radicals*, by the process of *electron transport*. This process of electron transport, now located at the end of *Krebs cycle*, evolved into a superb process for using oxygen to extract far more energy from each food molecule. The legacy of all this, billions of years later, is that the modern dancer can call on two major energy supplies, the original anaerobic, and the more modern aerobic. This section will deal with aerobic energy supply.

Aerobic fitness implies muscular work done utilizing oxygen to liberate energy from the muscle fuels. This brings us to a major division, involving supply and demand. Oxygen supply, and more specifically its absorption and transportation, is carried out by the cardiorespiratory system of lungs, heart, blood vessels and blood. The demand comes from the muscles, which utilize the oxygen by taking the blood into their network of muscle capillaries and passing it deep into the interior of the individual muscle cells, to the energy production pathways of Krebs cycle and electron transport.

2.2 Measurement of Aerobic Fitness

There are several ways to measure aerobic fitness, from full-scale laboratory physiological assessment, down to simple step tests which can be done at home.

LABORATORY TESTING

In the laboratory, two values are usually measured, which together give an overall rating of aerobic fitness. These are the maximal oxygen uptake (usually abbreviated to $\dot{V}O_2$ max) and the Onset of Blood Lactate Accumulation (or OBLA), often more conveniently called the *anaerobic threshold*—and this relates to the percentage of the $\dot{V}O_2$ max which can be sustained for a reasonable length of time. Given that the $\dot{V}O_2$ max itself can be maintained for only a very few minutes, it is much more useful to know what level of oxygen uptake can be sustained for as long as the dance or the exercise lasts, and it is this that the anaerobic threshold tells us. The anaerobic threshold is measured by noting the level of exertion at which blood lactic acid begins to rise significantly.

The $\dot{V}O_2$ max is measured on the form of *ergometer* which is most suited to the sport or the activity. For runners, this is a treadmill, for rowers and canoeists a rowing and canoeing machine respectively, while for cyclists it is a cycle ergometer. We tend to test dancers on a treadmill, as running is the nearest to dance that we can get in the laboratory (Fig. 5.2). There are also now available very light forms of oxygen measurement apparatus, worn as a face mask, which can be utilized during an approximate run-through of a dance sequence, thus opening up very promising prospects for further investigation of all forms of dance.

For the $\dot{V}O_2$ max test, the dancer is given practice at running on the treadmill, to warm up, and in particular on how to get off it should sudden fatigue set in. Then a set of appropriate speeds is chosen, and he/she is 'connected up'. This implies putting small elastoplast-like electrodes on the chest—one below where the heart beats, and two up by the collar-bones. These record the electrical signals from the heart. Then a mouthpiece is put in his/her mouth, for breathing in and out of, so that

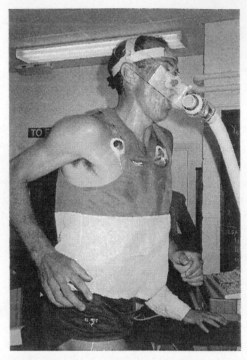

Fig. 5.2   A maximal oxygen uptake ($\dot{V}O_2$ max) test on a treadmill

the volume of expired air can be measured, and the expired air can be
analysed for its oxygen and carbon dioxide content. Finally, a nose-clip is
put on (such as synchro-swimmers wear) to ensure that all the expired
air is collected via the mouthpiece (Fig. 5.2). Then the treadmill is set
going for about five minutes at a low pace to settle the dancer, and to
make sure the heart rate and the gas collection are satisfactory. Then the
treadmill speed will be raised a little every three minutes or so until the
dancer signals that he or she simply cannot go on any longer.

Throughout the test, the expired air is analysed for its content of
oxygen and carbon dioxide, and the maximum uptake of oxygen that is
reached is calculated and related to body weight to give the $\dot{V}O_2$ max
figure in millilitres of oxygen per kilogram per minute (ml/kg/min). If an
'anaerobic threshold' (OBLA) estimation is wanted, a few small finger-
prick or ear-lobe blood samples are taken at the different treadmill
speeds, and analysed for their content of lactic acid.

Consider a female dancer with a $\dot{V}O_2$ max of 45 ml/kg/min. This is
what she might maintain for two or three minutes. If she was reasonably
fit, with an anaerobic threshold occurring at 35 ml/kg/min, this would

mean that she should be able to work at a rate of 35 ml/kg/min for an hour, for example. If her aerobic fitness had fallen, through illness or injury, her anaerobic threshold might drop to 30 ml/kg/min or even lower, even though her $\dot{V}O_2$ max might not have changed by anything like the same percentage. The $\dot{V}O_2$ max is more a measure of potential fitness, and the anaerobic threshold is more a measure of current state of training or fitness.

The spectrum of aerobic capacities varies from a $\dot{V}O_2$ max of about 42 and 38 ml/kg/min for untrained 25-year-old men and women, up to values of about 90 and 80 ml/kg/min in similarly aged cross-country skiers and road cyclists. Some values for dancers are given in Table 5.1.

As with most of their physiological values, most of the current data regarding aerobic fitness of dancers have been derived from ballet. For example, male and female professional ballet dancers have shown $\dot{V}O_2$ max values of 56 and 51 ml/kg/min respectively (Schantz and Åstrand 1984), which are considerably higher than those measured by Cohen *et al.* (1982). The latter authors found $\dot{V}O_2$ max levels in ballet dancers to be about 48 and 44 ml/kg/min for men and women respectively. They also noted that ballet class work—especially at the barre (e.g. pliés, tendus)—represented, aerobically, exercise of only low to moderate intensity.

Matters are slightly different during centre-floor work. Although for only brief periods of up to 3 minutes, intensities of centre-floor work can reach 70–80% of $\dot{V}O_2$ max (Schantz and Åstrand 1984), which are similar to cardiorespiratory responses during ballet stage performances (Cohen,

Table 5.1 Maximal oxygen intake ($\dot{V}O_2$ max) values obtained from British dancers and untrained individuals

Form of dance	Sex	Age	$\dot{V}O_2$ max (ml/kg/min)
Contemporary[a]	Males	26.6	55.7
Ballet[a]	Males	25.8	53.2
Dance students[a]	Males	23.0	49.4
Dance students[a]	Females	21.3	46.0
Contemporary[a]	Females	27.1	43.5
Ballet[a]	Females	25.9	39.1
NSCD[b]	Males	20.2	54.9
NSCD[b]	Females	19.4	43.8
Untrained	Males	25.0	42.0
Untrained	Females	25.0	38.0

Sources: [a]From Brinson and Dick (1996)
[b]Northern School of Contemporary Dance (1997), unpublished data

Segal and McArdle 1982). Given that fairly strenuous exercise intensities, for at least 20 minutes, are needed to stimulate an increase in aerobic fitness, it is probable that most ballet activities do not provide an adequate stimulus to cardiorespiratory or aerobic fitness. This was supported by Rimmer, Jay and Plowman (1994) in a study on rehearsals for 'Sleeping Beauty'. Kirkendall and Calabrese (1983) also found that the relatively small increments in aerobic fitness in professional dancers were not related to their class work, but to the duration and frequency of their performances. It is worth noticing that contemporary dancers generally have higher $\dot{V}O_2$ max values than ballet dancers (Kirkendall and Calbrese 1983; Chmelar, Schultz, Ruhling *et al.* 1988), although it is not clear whether this is a result of selection or training (or both).

Field Testing

A field test is merely one which does not require a laboratory and its highly sophisticated equipment. The main feature of such assessments, especially the simpler tests, is that each time the test is done, great efforts should be made to ensure that the conditions are the same as, or as similar as possible to, the previous tests. Otherwise, if the test is not exactly comparable, neither are the results. This includes repeating the test at the same time of day and, in women, at the same time during the menstrual cycle. There is a number of field tests that a dancer can use to estimate his or her levels of aerobic fitness.

1. The simplest field test is the *resting pulse count*. By and large, the fitter one is, the larger one's heart relative to body weight; the larger the heart, the bigger the *stroke volume*, or the amount of blood at each beat. And the larger the stroke volume, the fewer beats required to pump an adequate volume of blood at rest, hence the lower the resting pulse count. Many sport competitors keep a training diary, in which they record their morning resting pulse and notice that it gradually declines, over the months and years. Perhaps from a 'normal' 75 beats per minute it goes down to 70, then 65, then 60, and possibly lower. Olympic-level marathon runners may demonstrate resting pulse rates as low as 30–35 beats per minute.

The best place to find the pulse is on the inner surface of the wrist, just below the base of the thumb. If you are counting someone else's pulse, don't use your own thumb to count it, as the thumb often has a palpable pulse of its own, and you could count your own heart rate. Another convenient pulse is to be found in the carotid artery in the neck, just in front of the angle of the jaw. For resting pulse rates, it is best to count for a full minute, shortly after waking and before morning coffee or tea (or cigarette!).

2. Different *step tests* are also useful, especially to compare a subject at a given time with himself on a future occasion; in other words they are at their best when comparing one's own fitness levels over time.

One such is the *Harvard step test*, which is easy to perform, and all you need is a 50 cm (20 in.) step for men and a 45 cm (18 in.) step for women, together with a metronome and a stopwatch. The step may be a stool or a chair or a firm box. For dancers, the length of the test would be five minutes, with a step rate of 30 per minute, that is a metronome setting of 120. The procedure is to give the subject a practice at the stepping and the rhythm. Then, after a brief rest, start the test and the stopwatch, and ensure that the subjects stand fully upright on the step each time and that they keep up with the rhythm for the five minutes. If they fall behind the rhythm for more than 15 seconds, note the time, and stop the test. Either way, when the subject stops, sit them down, and start looking for the pulse—in the wrist or at the angle of the jaw. Wait for one minute after stopping the test, then count the pulse for 30 seconds.

Now, you have two figures. The 30-second pulse count (usually between 40 and 65), and the stepping time which will amount to 300 seconds. If the subject did not step for the full five minutes, then record the time (converted to seconds) for which they did step. Then put the two figures into the formula below, to find the fitness index (FI).

$$FI = \frac{(\text{time in seconds}) \times 100}{(30 \text{ secs pulse count}) \times 5.5}$$

For example, for a 30-second pulse count of 54 after 5 minutes of stepping:

$$FI = \frac{(300) \times 100}{54 \times 5.5} = \frac{30\,000}{297} = 101$$

Here, the fitness index works out at 101. In this test, the higher the index, the better. And, roughly, a score of 80–99 is a reasonable level of fitness for a dancer; 100–119 is creditable, and 120–139 is good, with 140–159 very good indeed, and above this would be into the range of high-level athletes. However, the main use of the step test is to measure your own improvement.

3. There are run tests too that can be used to assess aerobic fitness. One is the *multistage shuttle-run test*, which works by subjects running between two markers 20 metres apart, in a studio or gymnasium. Timing is from a recorded tape in a cassette player, with the sound signal getting progressively faster. The exercise level the subject reaches gauges the fitness level. There are different versions of this test, but the best one is with the

tape and instructions put out by the National Coaching Foundation, in Beckett Park, Leeds LS6.

4. Lastly, there is a 6-lap run (1.5 miles, or 2.4 km) known as the *Cooper test*. For this one really needs a running track, and ideally the weather and underfoot conditions should be the same at each test, which consists simply of running six laps as fast as possible, timed with a stopwatch. The trick here is to learn to pace oneself over the distance, but having achieved this, with a little practice, it again is a good test for recording improvements in aerobic fitness. It also has the advantage that there are tables of normal values, in minutes and seconds for both men and women (Table 5.2). Dancers would be expected to be at least in the category of 'good' or better.

Table 5.2 Classification of aerobic fitness based on the Cooper running test. Figures are minutes and seconds

	Age (years)	Poor	Fair	Good	Very good	Excellent
Men	17–29	14.30+	12.00+	10.15+	8.15+	7.30+
	30–34	15.00+	12.30+	10.30+	8.30+	7.45+
	35–39	15.30+	13.00+	11.00+	9.00+	8.00+
Women	17–29	17.24+	14.24+	12.18+	9.54+	9.00+
	30–34	18.00+	15.00+	12.36+	10.12+	9.18+
	35–39	18.36+	15.36+	12.54+	10.30+	9.36+

2.3 Factors Affecting Aerobic Fitness

The main factors that affect aerobic fitness are associated with oxygen supply, and more specifically with the absorption and transportation of oxygen. They form the *cardiorespiratory* (or *cardiovascular*) system, which include the *lungs, heart, blood* and *blood vessels*. However, 'supply' is normally matched by 'demand', which in this particular case comes from the muscles. Through their network of muscle blood capillaries, oxygen is delivered deep into the interior of the individual muscle cells (with the help of *myoglobin*), to the energy production pathways of Krebs cycle which takes place inside the *mitochondria*. Appropriate aerobic training can result in significant myoglobin increases from 2 to 7 grams per 100 ml of blood, and in doubling of the size and number of mitochondria. However, none of these muscle changes can be found, if the oxygen supply is not adequate. Therefore, this section will concentrate on the oxygen-supply elements, namely the *lungs, heart, blood* and *blood vessels*.

Factors that can also influence aerobic fitness are *muscle fibre profile, age* and *gender*, and they are discussed elsewhere in this book. *Training at altitudes* of above 6000 feet (2000 m) and the use of certain doping agents (such as the hormone 'erythropoietin' which stimulates the bone marrow to produce more oxygen-carrying red cells) can also affect levels of aerobic fitness. However, these techniques—apart from the fact that some may be illegal—are of little practical value to dance and dancers.

LUNGS

In the lungs, the air passages or bronchi divide like a tree into ever decreasing branches, twigs and twiglets, until the air sacs or alveoli (like leaves) are reached, where the gas exchange takes place. Oxygen is taken in and quickly absorbed by the red blood cells in the capillary blood vessels which invest the alveolar walls. The total area of the alveoli available for this diffusion amounts to over half a tennis court. The red cells take about three-quarters of a second to traverse an alveolar wall at rest—and about a quarter of a second during vigorous dance. The oxygen needs about a quarter of a second to be fully taken up by the red cells, so there is just time enough! At the same time, carbon dioxide, the end product of Krebs cycle, is exchanged and breathed out.

Dancers occasionally ask if there is any point in deep breathing before going on stage, but as the blood at rest is virtually saturated with oxygen, extra breathing will not result in any more oxygen being absorbed. It will blow off more carbon dioxide, but that is not a particular advantage. However, slower deeper breaths may be part of a pre-performance psychological ritual, which could indeed be beneficial in coping with stress and nervousness.

At rest, about 10 litres of air are breathed in per minute. During a hard rehearsal session this can readily rise to 120 litres per minute or even higher—up to a maximum of about 200. About 30 to 50 litres a minute is as much as can be breathed in through the nose. The main function of the nose in breathing is to warm the air, and to moisten it to some extent. Warm moist air is what the lungs like; in some dancers the lungs' objection to cold dry air is to react by constricting the air passages in the condition known as 'exercise-induced asthma', which is extensively discussed elsewhere in the present book.

The main detrimental effects of smoking are the long-term risks of lung cancer or of increasing the chance of coronary heart disease. However, there is another much more immediate effect which concerns the dancer, namely the effect of the carbon monoxide in the tobacco smoke. At a level of about two cigarettes an hour, the inhaled carbon monoxide cuts down by about 8% the amount of oxygen the blood can carry. A dancer would not notice this in bursts of anaerobic high-intensity work, but might notice the effect in a sustained level of fairly hard aerobic work over 10 minutes or longer.

If those dancers who do smoke could refrain from doing so for at least four hours before a hard rehearsal or performance, they would give their blood a chance to clear at least some of the carbon monoxide. Alternatively, one might consider smoking small cigars or a pipe, where the smoke does not need to be inhaled. Because of the different way that pipe or cigar tobacco is cured, leading to its much greater solubility in water, the nicotine is absorbed through the cheeks and other mucous membranes of the mouth. Hence the short-term problem of carbon monoxide is greatly diminished, and the longer term cancer and heart disease risks are also much lessened.

THE HEART

At rest, the heart may pump about 5 litres of blood per minute, and during strenuous exercise this may rise to upwards of 20 litres per minute, depending on size and state of aerobic fitness.

The heart increases its output by two means. First, it increases its rate, from a resting level somewhere between 50 and 80 to about 200 beats per minute, in dancers in their 20s. Second, the volume of blood expelled at each beat, known as the *stroke volume*, increases from a resting level of, say 85 ml, to an exercising volume of 130 ml. As a result of such increased outputs, you can feel the heartbeat thudding against your chest wall—and can often see it, even through a leotard or T-shirt.

With aerobic training, the heart muscle, the *myocardium*, responds to these increases of *cardiac output*, like other muscle, by becoming larger and stronger. The myocardial walls become thicker, and the chambers increase in volume. Thus the whole heart increases its size, which is reflected in an increase in its stroke volume, both at rest and during exercise. The exercising volume of 130 ml just indicated above may increase to 160 ml or more. And the resting volume may increase from 85 ml, for example, to 100 ml. Thus to provide the same 5 litres of blood per minute at rest, the larger heart will beat slower. In general, as dancers (and others) become aerobically fitter, their resting heart rates will gradually drop, to below 60 or even below 50. It is interesting to note that no information is available regarding heart sizes in dancers and other active individuals before they engaged in specialized training, leaving a question mark over the contribution of heredity.

The maximum rate of the heart does not rise with training. Indeed, if anything, it tends to fall by some 5 to 10 beats per minute. This may be related to a problem that the heart has at high rates, not in pumping blood out, but in getting blood in. It is easy to imagine a heart, the size of a large fist, pumping blood out—but it is dependent on a good venous return to get the blood back. This 'venous return' is aided by the diaphragm, which contracts to cause negative pressure inside the thorax, leading to air rushing into the lungs. But the same negative pressure creates a suction effect on the great veins, pulling the blood back to the heart. This is one reason why sleepers breathe deeply at night—although their requirement for oxygen is at its lowest. They breathe deeply to keep the blood coming back to the heart.

So, what about venous return and filling for dancers in their 20s and an average maximal heart rate of around 180? Over two thirds of the time from one *systole* (contraction or emptying of the heart) to the next is taken up with filling, and a heart rate of 180 implies three beats per second, or 0.3 seconds per complete cardiac cycle of systole and *diastole* (filling). So at 180, there are about 0.2 seconds available for filling, which is just about the minimum requirement. That is why maximum heart rate does not rise with training.

This 'filling problem' of the heart in diastole has another important implication for strenuous exercise. If a dancer stops very abruptly following a hard routine, which has lasted more than a minute or two, he or she may feel slightly faint for a short period. Indeed, if the studio is particularly hot, the dancer may actually faint. This is because, on too sudden a cessation of vigorous effort, there is too marked a drop in venous return, giving a sudden, though transient, drop in blood pressure, which affects the brain, and causes the feeling of faintness. This is why the collapse of a dancer at the end of a hard routine is much less serious than such a collapse during a bout of very hard effort. And this is another very good reason for a brief warm-down after hard effort.

BLOOD AND BLOOD PRESSURE

The average man has about a gallon (4.5 l) of blood, with women about 10% less. Regarding aerobic fitness, the important measure is the quantity of *haemoglobin*, the iron-containing component of the red blood cell, which carries 99% of the oxygen (the rest is in solution in the plasma). Haemoglobin also carries about 30% of the carbon dioxide back to the lungs. The range of haemoglobin in normal men is between 14 and 16 grams per 100 ml of blood, and in women it is between 12 and 14 grams. If the values are a few grams below these lower values, then a state of *anaemia* may be said to exist.

Many men and women endurance athletes do have haemoglobin levels at the bottom of the normal range, and this is sometimes referred to as *sports anaemia* (Åstrand and Rodahl 1986). This arises because one of the normal changes of aerobic endurance training is an increase in the volume of blood of the order of from 20% up to 35% or over. However, the plasma volume increase is not quite matched by the increase in red cells and haemoglobin, whose concentration therefore decreases and the blood becomes 'thinner'.

No such information is available for dancers. This is partly related to the nature of most dance activities which, as discussed earlier in this section, seem not to provide adequate stimuli for aerobic fitness improvements (Rimmer, Jay and Plowman 1994). The relatively small increments in aerobic fitness found in professional dancers are more related to the duration and frequency of their performances, and not on the levels of aerobic work during classes (Kirkendall and Calabrese 1983).

The condition of *march haemoglobinurea* (first noted in marching soldiers) may occur in athletes who work on firm surfaces, such as basketball and volleyball players, runners, and dancers. In this condition it is noticed that the urine is discoloured a slight brown or reddish tinge after a hard or long workout. This is due to the pounding effects on the capillaries and *venules* of the soles of the feet whereby a small fraction of the red cells are disrupted, and release their haemoglobin content free into the blood, and it filters out into the urine. The condition is more prevalent in men than women, and seems to cause no harm whatever, although initially its presence may be a source of worry.

Another response to exercise is that of *blood pressure*. The blood pressure in the general circulation has a high value (the systolic pressure) of around 120 millimetres of mercury (mm Hg), representing the pressure at the time when the left ventricle is pumping the blood into the aorta and the general circulation. This pressure then falls to its lowest value (about 80 mm Hg) when the heart is refilling itself. This is why blood pressure is written as two values, in the form of 120/80. When a reasonably vigorous exercise routine begins, blood pressure rises by about 30 or 40%, then gradually falls back to normal in about half an hour, as the body heats up and the skin vessels dilate, so lowering the resistance to blood flow, and lowering the pressure. Appropriate aerobic exercise and training programmes often result in a modest drop of resting blood pressure over time.

BLOOD VESSELS

The network of *arteries, capillaries* and *veins,* respectively taking blood to the tissues, exchanging substances, and returning blood to the heart, is known as the *vascular* system. At any one time, 80% of blood is in the veins at low pressures. Arteries are the high-pressure distribution system. Yet the whole point of both arteries and veins is to ensure the passage of blood through the capillaries, a maze of tiny vessels, each scarcely wider than a single blood cell. For it is at the capillaries that all the meaningful exchanges take place between blood and the tissues they serve. All the glucose, amino acids, fatty acids, hormones, vitamins, minerals together with oxygen diffuse through the capillary walls into the surrounding *interstitial fluid*, to be taken up by all cells, including muscle cells. And all the waste metabolites, including carbon dioxide and lactic acid, are taken away from the tissues, to be disposed of by liver, kidneys and lungs.

Just after a bout of strenuous exercise, including a warm-up, begins, there occurs what is knows as the *vascular shunt*, which is a major rerouting and shutdown of blood from the organs of the abdomen and pelvis, to increase the volume available for muscle. At rest, the liver and kidneys account for about half of the entire output of the heart, but at the start of strenuous physical work, the blood flow through hepatic and renal and other visceral arteries is much reduced, to be available for use by the exercising muscles. As part of this process, the liver reduces its volume by about 25%, and in dancers or athletes who are exposed to a higher work rate than usual, the receptors on the liver's outer capsule signal a sensation which is felt as 'stitch'. However, in the fit and well-trained performer, the liver seems to get used to giving a blood donation before work, and that particular form of stitch ceases to occur.

The vascular shunt puts about half a litre or more of blood into the four and a half litres or so already in circulation. And the shutdown of blood to the abdomen and pelvic organs in general, together with the relaxation of stomach and intestines, and a tightening of their sphincters, all combine to produce the feeling of 'butterflies' at the start of exercise. This is controlled by the sympathetic nervous system, and is part of the 'nerves' felt before performance, and in rehearsal, as described in the previous chapter.

The total blood flow through the whole body musculature at rest may be of the order of one litre per minute (only a fifth of the cardiac output, for almost half of the body's mass) but during a vigorous routine this may rise 20 times. The red cells squeeze their way along the capillaries, in close contact with the vessel walls, the better to unload their oxygen, and they must be in contact for about one third of a second to off-load the oxygen. Thus, as the muscle, through training, becomes capable of generating more energy, and hence needs more blood, there is no point in increasing the speed of the blood in the capillaries—and decreasing the time for gas exchange. What must, and does, occur is the development of more capillaries.

Untrained muscle has on average about 560 capillaries per square millimetre of cross-section area. With training and exercise this number may double, or increase even more, correspondingly increasing muscle blood flow. The increased flow not only brings more oxygen and nutrients to the muscle, it also more quickly removes waste products, such as carbon dioxide and lactic acid. Importantly too, the capillaries are the site of heat exchange, as blood leaving working muscle is hotter than blood entering it. The warmed blood goes back to the heart, and a proportion of it is then pumped out to the skin, where the heat is radiated away from a hot red skin, or used to evaporate sweat from a wet skin.

2.4   Training for Aerobic Fitness

The ability to consume large volumes of oxygen during increased physical effort has been associated with the limits of human endurance and cardiorespiratory fitness. In dance, although increased cardiorespiratory fitness does not of course guarantee a better performance, it is nevertheless an important factor in coping with the long hours in the studio, facilitates recovery after physically demanding sessions, probably ensures lower injury rates, and, therefore, more years of successful performance.

Training the aerobic system involves working it hard enough to elicit an adaptation or training stimulus. In practice, this means raising the heart rate to an appropriate level, which is maintained for a suitable time. The problem lies in deciding what is an appropriate level.

For most dancers in their 20s or 30s, two or preferably three training sessions a week of about half an hour each at a heart rate of around 150 per minute will produce an acceptable increase in aerobic fitness. A very rough guide to more vigorous training for those who already are reasonably well trained is to add 25 to the dancer's age, and subtract that from 220 to give an approximate training pulse rate. For a 25 year old this would be 170.

Many dancers of all ages train to specified heart rates, which they measure with a heart-telemeter watch. This is a small elastic strap around the chest, picking up the heart rate and transmitting it to a wrist-receiver, which may be programmed to give a signal if the heart rate is too high or too low for the training effect. In general, when training for aerobic fitness and endurance, the tempo does not have to be maximum for a maximum training effect. The dancer does not have to be exhausted at the end of such a session. Serious competition runners try to work as near the 'anaerobic threshold' as possible, without going over it, and here they need the services of a laboratory to inform them at what heart rate they can expect to enter their threshold area. But for most other sports and activities, such as dance, such high precision is not necessary.

A harder question to answer for most dancers, as for most competitors in the non-track sports—such as gymnastics and judo—is what is the best form of training? Running itself is an excellent aerobic exercise, as are various forms of gym- or studio-based 'aerobics', provided the standard is high enough. With running, it is important to wear a good pair of trainers, to start gradually and work up to between 20 and 30 minutes, and to run on an even surface, preferably a good stretch of firm grass. Hills are useful, but run down them gently, or you may find yourself inordinately stiff two days later.

It is worth getting to know a route, timing yourself over it regularly and recording your time, which should gradually get less as the months go by. Very roughly, one run (or other exercise) session per week will maintain a fitness level which it has taken three (or perhaps two) weekly runs or sessions to attain.

If space or time are at a premium, skipping can form an excellent aerobic training mode. It must be done on a cushioned surface, such as carpet, with alternate leg skips at a rate of about 1000 skips in eight minutes, that is 120/minute. In the first week or two it is best to stick to one set of 1000. Then do two or three weeks of two sets. And then on to three sets of 1000, which is an ample aerobic stimulus. If the rate is slightly too high, drop it. And if it is too low, increase the rate. But keep the times constant at sets of eight minutes.

Similarly, exercise cycles can be useful, especially to mix in with other activities. For example, one session of cycling, one of skipping and one of running would make a good mix, fitting into the modern vogue for 'cross-training'. You should treat the exercise cycle like the run, in terms of duration, although the heart rate should be 5 to 10 beats higher on the cycle. Galanti *et al.* (1993), working with jazz dancers, noted improvements in aerobic fitness with routines whose intensity was pitched at an optimal level to provide a genuine training stimulus. Similar results were obtained from a preliminary set of data where appropriate extra-curricular exercises increased aerobic fitness in female ballet students (Dowson, Evans, Randolph *et al.* 1997).

3 ANAEROBIC FITNESS

3.1 Introduction and Definition

Just as 'aerobic', meaning 'with air', is taken to mean 'with oxygen', so 'anaerobic' means 'without air', namely 'without oxygen'. *Anaerobic fitness* is *the ability to produce an appropriate energy supply, which does not require oxygen, for muscle contraction processes.*

In dance, as in other activities, there are two main anaerobic requirements. One is when a very large surge of power is required, as in the act of a lift or in grand allegro, both lasting from one to a few seconds. The need here is for sheer power, for which the energy source happens to be anaerobic, mainly from *phosphocreatine*. The other prime anaerobic situation is when a high power output must be sustained, as when holding a partner in a lift, or in a series of adagios, or in an acrobatic jazz or modern sequence, all lasting up to around 30–60 seconds, and energized primarily by *glycolysis* (more information about phosphocreatine and glycolysis in Part I, Chapter 1). The need in the former would be termed *anaerobic power*, and in the latter would be termed *anaerobic endurance* which, in turn, may be seen as the opposite to *muscular fatigue*.

Anaerobic endurance should be differentiated from aerobic endurance, as the former refers to a much higher order (or rate) of work than that achieved during aerobic conditions. Anaerobic endurance may also have a 'local' nature, hence, the term *local muscular endurance* is very often used. Indeed, through long specialized practice, it is possible to develop considerable local endurance in selected muscle groups (e.g. the finger flexors used by guitarists, or the gastrocnemius—calf—muscle used by dancers), without causing any noticeable training effect on the cardio-respiratory system. In general, and in a somewhat imprecise way, anaerobic fitness describes a type of physical fitness lying in the centre of a continuum between aerobic fitness and muscle strength.

3.2   Measurement of Anaerobic Fitness

Anaerobic fitness is notoriously hard to measure, mainly because of the difficulty in knowing when to stop the test. Phosphocreatine is quickly exhausted in a few seconds, but the contribution from glycolysis falls off gradually. After about 30 seconds of maximal work, aerobic energy may be accounting for between 10 and even 25% or more of the energy, and this proportion continues to increase (and the work output continues to fall) the longer the test continues. There is no sudden end point when the physiologist can say 'that is the end of the anaerobic energy supply'. And it is almost equally difficult to separate phosphocreatine energy from glycolysis energy. Furthermore, measurement of anaerobic fitness is less reproducible than aerobic fitness and strength, probably because of variability in motivation for maintaining maximal (and often painful) muscle contractions. Nevertheless, there are some useful tests of anaerobic power and endurance. Remember that it is phosphocreatine which produces the fairly instantaneous high peak of anaerobic power, and glycolysis which fuels anaerobic endurance for half to one minute of intensive physical effort. Therefore, anaerobic tests tend to be described as power tests and endurance tests.

ANAEROBIC POWER TESTS

The Margaria Stair-Test. This test was one of the first in the field, developed by the Italian Margaria and his colleagues (1966). For the purpose of the test, the subjects accelerate over 2 m towards a staircase, and run up the stairs two at a time to a height of about 1.75 m. Timing mats or photocells time their rate of ascent, and the subjects are weighed. The results are then fitted into the formula:

$$\text{Power (in Watts)} = \frac{\text{Body weight (kg)} \times \text{Height ascended (m)}}{\text{Time (seconds)}} \times 9.8$$

To give an example, for a dancer of 70 kg in body weight, a stair height of 1.75 m and a 'running-up' time of 1.5 seconds, the power generated would be:

$$\text{Power} = \frac{70 \text{ (kg)} \times 1.75 \text{ (m)}}{1.5 \text{ (seconds)}} \times 9.8 = \frac{1200}{1.5} = 800 \text{ Watts}$$

The Sergent Jump Test. Another test of anaerobic (peak) power is the vertical jump test, often called after Sergent who developed it. The test is to stand sideways on to a wall or mounted blackboard, and to reach up as high as possible with heels on the ground to make a mark, with a chalked or licked finger. Then to crouch down and jump up to make another mark on the wall as high as possible, with three attempts. The best difference between the two marks gives the height jumped, and this in itself is used as the test result. But better information is gained by using the body weight in the following formula, whereby the anaerobic power can be calculated:

$$\text{Power (Watts)} = 21.67 \times \text{Body weight (kg)} \times \text{Height jumped (m}^{0.5})$$

The $m^{0.5}$ refers to the square root of the height jumped in metres. That is, 65 centimetres, for example, must be expressed as 0.65 metres, and the square root of 0.65 can easily be found from the calculator. Therefore, using the above formula, what is the power of a dancer weighing 75 kg, whose best height between his two marks is 65 centimetres (26 in.)?

$$P = 21.67 \times 75 \times \text{square root of } 0.65 = 21.67 \times 75 \times 0.806 = 1310 \text{ Watts}$$

ANAEROBIC POWER AND ENDURANCE TEST

The Wingate Test. This is a more sophisticated test than those described above, in which both anaerobic power and anaerobic endurance can be assessed. It is known as the *Wingate* test after the Israeli institute where it was developed (Bar-Or 1987). This consists, for a dancer, of sitting on a laboratory cycle ergometer, being suitably warmed-up and strapped on, and pedalling as hard as possible for up to 30 seconds against a resistance that is proportional to body weight. A specially mounted sensor records the speed of the flywheel, and the computer is programmed with the load. The result is a printout which shows the power in Watts rising over the first 4–10 seconds, then gradually falling until the end of the 30 seconds (Fig. 5.3). For male ballet dancers, one might make a case for

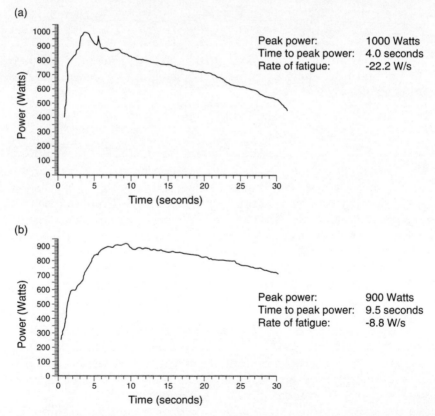

Fig. 5.3 Typical curves obtained from two separate 30-second Wingate Anaerobic Tests. These curves belong to two professional male dancers, principally involved in 'modern' productions. Note that dancer (a) achieved higher peak power and in less time than his colleague (b)

their doing an 'arm-based' Wingate test, to measure upper body peak power and anaerobic endurance in terms of lifting and holding a partner, as is done with the ice-skaters and ice-dancers.

The *peak power* in the first few seconds is reasonably representative of phosphocreatine energy, and the average power over the full 30 seconds gives a reasonable measure of anaerobic endurance. The latter is often expressed as a rate of power decline per second, also known as *rate of fatigue*. A decline of only 10 Watts per second is extremely good; 15 still very good, 20 fair and over 25 indicates that anaerobic endurance is not very good.

In general, variations between individual dancers may be reflected by different shaped power curves. Individuals with high peak power outputs soon lose their ability to work at relatively high levels, which is then demonstrated by a noticeable drop in performance (Fig. 5.3a). These individuals are better suited for just a few very intense physical efforts of an 'explosive' nature. In contrast, dancers with lower peak power outputs often show good anaerobic endurance as they are able to maintain relatively high outputs for longer periods of time (Fig. 5.3b). Such dancers are better equipped to perform repetitive muscle contractions at reasonably high intensities.

Often, a *recovery index* is also obtained from, for example, two successive 15- or 30-second tests, four minutes apart, with the total work of the second test being expressed as a percentage of that of the initial test. Top-class squash players and footballers perform more than 95% as well on the second test, while dancers have shown values ranging from 65 to 80% (Koutedakis and Sharp, unpublished data).

Very few reports have been published in which anaerobic tests, such as the Wingate test, have been applied to dancers. Table 5.3 displays peak power and mean or average power from the limited data on dancers and from some British elite rowers and gymnasts by way of comparison. Peak power is self-explanatory, and mean power relates to anaerobic endurance being the average power sustained over the duration of the test.

From Table 5.3 it can be seen that the dancers show lower peak and mean power outputs than the athletes, although in fairness the rowers are considerably heavier, as well as very highly trained, as are the gymnasts. Within the dance group, the contemporary men and women dancers show higher anaerobic values than their ballet colleagues, as was also shown above regarding aerobic fitness. A significant number of contemporary dancers have an athletic background (e.g. in gymnastics, diving or athletics), which may explain this difference.

The values which correspond to the British dance students (Table 5.3) are slightly lower than the equivalent reported from USA (Rimmer, Jay and Plowman 1994). These authors found peak power to be 725 and

Table 5.3 Average values for peak power (PP), mean power (MP) obtained from British elite sports men and women and dancers

Activity	Sex	PP (Watts)	MP (Watts)
Rowing	Males	1140	880
Rowing	Females	690	595
Gymnastics	Males	790	690
Gymnastics	Females	580	500
Dance (contemporary)	Males	740	580
Dance (contemporary)	Females	465	359
Dance (ballet)	Males	680	580
Dance (ballet)	Females	410	329
Dance (students)	Males	650	510
Dance (students)	Females	477	374

Source: From Brinson and Dick (1996)

503 W respectively in men and women (compared to British 650 and 477), with mean power outputs of 568 and 372 W respectively (compared to British 510 and 374). This difference may be due to the fact that the British students were, on average, 5 years younger than their American counterparts.

ANAEROBIC ENDURANCE TESTS

Lactic Acid Measurements. A major consequence of anaerobic work lasting longer than a few seconds, involving glycolysis, is the build-up of the glycolysis end product pyruvic acid, in quantities too great to be released down through Krebs cycle. Under this circumstance, the pyruvic acid is transformed to lactic acid, and lactic acid dissociates into a proton [H$^+$] and lactate. It is this proton which ultimately interferes with the muscle's metabolism and contraction. Thus, anaerobic performance, expressed as fatigue resistance during maximal muscular effort, mainly depends on the degree of lactic acid buffering and dispersal. Lactic acid may ultimately increase to levels too unfavourable for glycolysis to continue.

In athletes and dancers, lactic acid is measured from a fingertip or ear-lobe needle-prick blood sample. Again, there is little information available on lactic acid levels in dance and dancers. For instance, Rimmer, Jay and Plowman (1994) noted that dancers do achieve a moderate anaerobic training effect in the classical discipline. In 1984, Schantz and Åstrand (the latter the doyenne of all exercise physiologists) found that a normal ballet class elicited a mean lactic acid blood level of 3 mM/litre in women, while a choreographed solo part raised this to 10 mM. This latter value is as high as top-class squash and hockey players achieve, and many professional footballers and rugby players. It also provides further evidence that dance should be regarded more in the light of a multiple-sprint sport than an aerobic activity—perhaps it is more like basketball or volleyball, with a touch of gymnastics.

It has also been found that professional female ballet dancers have shown lower levels of lactic acid, 4 minutes after finishing a Wingate test, than professional contemporary dancers or dance students (Chmelar, Schultz, Ruhling *et al.* 1988; Dahlström, Inasio, Jansson and Kaijser 1996). This may, partly, be explained by the fact that (1) slow fibres are far more aerobic than their fast equivalents, which is why lactic acid levels are in general inversely related to the percentage of slow (aerobic) fibres in the working muscles, and (2) Dahlström and colleagues (1997) reported a high proportion of such slow fibres in ballet dancers of both genders.

A widely held belief among athletes as well as dancers is that high levels of lactic acid lead to muscular soreness and stiffness. However, these muscle complaints are related far more to the type of exercise than to lactate levels. For example, eccentric muscle work, where a muscle is lengthened as its tension increases (as in jumps, rebounds, and downhill running) is strongly associated with delayed-onset muscle soreness, that is coming one or two days later. The two current authors noted that lactic acid is over 50% back to resting levels about 30 minutes after the end of about 8 minutes of very strenuous exercise, and back to the normal resting value about an hour afterwards, especially if the exercise is followed by about the same length of 'active' cool-down (Koutedakis and Sharp 1985). We tended to find that to maximize the rate of removal of lactic acid, runners should continue at about 65% of their training rate, canoeists should paddle at about 60% of theirs, with cyclists at about 50% and rowers nearer 40%. One might deduce that dancers should continue at around 55–60% of the rate of work that generated the lactic acid in the first place. The object of all this is to prevent lactic acid from being sequestered in the muscle, so that it is released into the bloodstream for buffering, dispersal and disposal.

3.3 Factors Affecting Anaerobic Fitness

In the energy section in Part I, the main energy sources were described, including the two anaerobic sources, *phosphocreatine* and *glycolysis*. There are two main situations when muscle turns to anaerobic sources of energy. First is at the start of exercise—as at the very start of a class. The first 20 seconds or so of work are anaerobic even if the exercise is fairly light, simply because there is a lag in the aerobic system (a lag before the stimulus gets through to heart and lungs and circulation to indicate that exercise has begun). This induces an 'oxygen deficit', which if it is fairly large (if the exercise level is moderately hard) will induce a feeling of 'second wind' when it is repaid. Thus the start of any exercise involves a brief flurry of anaerobic work creating an oxygen deficit, unnoticed if the exercise is light, but felt with relief as a second wind if the exercise is moderate in intensity. However, if the energy demand is both rapid and high, then it should be made quite clear that the reason muscle turns to its anaerobic sources of energy is nothing at all to do with a lack of oxygen. Instead, it arises from the need to generate far more energy than the aerobic system can possibly supply, no matter how much oxygen is delivered. In general, it is phosphocreatine that powers the act of lifting or grand allegro; glycolysis that powers holding the partner in a lift, or adagios, or an up-tempo jazz sequence. And it is Krebs aerobic cycle that powers the corps de ballet in Giselle, or dancers in an old-fashioned waltz or a polka.

3.4   Training for Anaerobic Fitness

Because of the nature of dance training, the *phosphocreatine* system tends to be reasonably trained in centre-class work as well as in rehearsal and performance. The *glycolysis* system also tends to be reasonably trained— as exemplified by the lactic acid levels of 10 mM already referred to. However, this is not always possible due to various facts of life. For example, the time lead-up to performance is often very short, with the dancer not only having to learn the new choreography, but also having to try to get fit in a very few rehearsals. This is less apparent in student or company dancers who may not need to seek additional employment, and who have access to more classes. But independent dancers, who do not benefit from regular free classes, and may need to do other work, may struggle to maintain fitness, especially anaerobic. For them, it may be even more important to undertake regular fitness training, which may then allow them to concentrate more on the choreography, and, hope-fully, suffer less injury (Wyon, personal communication).

   Anaerobic fitness is ideally gained by the interval mode of training, which for dance would take the form of fast shuttle runs or moves or step sequences on a sprung floor in an area roughly 10 × 6 metres (30 in. × 20 in.). More specifically, for *phosphocreatine* training, the work rate should be maximal, but the work periods very short, say 5–7 seconds, with 45–60 seconds actively-moving rest. Six repetitions (reps) of this should form a set, working up to a volume of three sets, with a 5–10 minute active rest (jog, etc.) between sets. This should be done three or four times per week, say for four to six weeks, and it should always be done both when the dancer is fresh, to get the best quality work, and when thoroughly warmed-up, to minimize any risk of injury.

The aim here is to stress a pathway which is not associated with fatigue, so dancers should not worry in the least if they do not feel tired after each set. Feeling tired here is not the object, but performing high-quality work is. This type of regimen should make an appreciable difference to anaerobic peak power.

Glycolysis training is similar in outline, but otherwise markedly different—the object here is indeed to feel exhausted, so this training mode should be done at the end of the working day, and probably two to three times a week but not on consecutive days. The work should be done at around 85–90% of maximum effort, initially for periods of up to 30 seconds, with one minute's (active) rest, and perhaps six repetitions of this in a set. After about two weeks of this 30:60 ratio, the rest intervals should be brought down to 30 seconds, giving 30:30 work to rest ratio, and the number of reps should then gradually be increased up to 10, and kept to a single set.

Other modes of glycolysis work could involve skipping—but much faster than the aerobic skipping mentioned previously. Anaerobic skipping should be done, with alternate feet, at a rate of about 180 skips per minute, for 30 seconds, with two minutes of walking/jogging/slow running in between each rep. And working up to 10 reps in a set, with just one set.

Even step-ups can be pressed into service for anaerobic fitness, at a rate of 60 steps/minute onto a step of reasonable height to allow such a pace, with five reps of this in a set, and two minutes jog/walk between reps. If this goes well, then a second set may be added in a couple of weeks later, with a 10-minute jog/walk between the two sets, but do work up gradually. Again, four to six weeks of one or a mix of these training modes should make a substantial difference to anaerobic endurance and recovery. It is worth repeating that these regimens are very exhausting, and should end the day's physical work. They should generate the synthesis in muscle of more of the enzymes which promote glycolysis, and they should also increase the rate at which lactic acid is buffered and removed. Thus they should increase anaerobic endurance in terms of higher sustained power output, without increasing fatigue (i.e. fatigue will feel much the same—but after having completed more work!).

In all the above training, the one factor always to remember is that exercises should be varied and moved around according to work, illness, aches and pains. A good schedule should be capable of being accommodated into one's living/working pattern, and of accommodating that pattern in turn.

4   MUSCULAR STRENGTH (AND POWER)

4.1   Introduction and Definition

Although many books and research articles have been published on muscular strength and power, very little exists that is directly relevant to dance and dancers. This partly reflects the scientifically unfounded fear, still alive and kicking amongst dancers (!), that strength and strength training would destroy their artistic prospects and would drag them away from the aesthetic standards of the profession.

There are no published reports which support such 'fears'. In contrast, the introduction of strength training for male and female dancers may, among other benefits, reduce injuries and improve balance between antagonistic muscles. Additionally, questions often debated, such as 'when should a young dancer attempt pointe', may become less subject to a teacher's intuition or parental pressure, if knowledge on the muscle strength and ability of the ligaments to sustain the load of the whole body is available before the technique is attempted (Micheli, Gillespie and Walaszek 1984). To obtain these benefits, however, an educational programme to dispense with the myths is required.

Strength is the ability to overcome external resistance, or to counter external forces, by using muscle. This is the result of the unique characteristic of the muscle cell, whereby it can convert the chemical energy of ATP into mechanical work. Therefore, *muscle strength* can be simply defined as *the maximum force that can be exerted in a single voluntary contraction*. In real life, however, matters are slightly more complex than that as muscle can perform maximal efforts during different actions (i.e. isometric, concentric, or eccentric) at a wide range of speeds. Thus, in order to successfully compare different sets of strength data, we must ensure that they have been obtained under similar conditions. *Maximal strength, speed-strength* and *strength-endurance* are the most common categories of strength.

In this section, we will attempt to introduce the concept of strength and of strength training to dancers. Where possible, the limited data on dance will be used to support the claim that an optimal muscular strength is necessary for successful dance careers. No mention will be made of the various body-conditioning techniques currently in use by the dance world, given that—although they command a strong, cult-type following—they are not adequately supported by scientific findings.

4.2 Measurement of Strength

Strain gauges and computerized equipment with accommodating speed and resistance facilities (i.e. *isokinetic machines*, Fig. 5.4) have been extensively used to obtain data regarding the tension developed by various muscle groups in males and females. Thus, isokinetic assessments on runners have revealed, not surprisingly, that elite sprinters are stronger than their long-distance counterparts. Male long-distance runners may demonstrate peak muscle strength (or *torque*) of around 220 and 120 Newton-metres (N.m) for quadriceps and hamstrings respectively. The equivalent values for female distance runners are approximately 160 and 85 N.m. On the other hand, male and female sprinters demonstrate

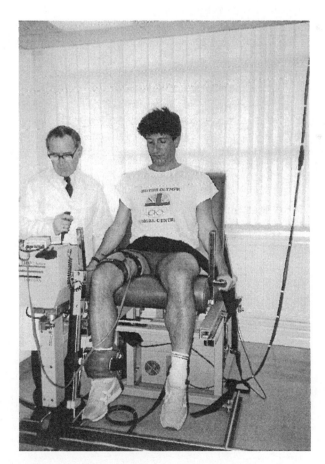

Fig. 5.4 Leg-strength assessment on an isokinetic machine

values in excess of 330 and 220 N.m for their quadriceps, and 160 and 110 N.m for their hamstrings respectively (Table 5.4).

Dancers generally show lower strength values than athletes (Kirkendall and Calabrese 1983). Within the danceworld, contemporary male and female dancers are stronger than their counterparts in ballet, and in many cases contemporary dancers can easily compare in strength with some athletes. Ballerinas appear to have the least muscular strength. They normally demonstrate only 77% of the weight-predicted strength-norms (Reid 1988). It is worth stressing here that, unlike most professional ballet dancers, individuals involved in other forms of dance often have a multidisciplinary background (e.g. former gymnasts, divers, etc.) which may explain certain elements of 'athleticism'. However, regardless of the training and background, male dancers should always demonstrate significantly greater strength compared to their female colleagues (Westblad, Tsai-Fellander and Johansson 1995).

Dance-related adaptive changes can be seen in muscle strength measurements of various muscle groups, such as the spine muscles of Flamenco dancers, while information on possible muscle imbalances is extremely useful for both dancers and their teachers. Furthermore, and contrary to the common belief that one side of the body is stronger than the other, strength measurements in male and female dancers revealed no differences between left and right legs (Westblad, Tsai-Fellander and Johansson 1995). In a recent study, designed to test whether different

Table 5.4 Typical peak strength values for the muscles involved in knee extension (i.e. quadriceps) and knee flexion (i.e. hamstrings) in athletes and dancers[a,b]

Activity	Sex	Knee extension (N.m)	Knee flexion (N.m)
Rowers	Males	350	165
Rowers	Females	212	89
Sprinters	Males	330	220
Sprinters	Females	160	110
Squash	Males	280	136
Squash	Females	168	79
Runners (long-distance)	Males	220	120
Runners (long-distance)	Females	160	85
Dancers (contemporary)	Males	196	94
Dancers (contemporary)	Females	133	68
Dancers (ballet)	Males	181	89
Dancers (ballet)	Females	118	59

[a] All data collected using isokinetic dynamometers in the concentric mode and at the angular velocity of 60 deg/sec
[b] Data from Brinson and Dick (1996); Koutedakis (1994)

modes of activity and forms of preparation affect certain basic strength and muscle contractile characteristics, no statistical differences were found between professional dancers, Olympic bob-sleighers, Olympic rowers and non-athletes (Table 5.5). This indicates that, at the muscle level, there are no obvious functional differences in individuals partici-pating in different physical activities.

Not only sophisticated and hi-tech equipment is valid for muscular strength measurements. Simple mechanical *dynamometers*, such as the handgrip dynamometer (Fig. 5.5), are equally useful. It has been estab-lished, for example, that handgrip strength is a reasonably valid indicator of the strength status of almost the entire body musculature; high levels of handgrip strength are normally accompanied with equally high strengths of different muscle groups such as back and thigh. Low purchase cost, easy use and storage, and speed of data collection are recognized advantages supporting the use of simple mechanical dynam-ometers.

Table 5.5 Averages for the combined left and right leg peak strength (expressed in N.m per kg body weight) for quadriceps and hamstrings, at three different speeds (angular velocities). Note that as the speed increases, there is a propor-tional decrease in muscle performance in all subjects (i.e. professional dancers, Olympic bob-sleighers, Olympic rowers and non-athletes). No statistical differ-ences were found

Angular velocity	Muscle group	Professional dancers ($n = 20$)	Olympic bob-sleighers ($n = 11$)	Olympic rowers ($n = 14$)	Non-athletes ($n = 10$)
1.04 (rad/sec)	Quadriceps (N.m/kg)	3.2	3.2	3.1	2.9
	Hamstrings (N.m/kg)	1.6	1.8	2.0	1.4
3.14 (rad/sec)	Quadriceps (N.m/kg)	2.1	2.5	2.2	2.1
	Hamstrings (N.m/kg)	1.3	1.6	1.4	1.2
4.19 (rad/sec)	Quadriceps (N.m/kg)	1.8	2.1	2.0	1.8
	Hamstrings (N.m/kg)	1.2	1.6	1.4	1.3

Source: Data from Koutedakis, Agrawal and Sharp (1998)

FACTORS AFFECTING MUSCULAR STRENGTH

Mechanical (e.g. lever length, inertia, momentum) factors as well as age, gender, fatigue, motivation, and drugs can influence strength. However,

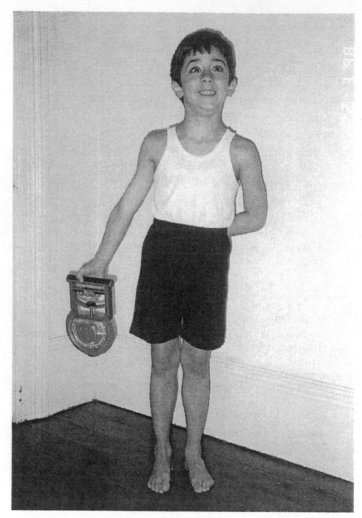

Fig. 5.5   Handgrip strength measurement in a child

those that principally affect strength levels are *peripheral* (i.e. muscular) or *central* (i.e. nervous system) in nature, *with type of muscle contraction, muscle area, muscle fibre profile*, and *muscle co-ordination* being among the most common factors.

- The *type of muscle contraction* can affect strength outputs of the same muscle. For instance, *eccentric* action of quadriceps muscle gives on average 20–30% higher values compared to its *concentric* contractions.

It is therefore easier to go down the stairs than to climb up, as the eccentric action of the muscles during the former case requires 20–30% less effort.

- *Muscle area* is often associated with *hypertrophy* (as the enlargement of muscle is called). Enlargement of muscle means greater fibre diameters and, thus, higher potentials for increased maximal strength values. However, as will be discussed in the following sections, hypertrophy is not a necessary consequence of augmenting strength, which may be seen as an advantage by many dancers.
- Fibre type ratio can also affect muscular strength, and as discussed earlier in Part II, the dancers' *muscle fibre profile* is genetically determined. However, it should be remembered that muscular strength depends on the fibres' diameter, not the fibre type. Since slow (or type I) fibres tend to have smaller diameters than fast (or type II) fibres, dancers with high percentages of slow fibres produce lower strength values and also demonstrate smaller muscle bulk.
- *Muscle co-ordination (or synchronization)* has an increased central (i.e. neural) element and is often regarded as synonymous with technique and skill during the execution of a movement. It can positively affect levels of muscle strength by controlling the recruitment of the right number of muscle fibres at the right time. The contribution of this factor is particularly important in the early stages of a strength-training programme, and it will be further discussed in the following sections.

4.3 Strength, Strength Training and Dance

Although strength training and its effects were known in classical Greece, the 'know-how' was sadly lost after the last Ancient Olympic Games in 393 BC. For many centuries, people forgot its significance for both health and physical performance, although some primitive forms of strength training were sporadically used for military purposes. During the last 60 years, strength training has been reintroduced as a significant form of exercise, as scientific information on the development of effective programmes for all has become available. In fact, the American association for the prevention of heart-related diseases suggests strength training even for cardiac patients. In general, the main objectives of any strength-training programme include:

- Facilitation of neural pathways
- Increasing muscle fibre recruitment

- Increasing synchrony of motor units during contraction
- Switching on and/or accelerating muscle–protein synthesis

Strength has not generally been considered as a necessary ingredient for success in dance. This is partly because of the widely accepted myth that increased muscle strength is associated with large increases in muscle size, an unwelcome feature for many male and particularly female dancers. The fact that marked improvements in muscle strength can occur without corresponding changes in muscle size is a relatively unknown concept within the profession.

Another myth is that strength and strength training will destroy flexibility, an anathema to dancers and their teachers. Again, there is little scientific evidence to substantiate such claims. If such incidents did ever happen, they were probably the result of incompetent training design, rather than the effect of strength increases. Both strength and flexibility should be regarded as of equal importance since a flexible body without strength is a useless dance instrument, whereas a strong body without flexibility can limit dance performance. But, *does dance alone promote strength enhancements?*

DOES DANCE ALONE PROMOTE STRENGTH ENHANCEMENTS?

This question was recently investigated by examining the effects of a 3-month supplemental strength-training programme on handgrip and upper-body strength in 15 professional male ballet dancers (Koutedakis, Cross and Sharp 1996).

For the purpose of this study, the volunteers were randomly separated into experimental and control groups. The latter group was involved in no extra exercise apart from dance. At the end of the training programme, the experimental group demonstrated a significantly lower percentage of body fat, and significant increases in grip strength, elbow flexion and extension strength, and in maximal 'bench-press' exercise. All these increases were similar at approximately 15%. No significant changes were found in the control subjects. It was argued that ballet exercises alone confer no strength benefits on relatively active individuals, while weak dancers are more likely to benefit from strength-training programmes than their stronger counterparts. These findings also support previous research on male and female dancers (Groer and Fallon 1993; Stalder, Noble and Wilkinson 1990), in which supplementary strength training contributed to improvements in leg strength, endurance and speed, without interfering with the dancers' artistic qualities. However, the main benefit of such research projects is that they dispel myths associated with strength and strength training.

4.4   Adaptations to Strength Training

For optimal results, training and exercise must be specific to the desired outcome, since the body can be subjected to large variations in exercise intensity and duration. Thus, at one extreme, resistance (or strength) training can involve very heavy weights with minimal repetitions in relatively short periods of time. At the other extreme, light weights can be lifted in sets of many repetitions during prolonged sessions. However, such variations dictate which type of muscle fibre will be recruited and, therefore, the expected adaptations. In general, the possible adaptations to strength training can be neural, muscular and/or metabolic.

NEURAL

Strength levels may increase by up to 50% without the presence of any muscular size changes (i.e. *hypertrophy*). Many researchers believe that an elevated neural involvement may account for some of the exercise-induced changes in muscular strength (Ploutz, Tesch, Biro and Dudley 1994), suggesting that, at least in the early stages of such training, hypertrophy is not a prerequisite for strength gains. This elevated neural involvement is necessary for the body to ensure that optimal muscle fibre recruitment can take place, or that most of the motor units can be effectively mobilized. As a result, strength can increase without concomitant changes in muscle shape.

Neural adaptations have been frequently invoked to explain increases in strength in novices, or in individuals participating in strength and power sports (e.g. Olympic weightlifting), associated with little or no change in muscle fibre size. The combination of high intensities ($> 70\%$ of maximal) and low volumes of work, two to three times a week for six to eight consecutive weeks, is the suggested way to achieve this adaptation. The number of sets should not be greater than 5–8 per muscle group with a full recovery period (5–6 minutes) between each set. After that, dancers may be able to maintain a satisfactory level of muscular strength by introducing just one strength session per week. However, as training proceeds and work volumes increase, hypertrophy of the exercised muscles does play a more dominant role.

MUSCULAR

Strength gains are related to muscle *hypertrophy* following intensive strength training for about three months, accompanied by an adequate protein diet. Hypertrophy mainly occurs as a result of an increase in fibre size, but may also be due to an increase in connective tissue around the muscle fibres and in the capillary blood vessels, and arguably to a small increase in fibre number. Indeed, synthesis of actin, myosin and other proteins is a response to resistance training, particularly in fast (type II) fibres, although slow (type I) fibres do have the capability to hypertrophy with such training.

Maximal *eccentric* (muscle lengthening) actions produce greater hypertrophy than exercise consisting mainly of *concentric* (shortening) contractions. It is thought that the higher forces experienced during eccentric exercises may provide greater physiological training stimuli. This may be of great practical value in dance since a large number of routines (e.g. jumping, pirouettes) have the element of eccentric muscular action and, therefore, are likely to induce muscular hypertrophy, particularly in the legs.

Although not directly relevant to dance, it may be worth knowing that strength-training programmes could also lead to improvement in the endurance of fast muscle in both men and women (Kraemer, Palton, Gordon *et al*. 1995). However, while transformation within the fast muscle fibre subtypes may occur with training, no transformations between slow and fast fibres have been reported yet as a consequence of strength exercise.

Should a dancer wish to increase muscle size, then the combination of moderate intensities (about 60–70% of maximum) and high volumes of work, three to four times a week for more than eight consecutive weeks, is the suggested way. Using lighter loads allows the dancer to perform more repetitions than is typical of a programme for pure strength, but they should be heavy enough for about 10–15 repetitions. Usually, the number of *training sets* is not greater than 10. However, it is not uncommon for some athletes (e.g. body builders) to perform more than 20 successive sets that focus on one muscle group during a single training session. The rest period is of short to moderate duration (2–4 minutes), since it is important to begin the next set of exercises before full recovery has been accomplished.

METABOLIC (OXIDATIVE)

Strength training may also promote adaptations related to aerobic function at fibre level. Favourable changes may include:

- Increased capillary density
- Raised percentage of the more aerobic type IIa fibres
- Increased levels of aerobic enzymes
- Elevated muscle glycogen stores

Ironically, most of these changes are related to production and removal of lactic acid from the working muscles. For example, strength training of moderate intensity (e.g. 60–70% of maximum), high volumes (i.e. many sets) and short rests (i.e. < 1 minute between sets) normally result in high lactate concentrations, with consequent increased capillary number which facilitates blood perfusion and lactate removal. In general, high-repitition lower load weight training protocols are thought to be more appropriate for such changes (Kraemer, Fleck and Evens 1996).

4.5   Strength Levels and Injuries in Dancers

Until recently, dancers have not received the same medical attention as sport competitors, as it has been assumed that dancers' movements are not capable of generating sufficient power to cause the muscular injuries seen in sport. However, dancers do get injured and the effects of these injuries, on both their health and career, may be detrimental. Overwork, unsuitable floors, difficult choreography, and insufficient warm-up are among the factors that may contribute to such injuries (Sohl and Bowling 1990). Also, the young age at which serious dance training begins, the long and rigorous hours of practice, the thin ballet slipper, dancing en pointe and unusual dietary regimens may further contribute to injury patterns in varying degrees. But what about fitness, and more specifically, what about muscle strength levels in relation to incidence of injury in dancers?

LOWER-EXTREMITY INJURIES

A recent study investigated whether dancers with lower muscle strength demonstrate worse lower-extremity injuries than their stronger counterparts (Koutedakis, Khalouha, Pacy *et al.* 1997b).

Fig. 5.6 shows the relationships between days off dance due to lower-body (i.e. pelvis, legs, knees, and feet) injuries, and the sum of knee flexors and extensors peak strength outputs. The general trend would appear to be that the lower the thigh strength, the greater the degree of injury in both male and female dancers.

Fig. 5.6 also shows that the female dancers were both relatively weaker and showed more severe injuries than their male counterparts. It was suggested that the introduction of supplementary strength training might circumvent such problems and provide a relatively cost-effective way of reducing injuries in dancers. Indeed, it has been previously discussed that strength training is more beneficial to weaker dancers than to their stronger colleagues (Koutedakis, Pacy, Sharp and Dick 1996; Stalder,

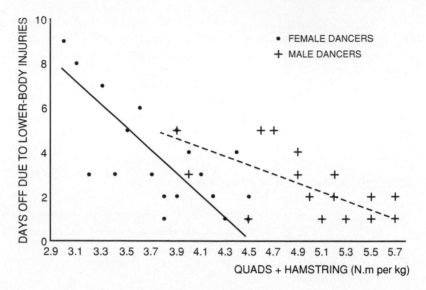

Fig. 5.6 Relationships between days off dance due to lower-body injuries, and the thigh strength (i.e. the sum of quadriceps and hamstring peak strength expressed in N.m per kg body weight) in male and female dancers. The lower the quadriceps and hamstring strength, the more likely it is for dancers to stay off action for a while due to a lower-body injury
Source: Modified from Koutedakis, Khalouha, Pacy *et al.* Thigh peak torques and lower body injuries in dancers. JDance Med Sci 1(1): 12–15. Reproduced with permission of J. Michael Ryan Publishing, Inc. (1997b)

Noble and Wilkinson 1990), and that such an activity does not interfere with the dancers' artistic and physical performance attributes.

Lower-Back Injuries

Lower-back injuries are frequent in both athletes and dancers. Factors which are thought to be linked to the genesis of lower-back problems include weak abdominal muscles, reduced range of movement in various joints, disc degeneration, inadequate lumbar flexibility, and short hamstrings. Although often overlooked, another factor associated with injuries in active individuals, including dancers, is the simultaneous presence of strong and weak muscles, especially antagonistic muscles in the same limb (Bejjani 1987).

Hamstring muscles are the antagonists of the quadriceps that extend the knee. Quadriceps and hamstrings, however, are not only knee extensors and flexors; they also act as hip flexors and extensors respectively, and play a major role in the development of an optimal lumbopelvic rhythm. Muscle imbalance may impair this mechanism, leading to increased local and general spine stresses, and thus to irritation and pain.

This was indeed the main finding of a study, the results of which appear in Fig. 5.7. It was shown that the smaller the ratio between hamstrings and quadriceps (knee Fl/Ext_{rat})—or the weaker the hamstrings compared to the quadriceps—the worse the degree of injury. It is interesting to note that similar patterns in lower-back injuries were found in both rowers and dancers. This is despite the fact that dancers and rowers are involved in very different activities, with different objectives and aspirations.

From the above it becomes clear that a safe and long-term solution to the increasingly frequent problem of lower-back pain is to undergo a strength-training programme aiming at restoring the balance between hamstring and quadriceps muscles. This was confirmed by the same study (Koutedakis, Frischnecht and Murphy 1997) where some of the subjects were retested after a 2-month period, during which a specific hamstring strength training had been introduced. The retest revealed that the knee flexion-to-extension ratio was higher (due to increased hamstring strength), whereas there were fewer days off activity due to lower-back pain.

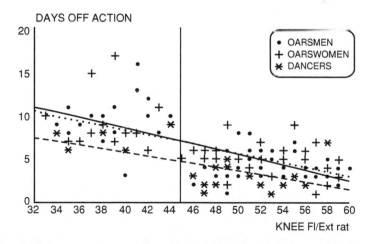

Fig. 5.7 Trends between days off serious physical activity (due to lower-back injuries) and balance between quadriceps and hamstring strength. The smaller the ratio between hamstrings and quadriceps (knee Fl/Ext_{rat})—or the weaker the hamstrings compared to the quadriceps—the worse the degree of injury in both dancers and rowers
Source: From Koutedakis, Frischnecht and Murphy Vol 18, International Journal of Sports Medicine (1997). Reproduced by permission of Georg Thieme Verlag

4.6   Power

Muscle power is simply the explosive aspect of strength (often called 'fast strength'). It is the functional application of both speed and strength, and is a key component in many human movements. Indeed, dance routines—where jumping is required—can only be performed successfully if dancers have sufficiently high levels of muscular power. However, as in the cases of aerobic and anaerobic fitness and strength, power is not likely to improve beyond certain levels by using conventional dance exercises alone (Rimmer, Jay and Plowman 1994), although both explosive strength and mechanical power in leg muscles have been found to be good in dance (ballet)-trained boys (Pekkarinen, Litmanen and Mahlamaki 1989).

Although the term 'strength' is often associated with slow speeds and the term 'power' with the high speeds of movement, this is not entirely correct. Strength is the capacity to exert force at any given speed, and power the mathematical product of force and velocity at whatever the speed or force. Power can be determined for a single body movement, a series of movements, or, as in the case of dance, for a large number of repetitive movements. Power can also be assessed instantaneously at any point in a movement or averaged for any portion of a bout of exercise.

4.7   Practical (Training) Considerations

STRENGTH

The most popular forms of strength training are probably weightlifting and the use of resistance machines. Exercises are designed to strengthen specific muscles by causing them to overcome a fixed resistance, usually barbells, dumb-bells or weight plates. They are generally conducted according to the 'split' system, whereby a single workout focuses on two or three major muscle groups. With this system, dancers may include most muscle groups within a three-day interval.

In order to demonstrate muscular strength gains, the training load must be progressively increased, in at least three evenly spread training sessions per week. However, satisfactory gains of strength can be *maintained* by as little as one session of resistance training per week (Bell, Syrotiuk, Attwood and Quinney 1993), allowing the main focus of training to be shifted to the development of other performance-related parameters, such as endurance, flexibility and/or technique.

Table 5.6 shows selected strength-training intensities and the associated training effects. A universal method for assessing the strength of a

Table 5.6 Strength-training intensities and training effects

Intensity (% maximal strength)	Training effect
80–100	1. Maximal strength
60–80	1. Hypertrophy 2. Explosive strength
40–60	1. Speed strength 2. Strength endurance
20–40	1. Strength endurance (some) 2. No training effects (mainly)

muscle or muscle group is by noting the maximum weight which can be lifted successfully in a single effort. This, the single-repetition-maximum (1-RM), can subsequently be used in a training prescription.

The importance of strength-training *periodization* increases with the level of fitness and performance (more about periodization can be found in the next chapter). It has been suggested that periodized training provides differential recovery for muscle fibres—according to whether light, moderate or heavy resistance is used—and may therefore provide a better stimulus for strength improvements (Ploutz *et al.* 1994). Furthermore, by altering the intensity and volume of exercise over time, the deleterious effects of overtraining may be avoided (for more information on overtraining and overwork, see Part III, Chapter 7).

POWER

Plyometrics is a muscle-conditioning system geared specifically to power enhancements. It involves stretching the muscle groups immediately prior to contraction, as occurs naturally when the dancer dips before leaping high. This pre-stretch induces a stretch reflex which phases into the contraction. This high-loading, high-velocity type of muscle action is thought to maximize the stimuli both biochemically in terms of protein synthesis, and physiologically in terms of possibly synchronizing motor-unit activation within progressively smaller windows of time. Plyometrics may also favourably alter the energy-storage properties of tendon, ligament and fascia.

The classic plyometric exercise is the depth-jump. For example, three boxes of appropriate height (30–40 cm) are placed one metre apart on a sprung surface. The dancer should stand on the first with knees slightly flexed and arms down, then jump down and immediately up onto the next box with a strong arm swing, and so on for up to 10 reps in a set. Up to five sets may be done in a training unit, with perhaps two units per week. However, to avoid injury it is absolutely vital to progress into plyometrics very gradually over several weeks, as the high eccentric work on landing induces unusual amounts of delayed-onset muscle soreness. Plyometric training further includes bounding and one- or two-legged hopping and fast catching and trunk-twisting exercises, often with various weights of medicine ball.

5   MUSCLE FLEXIBILITY AND JOINT MOBILITY

5.1   Introduction and Definition

Given that any human movement consists of well synchronized musculo-tendonous, neural and ligament functions, adequate muscle flexibility and joint mobility (MFJM) is commonly accepted as an important factor for optimal physical performance, and thus as a key component of overall fitness (Corbin and Noble 1980). Adequate MFJM is likely to assist performance in most sports by allowing a more efficient posture to be assumed, and by permitting application of forces over greater distances.

Dance is an expressive art that relies on human movement for com-munication. As levels of communication increase and greater precision and purity of movement are required, modern dancers are constantly confronted with new movement expectations and choreographic de-mands. Therefore, optimal levels of MFJM are a major factor of dance performance too, given that it facilitates greater versatility of movement. However, this physical quality is not only a dance- and sport-related characteristic. The very survival of many animals, such as the ultrafast cheetahs, is directly linked to MFJM, and special efforts are made by these animals to maintain adequate levels of this vital physical quality (remember the stretching exercises always performed by cats on waking).

The term *flexibility* derives from the Latin words 'flectere' (= to bend) and 'bilis' (= capacity or capability). Muscle flexibility refers to how supple, long and pliable particular muscles are, whereas joint mobility is more concerned with the active range of movement. For a more complete picture, the term MFJM will be used in this book with reference to the *individual's ability to move a joint through the required range of motion without undue stress to the involved musculotendonous unit*. Good MFJM usually indicates that there are no adhesions or abnormalities in or around the joint and that there are no serious anatomical or muscular limitations, while an event-specific flexibility has been thought necessary for success in sport (Chandler, Kibler, Uhl *et al*. 1990).

5.2 Types of Muscle Flexibility and Joint Mobility

MFJM exercises can be either *single* or *composite*. The former refers when only one joint is involved (e.g. stretching the calf muscle), whereas in the latter case the intended range of movement involves more than one joint or a series of articulations (e.g. spine). As it will be pointed out later in this section, the significance of this classification becomes more obvious during exercise training, where dancers should always introduce composite MFJM activities before they move onto those characterized as single.

HYPERMOBILITY

Hypermobility may be defined as *excessive mobility of a joint or a number of joints*, and is identified by unstable joints. It often prevents individuals from reaching the highest levels of professional dance or sport. For instance, mild hyperextension of the knee may be aesthetically desirable, but excessive range leads to symptoms in the posterior capsule and poor control. Similarly, a hypermobile foot is a disadvantage in point work.

This condition depends on certain inherited factors such as bone shape, cartilage thickness and ligament length. It may also depend on acquired factors, which are affiliated to past injuries, training and exercise, and which can be traced back as far as childhood.

When working with children, teachers and coaches must be exceptionally careful with the intensity and duration of, say, MFJM exercises, as unaccustomed loads may slightly, but significantly, alter joint-bone shape, cartilage thickness and ligament length. On the other hand, when dealing with individuals who already possess a degree of hypermobility, strengthening the surrounding muscles and the weak and relatively long ligaments is the recommended and safe way forward.

Carter and Wilkinson (1964) devised a test for hypermobility based on the degree of mobility at five given joints: knees, trunk, fingers, thumbs, and elbows. A score of 5 shows some hypermobility, while a maximum of 19 points indicates extreme laxity. The test is easy to administer since it does not require specialized knowledge or the use of instruments. In line with overwhelming anecdotal evidence, the application of this test has revealed that both trained and untrained females, including dancers, show a higher prevalence of joint hypermobility than their male counterparts (Decoster, Vailas, Lindsay and Williams 1998). Young dancers with a tendency to particularly lax joint structures should be identified early and protected from excessive stretching exercises.

5.3 Factors Limiting Muscle Flexibility and Joint Mobility

Individual differences are dependent upon conditions influencing the extensibility of the muscles and ligaments around the joint, and include heredity, age, gender, environmental temperature, warm-up, and psychological stress. Under normal non-pathological conditions, any combination of about 17 known factors can potentially affect the range of movement. These factors can be separated into (1) *joint* factors, which may contribute up to 85% of MFJM performance, (2) *muscular* (or *musculotendonous*) factors, which are responsible for about 10% of the total MFJM, and (3) *general* factors. The latter are often difficult-to-control aspects and account for the remaining 5% of MFJM (Table 5.7).

JOINT FACTORS

The anatomy of the joint, or, more specifically, the structure of the articulating bony surfaces, together with that of the cartilage that protects them from undue friction, is perhaps the most significant single factor that can influence the extent of MFJM (Fig. 5.8). These structures are genetically determined and account for about 45% of the joint's range of movement. Irreparable damage may occur if demanding flexibility training commences prior to the completion of bone development. It has been suggested, for example, that extreme hypermobility and joint laxity are due to intense flexibility training prior to the calcification of the growth plate (Hebbelinck 1988).

Table 5.7 Factors that can influence muscle flexibility and joint mobility

Joint factors	Muscular factors	General factors
Structure of bony surfaces	Muscle/tendon length	Age
Structure of articular cartilage	Fibrous connective tissue	Gender
Joint-capsule laxity	Elastic connective tissue	Body type
Ligaments	Muscle's fat content	Fitness levels
Synovial fluid	Stretch/relaxation techniques	Body fat
–	–	Environmental temperature
–	–	Psychological stress

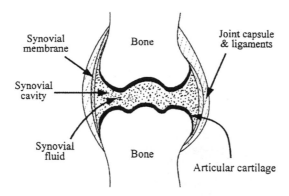

Fig. 5.8 Elements of joint anatomy which determine the range of motion of a joint

The joint capsule, length of ligaments and the amount of *synovial* fluid in the joint also influence MFJM (Table 5.7) and can account for about 40% of the joint's range of movement. Again, although these elements have strong hereditary links, uncontrolled flexibility training—especially during childhood—and/or injury can negatively affect them. This can then influence both MFJM levels and the 'health' of particular joints. Repetitive joint dislocation is a good example of unstable joint structures, mainly due to weak or relatively long ligaments caused, partly, by intensive flexibility work.

An issue worth remembering is that joint factors effectively determine the range of movement, as their contribution to total MFJM can be as high as 85%. Given that most of these factors are attributed to heredity, the effectiveness of exercises in individuals with 'unfavourable' joint characteristics may be debatable. This is, perhaps, why strict selection procedures (auditions) are available to ensure that young candidates have the required MFJM levels at the point of entry in dance schools (Nilsson, Wykman and Leanderson 1993) and gymnastics clubs.

MUSCULAR (OR MUSCULOTENDONOUS) FACTORS

MFJM also depends on the functioning of the muscle–tendon unit. The individual elements include muscle and tendon length, concentration of *fibrous* and *elastic* connective tissues, the fat content of the muscle, and the stretch/relaxation techniques utilized (Table 5.7). It is not clear whether the type of muscle (i.e. slow or fast) fibre also affects the levels of muscle flexibility and, therefore, joint mobility.

At least two of the muscle factors (i.e. the fibrous and elastic connective tissues) are hereditary. Yet the fibrous component of muscle can increase as a result of repetitive soft tissue injuries, given that following muscle microtrauma, the body uses fibrous connective tissue—also known as scar tissue—for the necessary repairs. It is this connective tissue, especially that found in the *fascial sheaths* of the muscles, that accounts for much of the limitation in MFJM (Holland, 1968). Nevertheless, muscle is a very adaptable tissue capable of increasing over 50% in length from the resting state, providing that there is not much fat within the muscle fibres to restrict elongation. This point, however, may not be entirely relevant to dancers as they normally demonstrate low muscle-fat content.

GENERAL FACTORS

The general factors that can affect MFJM appear in Table 5.7. Children are more flexible than older individuals, although large variations exist within members of the same age group (Fig. 5.9). Also, women are normally more flexible than their male counterparts and this ability is maintained at almost all stages of life (Fig. 5.10). Different hormonal and anatomical (i.e. skeletal) profiles between the two genders may account for these distinctions.

From the age of 20 and 25 for men and women respectively, MFJM may display 'descending patterns' along with many other fitness components. This is partly because ageing causes the *elastin* content in muscle

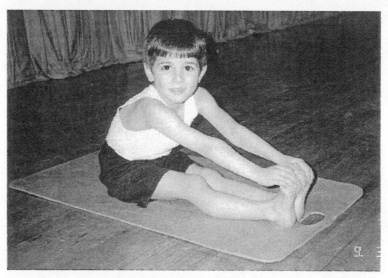

Fig. 5.9 Children are more flexible than older individuals, although large variations exist within members of the same age group

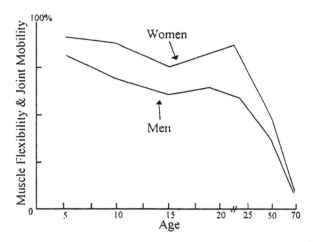

Fig. 5.10   Critical ages of MFJM development in normal men and women

and joint capsule to decrease. The decline seen in MFJM development between the ages of 10 and 15 is mainly due to unfavourable changes in body mechanics, occurring as a result of adolescent growth spurt. At this stage of life the proportions of legs and trunk change in relation to total body height, thus affecting levels of MFJM and, therefore, dance performance in both boys and girls. It is at this stage that many youngsters stop their formal dance education due to lack of confidence and enthusiasm. Appropriate counselling and training may restore confidence and minimize the effects of the growth spurt.

Body type, fat, fitness levels, environmental temperature, psychological stresses, and stages (or levels) of warm-up can also potentially affect the range of movement. While some of these factors (e.g. body type, environmental temperature, and psychological stresses) are difficult to control, others (e.g. body fat, fitness levels, and warm-up) clearly depend on the individuals concerned.

5.4   Injuries, Strength and Muscle Flexibility and Joint Mobility

INJURIES

MFJM has been the main physical fitness component which dancers have regularly sought to improve. However, while it is well established that inadequate MFJM detrimentally affects the quality of physical performance (Table 5.8), it is not yet clear whether poor MFJM contributes to

Table 5.8 Advantages of muscle flexibility and joint mobility

- Protects joints
- Increases the range of possible skills
- Improves the quality of action
- Permits compensatory movements when situations demand
- Maintains a healthy musculature
- Prevents injury?

certain action-related injuries. For instance, when MFJM levels were considered in rowers and dancers, no relationships were found with the frequency and severity of lower-back injuries (Koutedakis, Frischnecht and Murphy 1997). This is shown in Fig. 5.11 which illustrates a lack of significant trends between days off action, resulting from lower-back pain and sit-and-reach flexibility test scores in 48 elite oarsmen, 41 elite oarswomen, and 20 male professional dancers.

In contrast, Harrey and Tanner (1991) found that inadequate lumbar flexibility is one of the factors associated with the increased incidence of lower-back injuries in young athletes, while Knapik, Bauman, Jones *et al.* (1991) concluded that flexibility imbalances can lead to higher injury rates in active females. Sharkey (1997) reported that some injuries are more likely to occur as MFJM decreases.

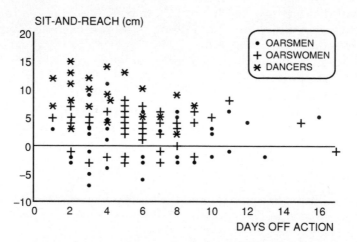

Fig. 5.11 Days off action due to lower-back pain versus flexibility scores (obtained with the sit-and-reach test) in 48 elite oarsmen, 41 oarswomen and 20 male professional dancers. No significant relationships were found
Source: From Koutedakis, Frischnecht and Murphy Vol. 18, International Journal of Sports Medicine (1997c). Reproduced by permission of Georg Thieme Verlag

The rationale behind such findings is that repeated demands on, say, a musculotendonous unit to exert force during increased physical efforts may cause it to shorten, thus decreasing the normal range of motion (Chandler, Kibler, Uhl *et al.* 1990). Furthermore, repeated physical demands on a musculotendonous unit cause a vicious circle of micro-trauma to the tight muscle, followed by scar formation, followed by more microtrauma with continued use. Optimal MFJM, therefore, can elimi-nate such problems, as the joints, ligaments and muscles of a 'flexible' dancer are able to withstand a stress considerably in excess of that which can be resisted by a less flexible person. However, findings like those stated above do not normally take into account the gender of the volunteers used in the corresponding studies, or indeed the levels of MFJM within certain populations.

With respect to gender, one point of MFJM increase—in a 9-point scale—has been associated with about 15% less injury in male athletes, but not in their female counterparts (Krivickas and Feinberg 1996). These authors also confirmed the long-held view that females are more flexible compared to males, and develop considerably fewer injuries. The most flexible women had 60% less injury than that of the most flexible men. Such findings may well support the idea that MFJM exercises in physi-cally active males are likely to reduce injuries, but will not guarantee a reduction of the severity or number of injuries in their female counter-parts.

MUSCLE STRENGTH

Many dancers, dance teachers, athletes, coaches and ordinary individuals still discourage strength training, because they believe that muscle strength gains may limit MFJM. Others preach the opposite, namely that noticeable increases in MFJM may have deleterious effects on muscular strength. Neither of these positions could be further from the truth, as strength bears a positive relationship to flexibility.

Male gymnasts, for example, have very well developed, and on some occasions bulky, bodies, yet they are not inferior to dancers in terms of MFJM. It may be that their frequent high resistance (i.e. strength) exer-cises—and the additional amount of muscle protein produced as a result—not only contribute to muscle fibre size, but also to its length. If muscle size is reduced, it can then affect the overall extensibility of the muscle. This is supported by considerable anecdotal evidence from ath-letics, where the 'bulkier' and stronger sprinters are normally more flexible than the leaner endurance runners.

In some extreme cases of muscle bulk, such as in bodybuilding, MFJM can indeed be restricted. Under these circumstances, strength training can be indirectly held responsible. In general, however, strength training and muscular strength developments do not result in restrictions of the range of movement. This is true in most physically active individuals including dancers. If anything, well-designed strength training may bring about some MFJM benefits.

It seems however that it also works the opposite way, namely that MFJM exercises—and more specifically stretching exercises—positively affect muscular strength. This is at least what happens in children where bone growth and the inevitable stretching of the body's musculature are followed by strength increases.

5.5 Measurement of Muscle Flexibility and Joint Mobility

As previously described, MFJM is a quantitative term that refers to the distance that a limb or segment is able to travel comfortably between the extreme angles. Although the contribution of MFJM to dance perform-ance varies with the type of activity, dancers should be individually tested to identify which muscles or joints are loose or tight. However, the test may give an inaccurate and relatively arbitrary set of values if not conducted correctly. Sound supervision and adherence to test protocols is also essential.

MFJM can be measured either directly or indirectly. Direct MFJM measurements are fairly accurate and involve the use of an apparatus on a specific joint. They may include different forms of the widely used manual *goniometry*, which includes *static goniometry* (for the assessment of a specific angle), and *dynamic goniometry* where the joint angle is assessed during dynamic activity. The apparatus frequently used are simple *goniometers*, *electrogoniometers* and *gravity* or *pendulum goniometers*. However, there is no universal agreement on the most reliable test protocol.

Indirect measurements of MFJM do not generally require the use of equipment, apart from a measuring tape. Tests usually consist of move-ment of a single or limited number of joints, while stabilizing the proximal portions of the body (e.g. sit-and-reach test). This type of MFJM assessment should not replace the more accurate direct ones. Here is some advice for those wishing to conduct MFJM measurements:

- Use a specific warm-up process related to the areas to be assessed
- Check the level of previous muscle activity. Exercise always creates some degree of fatigue, which in turn stimulates some unpredictable level of tension in the muscles and joints

- Assessments at one or two joints (sites) cannot be assumed to be true for other sites
- Keep the same conditions (e.g. testing time) for retesting
- Assess one individual at a time
- Provide no feedback on the individual's performance during testing
- If possible, use testing procedures that do not depend on gravitational assistance (e.g. 'sit-and-reach' test instead of 'touch-toes-from-standing')
- The mean of two to four readings should be obtained for each measurement
- Static measures of MFJM may not relate to dynamic situations

5.6   Training Muscle Flexibility and Joint Mobility

Improving MFJM is often recommended as a way to increase quality of movement. This is based on the fact that tight muscles, tendons or ligaments can restrict motion, in addition to creating a need for greater energy utilization to overcome this motion-resisting stiffness. Maintenance of optimal MFJM levels is equally important. If joints are kept in incorrect positions, connective tissue in tendons, muscles and joint capsules becomes dense and shortened, eventually restricting the range of motion. Fortunately they can be 'stretched'. Muscle and tendon stretching—and more specifically the 'stretch-shortening' cycle—is the basis of most movements in dance and sport, such as running and jumping (Fig. 5.12).

One of the questions frequently asked by many active men and women, is how many MFJM sessions per week (or per month) are required for optimal results. As with most other fitness-related components, 3–4 sessions per week are necessary when MFJM improvements are sought. For maintaining satisfactory levels of MFJM, one session per

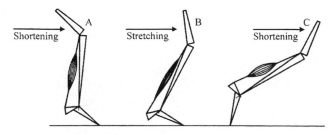

Fig. 5.12   An example of the stretch-shortening cycle in a musculotendonous unit

week is adequate. For elite performers, the time interval between consecutive sessions may be even longer. This is partly supported by some recent data (Koutedakis, Soulas, Sharp *et al*. 1999) where after 3–5 weeks of summer holiday, during which very little physical work was reported, MFJM measurements remained either unchanged or, in some cases, revealed some unexpected increases. It was hypothesized that the increased amount of work done prior to the holiday triggered a 'burnout' effect, which may then explain these controversial findings.

When exercises for MFJM improvements or enhancement are used, dancers should remember that these exercises:

- Are different from warm-up
- Are non-competitive
- Should be conducted with relaxation and in warm environments
- Should be used slowly and progressively
- Are not to be used if it starts to hurt
- Must be followed by cool-down procedures, as cooling of the tissues seems to stabilize the connective tissue structure at their new length (Lamb 1984)
- Should constitute separate sessions lasting 45–60 minutes each

BALLISTIC AND STATIC STRETCHING

Until recently, MFJM exercises consisted mainly of bobbing and jerking movements—sometimes without prior warm-up—lasting for only a few minutes. This ballistic type of MFJM exercise, which *inter alia* is likely to cause muscle soreness, has now been replaced by static stretching, whereby antagonist muscles are slowly placed in a position of maximal stretch for at least six seconds.

The main reason behind the changing of attitudes in MFJM training is the recognition of the *stretch reflex*, which could be illustrated by the doctor striking the patellar ligament. Stretch reflex is one of the body's protective mechanisms, where *muscle spindles* (Fig. 5.13) call forth a vigorous contraction of the stretched muscle, if stretching is too fast and too far. Thus, possible damage to muscle fibres, connective tissue and/or tendons is avoided. However, if a position of stretch is held for six seconds or more, a time is reached when the muscle spindles no longer feel tension. As a result, the muscle can be stretched a little further.

Such practices can effectively contribute to MFJM enhancements via the elongation of the connective tissue found in ligaments, tendons, and muscles, as well as via some muscle fibre lengthening. More specifically, appropriate static stretching forces connective tissues to undergo not only an elastic elongation, or temporary lengthening, but also a plastic elonga-

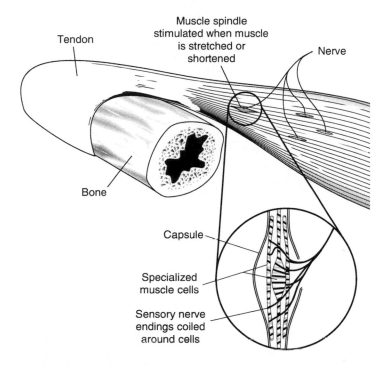

Fig. 5.13 Muscle spindles can sense sudden changes in muscle
Source: Modified from BR MacKenna and R Callander (1996). *Illustrated physiology*. Edinburgh, UK: Churchill Livingstone, p. 259, by permission of the publisher Churchill Livingstone

tion which is a more permanent state. It is also believed that these exercises may positively affect muscle protein balance, and therefore fibre size, mainly due to a retardation of protein breakdown and the stimulation of amino acid transportation. In general, static stretching is superior to ballistic for the following reasons:

- It requires less energy
- There appears to be less muscle soreness and connective tissue trauma
- The antagonistic muscles are fully relaxed

PNF

Over the last 10 years, a technique based on the principle of *proprioceptive neuromuscular facilitation* (PNF) has gained popularity as an alternative to the two traditional methods described above. It was originally developed in the 1940s for treating patients with neuromuscular disorders, as it facilitates the function of the muscle spindles, also known as *propriocep-tors*. Under specific conditions these proprioceptors cause muscles to relax, thus offering less resistance to stretch and, consequently, allowing an enhanced range of motion.

PNF, or 'contract–relax' stretching, is a form of static stretching technique that comprises isometric contraction of a lengthened muscle followed by further lengthening (McAtee, 1993). It has been shown that a combination of contract–relax with isometric contraction of the antagonists helps the involved muscles to relax, by overcoming the stretch reflex, so one can better stretch both muscles and tendons (Etnyre and Abraham 1988). *PNF* stretching exercises are beneficial for both men and women (Etnyre and Lee 1988), and consist of four different phases:

1. Gentle stretching of the muscle or the muscle group in question for up to 10 seconds.
2. Tightening of the same muscle(s) by developing as much isometric tension as possible for 10–30 seconds.
3. Relaxation of the tightened muscle for up to 10 seconds.
4. Repetition of stretching. Muscle(s) are stretched as far as possible, and stay in this position for 15–30 seconds.

Or

1. Gentle stretching of the muscle or the muscle group in question for up to 10 seconds.
2. Contraction of the antagonistic muscle(s)—without shortening—by developing as much isometric tension as possible for 10–30 seconds.
3. Relaxation for up to 10 seconds.
4. Repetition of stretching. The 'target' muscle(s) are stretched as far as possible, and stay in this position for 15–30 seconds.

For example, if the hamstring muscles are to be exercised using PNF, place one knee on the floor and stretch the other leg straight in front of you. Then, by moving your back slightly forward, apply a gentle stretching of the straightened leg's hamstring for about 10 seconds. Tighten the muscle of the back of the thigh by pressing the heel against the floor as hard as you can for 10–30 seconds. Following a 10-second relaxation period, keep your back straight and bend it forward over the straightened leg until you feel resistance. Maintain this position for 15–30 seconds.

All four phases (i.e. gentle stretching, tightening of muscle, relaxation, and full stretching of muscle) may be repeated several times on the same muscle or muscle group in order to get the maximal plastic elongation of the connective tissues. Throughout the flexibility routine the amplitude of an exercise has to be increased progressively. However, if dancers experience pain during the execution of PNF exercises, they should reposition the limb or use less force during the isometric contraction. If the pain persists, PNF should not be used until the cause of the pain is found.

5.7 Muscle Soreness and Muscle Stretching

Intensive physical activity and various forms of exercise may result in symptoms of muscular discomfort, soreness, or stiffness which can generally be classified as: (1) *immediate soreness* (which occurs during or immediately after exercise), and (2) *delayed localized soreness* (which appears 24–48 hours after exercise). Alter (1996) has described four possible causes which may, individually or collectively, explain the nature of muscular soreness:

- Torn tissue
- Connective tissue damage
- Metabolic accumulation (swelling)
- Localized spasm of motor-units

Regardless of the causes, current knowledge from muscle physiology tends to support the use of stretching exercises against the development of *immediate* or *delayed muscular soreness*. This can be achieved by holding the muscle in a static stretch, just to the point of discomfort, for 2-minute periods with 1-minute rest intervals, 2–3 times daily (de Vries 1986). During this period, stretching exercises stimulate the transport of *amino acids* into muscle cells, accelerate protein synthesis inside the cells and inhibit protein breakdown (Vandenburgh and Kaufman 1983). This in turn helps the body to nurse possible muscle microtraumas which may have occurred during intensive dance, and to minimize muscle soreness. However, some authors have provided data which contradict the claims that stretching can relieve muscle soreness (Buroker and Schwane 1989).

6 BODY COMPOSITION

6.1 Definition

Body composition is another fitness-related component, and refers to the internal makeup of the body. Its popularity has increased dramatically in the last two decades, in line with the extended application of methods connecting exercise medicine and science to performance. Fashion and the general trend for 'leaner' bodies have further contributed to the awareness of the whole concept.

The body is composed of five main *chemical components*: water, proteins, carbohydrates, minerals, and fat. These, in turn, form the four main *anatomical components* of the body, namely organs, bone, muscle and fat. The latter, however, is the main component that can be significantly changed through different dietary and physical training regimes, with effect to both its size and weight. The other three components (i.e. organs, bone and muscle) remain relatively unchanged in young and active individuals. So, a *two-compartment* model has been developed where body weight is taken to be the sum of fat weight plus fat-free weight. Body composition, therefore, is simply defined as *the ratio of fat to fat-free weight* and is often expressed as percentage body fat. The following terms are frequently used in connection with body composition:

- Lean body weight: Body weight—composed primarily of muscle, bone, and other non-fat tissue—minus the body fat; for our purposes, *lean body weight* is synonymous with *fat-free weight*
- Adipose tissue: The tissue that contains fat
- Essential fat: The fat required for normal physiological functioning; it is contained in bone marrow, muscle, central nervous system, liver, kidney, etc.; females have greater amounts of essential fat than males
- Storage fat: Mainly serving as nutritional reserve, this is the major fat depot that accumulates in adipose tissue; the quantity of storage fat is greater in females than males

---

Based on the above two-compartment model, body composition is also described as having *metabolically active* and *metabolically inactive* components. The former consists principally of lean body weight (i.e. muscle mass plus associated tissue components) which make up approximately 70% of the total body weight (Fig. 5.14). The metabolically inactive component constitutes the remaining 30% of the human body weight, of which about 20% is fat and 10% is bone. Changes in the metabolically active component are usually a function of changes in the muscle weight. Similarly, changes in the metabolically inactive component are normally a function of changes in fat weight.

FAT AND BODY DENSITY

Fat is stored in adipocytes (i.e. fat cells) which are generally located under the skin, especially at the back of the arms and on hips, thighs and

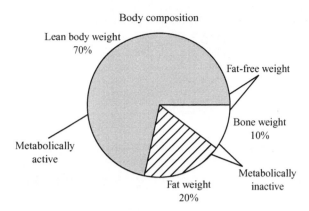

Fig. 5.14 Body composition and its main components

bust in women, and in the abdomen in men. Quantitative determination of stored body fat is defined by the number and size of adipocytes. Total body fat storage is often higher during the winter months, when fat serves as insulation against the cold. In the summer, the fat content normally declines in response to an increase in energy expenditure and a decrease in appetite.

Fat has a low content of water (and potassium) and has a density of about 0.900 grams per cubic centimetre, while fat-free tissues have high water (and potassium) content and a density of about 1.100 grams per cubic centimetre. Thus, the relative proportion of fat-free weight to body fat weight is reflected in *body density*. Body density decreases as the body fat proportion increases.

Fit and relatively young individuals (between 18 and 25 years of age) have higher body density values than children and the aged. This is partly because with each decade above age 25, the body normally loses about 4% (or about 3 kilograms) of its metabolically active cells, most of which come from muscle. As muscle is denser than fat, changes in muscle volumes inevitably affect total body density. It may be worth remembering that up to the age of 55–60, declines of metabolically active cells are followed by proportional increases of metabolically inactive tissues, particularly fat.

Densitometry is a technique for the estimation of total body density, and hence body fat percentage. A number of methods are available, but *hydrostatic weighing* (incorporating an underwater weighing device and measuring the loss of weight in water), and *volume displacement measurements* (using a body volumeter) are the most popular. The downside though is that such techniques are usually too cumbersome for the clinical setting or for mass testing.

6.2   The Effects on Health and Physical Performance

In the last 20 years it has repeatedly been confirmed that body composition—especially excessive body fat—is linked to a number of lethal diseases such as coronary heart disease, stroke, and several types of cancer, as well as high blood cholesterol, high blood pressure and osteoarthritis. Recent data have further demonstrated that the site where excess fat is deposited is as important as the fat itself. People most vulnerable to medical complications tend to have more of their fat deposited in abdominal areas rather than in the back, hip or thigh areas. The ratio of waist to hip and waist to thigh circumferences is a simple method of determining fat distribution, and whether excess fat is deposited in the high-risk area of the body. Dancers normally show low waist to hip and waist to thigh circumference ratios, indicating 'feminine' figures which are favoured aesthetically by the profession (To, Wong and Chan 1997), and which are healthier.

Body composition also plays an important role in sport and exercise. Appropriate active mass, coupled with the right levels of body fat, are essential ingredients for optimizing physical performance. This not only applies to activities involving specific weight categories, but also to activities where carrying excess fat is detrimental to performance, as in running- or jumping-based efforts. However, at least in female athletes, factors representing linearity of physique seem to be unrelated to physical performance (Claessens, Hlatky, Lefevre and Holdhaus 1994). It has been further found that although seasonal body weight alterations are mainly due to a significant reduction in fat mass, these weight restrictions appear to limit an increase in lean body weight which could be beneficial to athletic performance (Morris and Payne 1996).

There are no similar data in relation to dance. However, considering the well-established link between lean body weight (or fat-free weight) and physical performance, preliminary research has shown comparable lean body weights in dancers to that of untrained control subjects (van Marken Lichtenbelt, Fogelholm, Ottenheijm and Westerterp 1995). With dance performance in mind, do dancers need to pay some attention to their fat-free weight, and to what extent?

Body composition, and *somatotypes* in particular, constitutes vital data in 'talent' selection of young boys and girls for some sports and, of course, for dance. 'Talent' selection which incorporates such criteria is important, since there is little evidence to suggest that intensive training drastically alters the original body composition and somatotype characteristics (for more information on somatotypes see the end of this section). However, as levels of performance increase, these criteria become less significant when applied to members of the same discipline. For example, professional ballet dancers have many body composition factors in common, as indeed is the case with, say, Olympic weightlifters. It is this homogeneity that distinguishes dancers from other athletes.

Professional dancers and elite athletes appear to have constant body composition values throughout their careers. In fact, lean body weight in accomplished female ballet dancers can be adequately estimated from body weight alone, given the homogeneity of body size and body composition in female ballet dancers at this level (Hergenroeder, Brown and Klish 1993). However, when approaching their retirement age, both dancers and athletes show similar patterns of body composition changes dominated by gradual body fat increases. The reasons for these similarities can, perhaps, be traced to the ageing process, where increases in body fat and decreases in muscle mass are common features. Nevertheless, if body fat changes do emerge in professional dancers, they are relatively small and have little or no affect on their actual physical performance. Such changes, though, would threaten the 'aesthetic balance' which dancers faithfully observe.

6.3   Measurement of Body Composition

In the light of the evidence indicating an association between body composition and both health and exercise, calculations or predictions of the body's structural components have attracted the attention of many scientists since the 1940s. Most of them now agree that body composition estimates are a valid aid in classifying individuals who may be under- or overweight, and in recommending changes in body weight, assessing menstrual status in active females such as dancers (To, Wong and Chan 1997), and endorsing changes in dietary or physical training programmes.

There are several methods available that can provide authoritative information on body composition (Table 5.9). Most are laboratory-based,

Table 5.9   Selected methods for assessing aspects of body composition

Bone	Fat & fat-free body	Muscle
Computed tomography	Computed tomography	Computed tomography
Neutron activation	Neutron activation	Nuclear magnetic resonance (NMR)
Photon absorptiometry	Densitometry	Potassium 40 counting
Radiographics	Ultrasonics	Creatine excretion
	Skinfold measurements	Ultrasonics
	Bioelectrical impedance	

require a great deal of scientific expertise and experience and are expensive to run. However, there are some techniques which are quickly learned, require relatively inexpensive equipment, and can be satisfactorily used by dancers, athletes and ordinary individuals.

Although not without error, these simple techniques provide more accurate assessments of body composition than can be furnished by using the standard height–weight charts. The reason is that such charts cater for the average man and woman, rather than for individuals with specific needs such as dancers and athletes. Consequently muscular and athletic individuals are usually defined as 'overweight' when they actually carry low amounts of fat. On the other end of the spectrum, people with small amounts of muscle and bone are frequently designated as 'underweight' despite the fact that they may be carrying increased amounts of body fat. Before moving into two non-laboratory-based techniques, it may be worth emphasizing that most methods for estimating body composition in lean and fit individuals, such as dancers and gymnasts, are prone to greater error than in sedentary individuals.

SKINFOLD MEASUREMENTS

Estimation of body fat—and therefore body composition—from skinfold measurements is perhaps the best available method. It is based on the premise that areas of the body where adipose tissue tends to be deposited will be larger than average in persons with greater amounts of body fat. The use of a pair of relatively inexpensive skinfold callipers is necessary, and the main steps in measuring skinfolds are as follows:

- The skin and subcutaneous fat are grasped between the thumb and forefinger just above the measurement site, and held throughout the measurement
- The skinfold is then pulled away from the underlying muscle so that no muscle tissue is included in the fold
- The skinfold callipers are then applied to the fold about one-half inch below the thumb and forefinger
- The handle is released and the reading obtained in millimetres

When the skinfold values are added, the sum obtained is compared to a table of age- and gender-specific body-fat percentages. These tables have been derived from population-specific prediction equations applied to estimate *body density*, and hence *percentages of body fat*. In other words, there are two steps in the conversion of skinfold thickness into an estimate of percentage fat:

1. skinfold thickness → estimate of body density
2. body density → estimate of percentage fat

Fig. 5.15 shows typical sites for measurement of skinfold fat in men and women. Amongst them, *subscapular, suprailiac, biceps* and *triceps* are the most popular sites. To convert the skinfold thickness to an estimate of body density, these four skinfolds are added together and substituted in one of the following equations devised by Durnin and Rahaman (1967):

Men: body density $= 1.161 - 0.0632 \log_{10}$ (total of four skinfolds)

Women: body density $= 1.1581 - 0.0720 \log_{10}$ (total of four skinfolds)

Boys: body density $= 1.1433 - 0.0643 \log_{10}$ (total of four skinfolds)

Girls: body density $= 1.1369 - 0.0598 \log_{10}$ (total of four skinfolds)

The next step is to convert body density (BD) scores to an estimate of percentage fat. This can be achieved by using one of the following two equations:

Percentage fat $= [(4.95/BD) - 4.5] \times 100$ (Siri 1956)

Percentage fat $= [(4.570/BD) - 4.142] \times 100$

(Brozek, Grande, Anderson and Keys 1963)

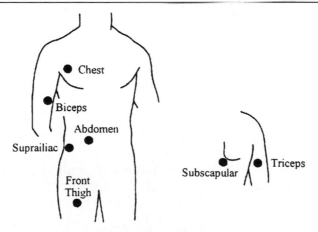

Fig. 5.15 Typical sites for skinfold measurements

When weight of body fat is known, then the lean body weight can be calculated from the total body weight. In general, body composition evaluation by the skinfold method is both valid and feasible for mass testing. It is not, however, as accurate as the laboratory method of, say, hydrostatic weighing although vastly more convenient, and considerably more accurate than the traditional method of using height–weight charts.

BIOLECTRICAL IMPEDANCE (BI)

Pioneered in the USA, this technique for estimating body composition is based on the concept that electrical current flows more easily through lean tissue than fat, as lean tissue has a greater water and electrolyte content, and therefore a greater conductivity. Subjects lie in a supine position with their arms away from the trunk, and four surface electrodes (two on the right hand and two on the right foot) are applied. A very small imperceptible electrical current is passed through the body, generated by a portable machine, which also incorporates built-in software to calculate percentage body fat. For BI measurements the following equation is used:

$$V = pL^2 \div R$$

where: V = volume of conductor
p = specific tissue resistance
L = standing height in centimetres
R = observed resistance in ohms

Although BI provides a simple, non-invasive and rapid means of estimating human body composition, it nevertheless has a number of inherent limitations, which may produce large errors. This was partly acknowledged by Hergenroeder and his colleagues (1991) in their work on the body composition of adolescent and young adult ballet dancers. Most of the researchers who have used BI conclude that further work is required especially with fit and relatively lean individuals. The main limitations of this method are:

- Lack of sensitivity to *age* and *gender*
- Oversensitivity to states of *dehydration* (or *overhydration*), as this influences the normal concentrations of body electrolytes
- *Ambient temperature*, which must be controlled to obtain valid measures

6.4 Body Fat in Dancers and Other Athletes

Table 5.10 shows the sex, age, body weight, and percentage (i.e. percentage of the total body weight) body fat in selected active and untrained individuals. The table confirms that active populations in general have lower percentages of their body weight as fat compared to healthy but untrained men and women. However, variability in body fat between individuals participating in the same physical activity does occur. This may partly reflect natural variation in patterns of fat distribution or could be related to individual eating and exercise patterns.

Table 5.10 also confirms that males have lower body fat values than their female counterparts. As Craig Sharp states in his chapter on Gender Differences (Part III, Chapter 11), until the age of around 10, there is little difference in body fat between boys and girls. However, when both sexes go through puberty, the boys tend to lower their body fat percentage, and the girls tend to gain fat. The difference in body fat between the 'average' young man and woman is of the order of 70 000 kilocalories (or

Table 5.10 Typical percentages of body fat (BF), age and weight in selected physically active and inactive men and women

Sport	Sex	Age (yrs)	Weight (kg)	BF (%)
Dancers (Ballet)	Males	26.0	64	10
Dancers (Ballet)	Females	25.0	52	17
Dancers (Contemporary)	Males	27.2	72	12
Dancers (Contemporary)	Females	26.3	59	20
Gymnasts	Females	15.2	45.3	13.4
Mid-distance runners	Males	25.7	62.9	7.3
Mid-distance runners	Females	24.1	52.8	14.8
Sprinters	Females	21.6	60.7	18.1
Ice dancers	Females	19.3	52.1	22.0
Squash players	Females	18.4	62.1	24.7
Sprinters	Males	23.4	82.3	9.1
Hockey players	Males	27.8	75.6	12.3
Road cyclists	Males	20.0	68.9	8.7
Lightweight rowers	Males	24.3	70.3	6.7
Rugby players	Males	20.6	64.4	21.0
Judoists	Males	21.8	72.2	16.0
Nordic skiers	Males	25.8	73.6	8.2
Untrained	Females	28.0	60.0	28.0
Untrained	Males	29.0	79.0	19.0

Sources: Data on athletes from Koutedakis (1994)
Data on dancers from Brinson and Dick (1996)

300 000 kilojoules), which is just about the energy cost of producing a full-term human infant.

Men demonstrate higher non-fat values than their female counterparts, and given that muscle is the main non-fat component, and that it uses relatively high portions of energy, differences in body composition partly explain why males expend more calories than women of similar weight. Body fat ratings for males and females are given in Table 5.11.

Body composition in dance has been viewed primarily in the context of ballet, where typical body fat values for females range from 16 to 18% (Clarkson, Freedson, Keller *et al.* 1985; van Marken Lichtenbelt, Fogel-holm, Ottenheijm and Westerterp 1995). The equivalent values in male ballet dancers range from 5 to 15% (Sawyer-Morse, Smolik, Mobley and Saegert 1989; Hergenroeder, Fiorotto and Klish 1991; Koutedakis, Cross and Sharp 1996). Very little information has been published in relation to other forms of dance. However, results obtained from ballet dancers may not be applicable to other dancers, as ballet dancers appear to be the leanest (Pacy, Khalouha and Koutedakis 1996).

Dancers, on average, do not demonstrate the lowest body fat values among active individuals (Table 5.10). This is despite attempts by sections of the profession to comply with the well-established 'aesthetic' standards, which dominate traditional dance education. For example, student ballet dancers are more preoccupied with thoughts of eating, body weight and body fat, use and abuse laxatives for weight control, and report disordered eating more than ordinary school students (Abraham 1996). Nutritional habits, body stereotypes, and, especially, limited awareness of aspects related to dance physiology, may account for this observation.

Very few studies on athletic populations have reported male and female body fat values less than 5% and 10% of total body weight respectively, indicating that a certain minimal level of fat is necessary. Indeed, very low levels of fat may result in abnormal biological function-ing and, perhaps, in decreased sport and exercise performance.

Sports amenorrhoea (or absence of periods) is one such abnormal

Table 5.11 Rating of percentages of body fat for males and females 20–30 years of age

Rating	Males	Females
Thin	7–10	12–16
Slim	11–14	17–21
Average	15–20	22–27
Plump	21–26	28–32
Fat	27+	33+

biological function which females should bear in mind. This condition is associated with low levels of the female hormone oestrogen, which helps to control bone calcium; low oestrogen may cause osteoporosis (or calcium and bone mineral loss) which increases the likelihood of stress fractures. Significant relationships were found between musculoskeletal injuries and low body fat in physically active individuals. Elite female middle/long-distance runners, gymnasts, and ballet dancers are prime candidates for developing osteoporosis of varying severity. More about osteoporosis and body weight control appears in Part III.

6.5   Body Shape (Physique)

It is obvious that body shape and composition are very closely related. If we add here the problems in categorizing weight into fat and fat-free mass, it perhaps becomes easier to appreciate why scientists have looked at alternative ways of describing body characteristics.

One such approach, described as the 'body profile analysis system', or *somatotype*, was originally developed in the 1950s for males only. According to this system, three basic builds (or physiques) were identified describing the degree of *roundness* (endomorphy), *muscularity* (mesomorphy), and *linearity* (ectomorphy) of the body (Fig. 5.16). These exhibit the characteristics of the extreme variants found in the population. Specifically, endomorphy is characterized by softness of the body and there is a predominance of the abdomen area over thorax; mesomorphy is characterized by large bones covered by thick muscle, while ectomorphy's common features include linearity, fragility and delicacy of the body. However, given that most humans share characteristics from more than one of these physique types, three numbers (on a seven-point scale) were used in order to quantify each of these characteristics, with 7 indicating a maximum and 1 a minimum of the component. For example, the rating 1–3–7 (for endomorphy, mesomorphy and ectomorphy respectively) shows a primarily lean individual with a hint of muscularity, while that of 3–7–1 represents a very muscular individual with his body weight being slightly above what one might consider as ideal. The rating 7–1–1 denotes a primary endomorphic individual and is normally reserved for obese men and women. However, this system is highly subjective and not suitable for athletic populations.

Heath and Carter (Katch 1993) refined the above method to accommodate individuals involved in sport and exercise. They extended the original seven-point scale to nine, while certain body measurements (i.e. weight, height, two limb girths, two bone girths and four skinfolds) were added to the original photography-only procedures. These measurements

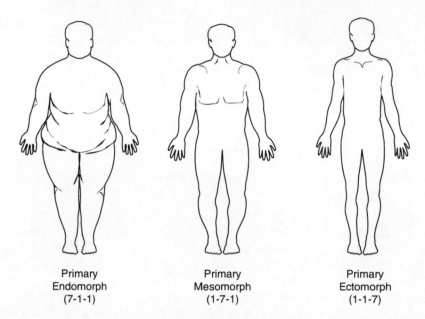

Primary	Primary	Primary
Endomorph	Mesomorph	Ectomorph
(7-1-1)	(1-7-1)	(1-1-7)

Fig. 5.16   The three basic physique types (or somatotypes)
Source: Redrawn in modified form from Applied Anatomy by J. Bloomfield, pages 2–31 Science and Medicine in Sport 1995. Reproduced by permission of Blackwell Science Ltd

are then used to calculate a body profile in terms of muscular and non-muscular components. The employment of a specially designed chart is necessary in order to determine the somatotype of each individual (Fig. 5.17).

Although somatotyping is of little practical value to dance teachers and sport coaches, it is nevertheless a useful research tool. It has been found, for example, that dancers and basketball players are predominately ectomorphic individuals, that sprinters tend to be mesomorphs, while a high mesomorphic component is an important factor determining strength (Bale, Colley, Mayhew *et al.* 1994). Research has also shown that endomorphic individuals are more likely to suffer from a cardiovascular disease than individuals classified either as mesomorphs or ectomorphs.

7   CONCLUSIONS

While aesthetic goals are of the utmost importance, dancers remain subject to the same unyielding physical laws as athletes. Assessment of physiological characteristics of dancers can help to quantify overall levels

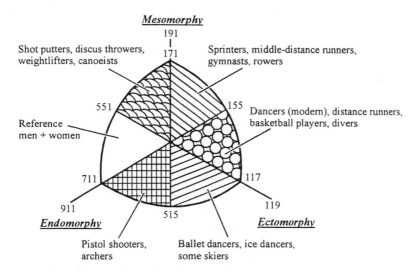

Fig. 5.17   Chart showing the three basic body-types and the areas where selected groups of active individuals are likely to appear based on their physique

of fitness. This knowledge will then assist dancers and their teachers to improve training techniques, to employ effective injury-prevention strategies, and to determine better standards of health and physical conditioning.

Physiological aspects of dance have been viewed primarily in the context of ballet. It has been shown that certain aspects of physical fitness are often neglected by factions of the dance profession, and that conventional dance exercises alone are not sufficient to promote fitness enhancements in male and female dancers. Training to elevate standards of fitness, especially strength, may help in coping with the increased number of musculoskeletal injuries. However, any change in the traditional training of dancers must be approached cautiously, and great care must be taken to ensure that the aesthetic content is not affected by new training techniques. Further scientific research on the physical and physiological aspects of all forms of dance is required.

8   FURTHER READING

Blakey P (1994) *Stretching without pain*. Stafford, UK: Bibliotek Books
Beachle TR (ed.) (1995) *Essentials of strength training and conditioning*. Champaign, IL: Human Kinetics

Bouchard C, Shephard R, Stephens T (eds) (1994) *Physical activity, fitness, and health*. Champaign, IL: Human Kinetics

Heyward VH (1998) *Advanced fitness assessment and exercise prescription*. Champaign, IL: Human Kinetics

Maughan R, Gleeson M, Greenhaff PL (1997) *Biochemistry of exercise and training*. Oxford: Oxford University Press

Shell CG (ed.) (1986) *The dancer as athlete*: the 1984 Olympic scientific congress proceedings, Vol. 8. Champaign, IL: Human Kinetics

Chapter 6

Fitness and Training

1 INTRODUCTION

For many animals the ability to survive depends on the ability to run or jump, either to escape danger or to capture food. For humans too, the ability to use our bodies in a versatile way has enabled us not only to survive through the millennia, but also to progress in a fashion unmatched by other species.

While *fitness* has been the key element behind both survival and progress, *training* is the result of a conscious and planned attempt by humans to become better. The latter is primarily based on the fact that, unlike machines which wear out from the moment they are first used, human bodies actually improve with use.

This has been known for more than 2000 years. In classical Greece, professional trainers were highly respected members of society, as were the masters of the 'art' of aesthetically improving the human body and its performance both in the athletic field and in life in general. Eminent philosophers and statesmen including Plato, Socrates and Alexander the Great had their own personal trainers who, through exercise and training, applied the *'healthy mind–healthy body'* relationship. By using the method of observation, these trainers had learned that appropriate diet, warm-up, control of fatigue, and *periodization*, or variation, of physical effort, were (and still are!) amongst the determining factors of human physical performance. They also observed that lack of well-designed training programmes could be detrimental to both health and performance.

When a dancer, or an athlete, repeats a specific exercise, the same muscle fibres and energy system are recruited over and over again as many times as are the number of repetitions of the exercise. If this is done on a regular basis, the body begins to adapt by making adjustments, also known as *training effects*, whereby the exercise stimulates the body—and more specifically the muscles involved—to undergo changes that permit more exercise in the future.

Dance training is a long-term process of physical, technical, intellectual, and psychological preparation by means of physical exercise. This long-term process covers an extensive period, which spans from childhood until the dancer reaches the highest level of performance. However, questions as to what type of physical work (and to what extent) could supplement traditional dance training have gone largely unasked. This is despite the fact that some preliminary data favour the use of athletic-type exercises for, say, injury prevention and fast recovery (for more information, see previous chapter).

This lack of enthusiasm may well be related to the fact that the principles and other aspects of physical training have always been associated with sport and therefore remain relatively unknown amongst dancers and their teachers. Therefore the purpose of this chapter is to introduce the basic theoretical elements supporting physical training, together with warm-up and fatigue, which are thought to be important parts of any physical training process. When these aspects are properly observed, then the designing of training programmes and schedules becomes an easier task, while the effects of training (or lack of it) can be effectively quantified and assessed for the benefit of the individual dancer and the profession as a whole.

2   PHYSICAL TRAINING

2.1   Principles of Physical Training

Physical training entails exposing the body to exercise stimuli of sufficient intensity and duration to produce a desirable and lasting effect. In the case of dancers and sport competitors, these stimuli should also derive from exercises that are mechanically as similar as reasonably possible to the event in question. Furthermore, all training programmes must be flexible enough to cope with illness, injury, emergency, different weather conditions, and change of location and individual lifestyles. *Specificity*, *reversibility*, *overload*, and *individuality* are the general principles that apply to all training regimens.

SPECIFICITY

According to this principle, *the effect of exercise is reasonably specific to its type*. If the aim is to increase force levels, exercises should be characterized by high loads and low velocities. Alternatively, if speed of movement is the intended adaptation, then lower exercise loads should be coupled with high-velocity muscular actions (Fig. 6.1).

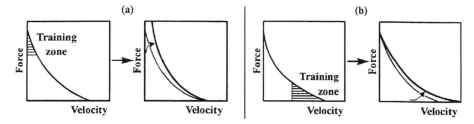

Fig. 6.1 Specificity of exercise training. If the aim is to increase force levels, exercises should be characterized by high loads and low velocities (a). If speed of movement is the intended adaptation, then low exercise loads should be coupled with high-velocity muscular actions (b)
Source: Redrawn from Dirix: The Olympic Book of Sports Medicine Vol. 1 (1988). Reproduced by permission of Blackwell Science Ltd

When designing an exercise programme, aspects such as energy sources (i.e. aerobic versus anaerobic), muscles involved, and levels of muscle involved (i.e. force production, speeds of movement, fatigue patterns) should be considered. Changes only occur if the different parts of the body are appropriately engaged in exercise. Thus, exercising the legs will not yield training effects in the arms or the upper body, while low-intensity strength training does not promote the body for situations in which high muscle force and power are required. In general, strong similarities should exist between the training conditions and those required on stage during dance performances.

REVERSIBILITY

All training effects are reversible, either due to injury, ageing, illness and bed-rest, or by infrequent and insufficient exercise training, as may occur during busy seasons and touring periods through lack of specific physical work. Literature indicates that dancers as well as sports people may demonstrate lower levels of fitness during stage performance and competition periods respectively, than at other less physically demanding periods of time (Koutedakis, Boreham, Kabitsis and Sharp 1992; Koutedakis, Soulas, Sharp *et al.* 1999). It has been argued that during such busy periods, stage and rehearsal commitments leave relatively little time for rest and specific physical fitness work, which then can lead to reduced levels of fitness. However, fitness gains decline more slowly than the rates at which they increase. Several factors may affect the rate of reversibility.

First is the duration of the physical training. As a general rule, the longer the training period the slower the detraining. A second factor is the type of muscle action. A combination of concentric and eccentric strength training, for example, will result in a slower reduction of maximal strength during detraining than will concentric-only exercises. Third is muscle fibre type. Fast (or type II) muscle fibre area is more affected by periods of little or reduced physical training compared to slow (or type I) fibres. The final item is linked to the performance-related component of power. While, say, four weeks of reduced training or inactivity result in minor reductions of muscular strength, the same conditions are associated with a pronounced decline in the ability to generate power (i.e. velocity of muscle contraction and strength combined).

OVERLOAD

Adaptation to training is dependent on overload, and thus training volume and load should progressively increase. As levels of a particular fitness component increase, a higher quality of exercise stress is needed to create 'overload'. Milon of Croton was the first known athlete who, perhaps unwittingly, implemented the principle of progressive muscle overloading as early as the late sixth century BC. He carried a bull calf on his back each day until the animal reached maturity.

At the beginning of this century, the principle of overload for training was reintroduced initially in the field of medicine and subsequently in sport and exercise. The pioneers DeLorme and Watkins (1948) suggested that, in order to improve strength and other fitness components, exercise resistance (or load) must be periodically increased. By ensuring that the magnitude of the training load is above the habitual level, the overload principle is also applicable to untrained individuals and novice dancers and athletes. Pregnancy could be regarded as a form of progressive resistance training, for both leg strength and aerobic endurance.

INDIVIDUALITY

Even at the highest level, each dancer has his/her own physical, physiological and psychological (personality) characteristics, which make them more (or less) suitable for a particular training programme. Wherever possible, the physiological status of each dancer should be assessed and individual training should be offered accordingly. It is, therefore, not recommended to devise a universal programme for a dance company with many different individuals. It is also unwise to mimic slavishly the training programmes or the technique of successful individuals in dance, or in sport, as these individuals most probably have a physiological and psychological profile that cannot be met by the majority.

2.2 Periodization of Training and Exercise

Training and exercise training may be arranged into several periods known as macro-, meso- and microcycles, the last consisting of 'training units'. Such *periodization* (or scheduling) has increasingly been part of serious athletic training over the past half-century, as it sets out the format and the time-scale of the complete training and competition plan. A similar approach, with some difficulty perhaps, may also be adopted by dancers, given that their life is a constant cycle of hard work (with fatigue), recovery (with regeneration), improvement in performance (for a brief period), and brief layoff (for mental and physical rest) to permit another cycle to repeat.

Schedules are organized around the *training unit* (or training session), which is an assignment aimed at the implementation of the four basic principles of exercise training, namely specificity, reversibility, overload and individuality. A number of training units form a *microcycle*, which usually for convenience lasts one or possibly two weeks. The microcycle has an overall goal, such as enhancement of stamina or leg power, and is planned so that an optimum effect is gained from each unit. Work is progressive, with the training volume increased through a microcycle, then the intensity is increased, then the volume again, in a rhythmic see-saw pattern.

Three or four (or more) microcycles together form a *mesocycle*, which is an intermediate period also with an overall goal (e.g. maintaining a fitness component and increasing another one). Each mesocycle would include training units that dovetail back to the previous mesocycle—and dovetail forward to the next mesocycle. Finally, a *macrocycle* covers anything from a few months to one year. However, yearly macrocycles are more frequently used, and they too have overall goals (e.g. improvement of jumping ability and/or better partnering and lifting techniques). The end of this cycle is often marked by a need to change the main training objective.

2.3 Components of Physical Training

A single formula for successful training to satisfy the needs of all individuals of varying age, gender and fitness levels does not exist. However, exercise scientists agree that a well conceived programme should incorporate at least four distinct components: (1) optimum exercise intensity, i.e. load; (2) appropriate volumes of training; (3) specific rest periods between exercises; and (4) adequate recovery from a training and exercise session.

EXERCISE INTENSITY

Exercise intensity may be defined *as the exertion level which can cause positive physical and/or physiological adaptations.* For instance, in order to obtain improvements in cardiovascular function of untrained 20–30-year-old individuals, a training intensity that forces the heart to work beyond the margin of 130 beats per minute is necessary. Many dancers use various forms of exercise pulse-meters, and very roughly, the training-zone heart rate should just exceed the sum of the resting heart rate and 60% of the difference between resting and maximal heart rates, with age-related maxima being estimated as 220 less the age in years.

Similarly, when an adult muscle is forced to contract at intensities which exceed 60% of its maximal force-generating capacity, adaptations occur which result in increases in strength. This normally accompanies better muscle fibre synchronization. A universal method for assessing the strength of a muscle or muscle group is by noting the maximum weight which can be lifted successfully in a single effort.

VOLUME OF EXERCISE

The volume of training for a given exercise, or session, may be defined *as the product of the number of sets, the number of repetitions, and the load in each repetition (sets x reps x load).* From these three elements, the load used in each repetition is of particular importance. It is indicative of the number of repetitions in each set and, hence, the final volume of a given exercise or training session. In strength training, for instance, relatively heavy weights cannot be lifted for a large number of repetitions in a single set. Therefore, high-volume training is usually done with low to moderate loads.

In sport the relative magnitudes of the three individual volume components are critical. Indeed, while weightlifters and bodybuilders both attain very high training volumes, the former meet their training demands by performing many sets of low repetitions, but with near maximal load. In contrast, bodybuilders usually exercise in fewer sets of many repetitions with lower loads. However, such a degree of specificity is not necessary in dancers. For them, maintenance of an individually tailored volume of physical exercise over and above their dance commitments seems more appropriate.

Each individual has a different capacity for training with various volumes. Some may make substantial progress with longer or more frequent periods of high-volume training sessions, while others may not. Dancers, therefore, should be careful when adopting the training cycles of other dancers or, particularly, of sport competitors.

REST PERIODS BETWEEN EXERCISES

Depending on the overall aim of a particular session, the rest periods between two consecutive exercises (or sets) may range from just a few seconds to several minutes. In dance, both experimental and anecdotal evidence supports the use of longer (i.e. greater than 3 minutes) rather than shorter rest intervals, in order to enhance the effects of subsequent bouts of muscular work. During these rest periods, muscles recover most of the ability to work effectively by replacing the energy used during the preceding exercise bout, and by removing the fatigue-causing metabolic by-products. However, it has also been argued that the development of fatigue, through the reduction or elimination of rest intervals, may accelerate the progress of selected fitness componets (Schott, McCully and Rutherford 1995).

DURATION OF A TRAINING SESSION

For minimum possible training effects, the duration of each training session for dancers should never be less than 30 minutes, which includes a 10-minute warm-up and cool-down period. On the other end of the spectrum, sessions that are longer than 90 minutes (including half an hour of warm-up and cool-down) are probably not much more effective than those sessions lasting between 45 and 60 minutes.

RECOVERY FROM TRAINING AND EXERCISE

Two workouts per week per muscle group are sufficient to induce an optimum adaptive response; more frequent sessions may 'overtrain' muscle. This is supported by Ackland and Bloomfield (1995) who proposed a two-day recovery period between resistance-training sessions. More data are needed with specific reference to dance.

3   WARM-UP AND COOL-DOWN

3.1   Introduction

The periods of general activity before the start and after the end of a class or rehearsal are generally known as *warm-up* and *cool-down* respectively. The former is connected with the starting of the 'biological machine' of the body, while the latter is more concerned with the safe return to resting levels of the action-stimulated bodily functions. Both warm-up and cool-down are associated with a number of physiological and psychological benefits such as injury prevention, control of muscle soreness, enhanced energy production and discharge of frustration prior to important performances. However, the actual warm-up and cool-down methods when and if used, are more frequently based on the trial and error experience of the dancer or teacher, rather than on scientific study and advice. Furthermore, there appears to be little consensus about the precise definition of warm-up or cool-down in dancers, while the relevant literature is rather slim. The aim of this section is, therefore, to stress the importance of these two components to dance and fitness, and underline their relevance to everyday dance activity.

3.2   Warm-up

DEFINITION AND EFFECTS OF WARM-UP

The term *warm-up* is usually understood *as a set of procedures aiming to start the 'biological motor' of the body*. Its importance was perhaps known in classical Greece, where a number of religious and bodily activities—such as covering the body with olive oil, massage and use of light exercise equipment—were always employed before athletic competition and, even, theatre performances. These preparation procedures were treated as part of the whole accomplishment and were closely observed by officials known as 'judges' who were protected by the 12 gods. Obviously, not everybody shares this view today.

   This is partly due to a legacy left by the research on the effects of warm-up in the 1960s and 70s. About 55% of the research projects found warm-up to be superior to resting, but 40–45% found no significant difference between different kinds of warm-up and rest in relation to exercise performance (Franks 1983). Since then, the investigative techniques have been greatly advanced and the most recent reports are overwhelmingly in favour of warm-up prior to any form of exercise.

Nevertheless, it is not yet clear to what extent warm-up exercises should be specific to the activity that is to follow.

Any warm-up is better than no warm-up (Romney and Nethery 1993). This is particularly the case if a dancer has been diagnosed as asthmatic. For instance, 15 minutes of continuous exercise at 50–60% of maximal aerobic capacity has a protective effect on post-exercise bronchoconstriction in athletes with exercise-induced asthma (McKenzie, McLuckie and Stirling 1994). Appropriate warm-up and stretching exercises may also reduce the negative effects of muscle soreness experienced the day after intensive muscular efforts (Rodenburg, Steenbeek, Schiereck and Bar 1994), especially when repeated powerful eccentric contractions as in jumping have been used.

An important benefit of warm-up is the increased anaerobic power outputs (Sen, Grucza, Pekkarinen and Hanninen 1992), which then enable most dancers to sustain higher performance levels during 'fast-moving' routines. This effect is probably due to three reasons, namely reduced muscular viscosity, increased rate of chemical reactions in the muscle, and increased speed of conduction of impulses by nerves. Further advantages of warm-up may include: increased thermoregulatory responses during exercise performed in cold environments (Torii, Yamasaki and Sasaki 1996); improved muscular strength output (Rosenbaum and Hennig 1995); better buffering of metabolic by-products linked to delayed onset of fatigue (Black, Ribeiro and Bochese 1984); and improved joint mobility and flexibility (Ferris 1988). Good warm up has even been suggested for active pregnant women, for all stages of their pregnancy (Newsholme, Leech and Duester 1994). Table 6.1 summarizes the most common physiological and psychological benefits of warm-up. It is necessary to raise muscle temperature by at least 2 °C before these changes become significant, which is about the level reached after several minutes of vigorous warm-up.

Warm-up and Muscle (Body) Temperature

Muscle functions as a 'chemodynamic engine' that transforms chemical energy into mechanical work. In this process large quantities of heat are liberated which eventually increase the temperature of the muscle itself, as well as that of the entire body. This temperature increase is the principal aim of warm-up. It is mainly achieved with the help of the cardiovascular (or cardiorespiratory) system through many physiological functions (Fig. 6.2). Hormones secreted into the bloodstream set the pace of the changes to come, by enhancing cardiac function and causing blood to be diverted from the organs to the working muscles. At the same time, muscle arterioles dilate allowing greater volumes of blood to pass

Table 6.1   The most common physiological and psychological benefits of warm-up (↑ indicates 'increases' and ↓ 'decreases')

A.		*Physiological benefits*
•	↑	Body (muscle) temperature
•	↑	Chemical (metabolic) processes
•	↑	Thermoregulatory responses during exercise
•	↑	Blood supply by reducing vascular bed viscosity
•	↑	Heart rate, which will prepare cardiovascular system for work
•	↓	Affinity of haemoglobin for oxygen
•	↑	Cost-effectiveness of breathing (i.e. more oxygen is extracted from a given volume of inhaled air)
•	↑	Tissue oxygen supply/utilization
•	↑	Energy generation and supply
•	↑	Aerobic capabilities (or stamina)
•	↑	Speed of nerve impulse
•	↑	Muscle contractility
•	↑	Neuromuscular co-ordination
•	↑	Muscular force (or strength)
•	↓	Viscosity of connective tissue and muscle
•	↓	Post-exercise bronchoconstriction in individuals with exercise-induced asthma
•	↑	Connective tissue and muscular extensibility
•	↑	Anaerobic power outputs
•	↓	Incidences of nausea during short but very intensive muscular work
•	↓	Feelings of muscular soreness
B		*Psychological benefits*
•	↓	Reaction time for visual and auditory stimuli with increase of body temperature
•	↑	Self-discipline
•	↑	Motivation
•	↑	Concentration
•	↓	Emotional stress
•	↓	Anxiety
•	↑	Establishment of 'reference points' (e.g. status of the body, light, environmental temperatures, etc.)

through. This results in increased blood flow and a simultaneous augmentation in the available oxygen. Elevation of muscle temperature is the result of these changes and the beginning of a range of welcome developments, all of which directly benefit quality of movement and, therefore, physical performance.

The most noticeable change with increasing muscle temperature is that metabolic processes in the cell can proceed at higher rates, as these processes are temperature dependent. For each degree of temperature

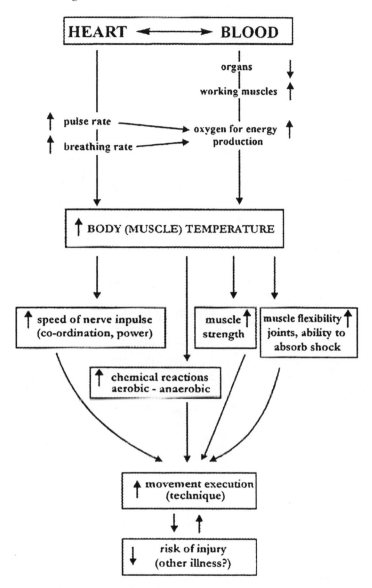

Fig 6.2 The role of the cardiovascular system in increasing body temperature (↑ indicates 'increases' and ↓ 'decreases')

increase, the speed of metabolism in the muscle cell accelerates by about 13%. This relationship between muscle temperature and metabolism is maintained up to about 40 °C, beyond which further increase in temperature is associated with the muscle's decreased capability to use oxygen.

Above 45 °C, and certainly above 60 °C, tissue proteins are denatured, in the same way as a poached egg changes in hot water.

There are not only physiological changes that occur as the result of variations in body temperature. There are also those related to motor skills and psychology (Norris 1994). For example, a distinct relationship between changes in body temperature and reaction time has been established. The poorest reaction time was measured early in the morning and late at night, when body temperature is normally at its lowest (Kelitman, Titelbaum and Feiveson 1938).

WARM-UP AND INJURY PREVENTION

Although many specialists advocate the importance of warm-up in preventing musculoskeletal injuries, relatively few scientific reports have actually confirmed it. One possible explanation may be that an injury can be only studied after its diagnosis. By that time, though, important information on warm-up and other pre-exercise preparations is either lost or impossible to obtain. Whatever the reasons for this lack of scientific data, there is overwhelming anecdotal evidence in support of warm-up having a preventive role against injury. It is also interesting to remember the close relationship between warm-up, injury and levels of movement execution (Fig. 6.2). Optimal warm-up can lead to better executed movements, which in turn can lower the risk of injury.

One of the few relevant reports is by Kujala and colleagues (1997) who suggested that pre-exercise stretching and adequate warm-up are important factors in the prevention of hamstring injuries. Warm-up has also been among the factors that prevent running injuries (van Mechelen 1992) which are similar in nature to those occurring in dance. This preventive mechanism of warm-up against injury may be based on the fact that physiological warming causes an increase in the length and elasticity of the muscle–tendon unit (Safran, Garrett, Seaber *et al.* 1988). However, not everybody agrees with this viewpoint (Williford, East, Smith and Burry 1986).

ACTIVE OR PASSIVE WARM-UP?

It seems that passive warm-ups (e.g. sauna, hot showers) do not have the same beneficial effects as the active equivalents. For instance, a 45-minute hot water bath immersion prior to exercise does not significantly affect muscular strength, and therefore does not appear to elicit any ergogenic effects (Stanley, Kraemer, Howard *et al.* 1994). Also, one of the negative effects of passive warm-up is that blood flow is directed away from muscles (Karvonen 1992).

With passive warm-up, there is a great possibility that blood flow to the heart muscle itself might be inadequate during the first minutes of intensive activity, thus inhibiting the optimal function of the heart and therefore postponing the gradual rise of body temperature. Furthermore, evaporation of reduced amounts of sweat in response to passive warm-up may either inhibit the mechanisms for body-temperature increases, or minimize its effects by causing a drop in the overall temperature. Instead, jogging, callisthenics, stretching and practising the skills which dancers are about to carry out are more suitable for preparing the body. An exception might be massage which, in addition to saving energy, also contributes to the psychological 'feel-good' factor.

WARM-UP PRINCIPLES

Warm-up methods have been greatly developed in the last 10–15 years, but the principles surrounding them have remained the same and include:

- Warm-up should preceed every class, rehearsal or stage performance
- The duration of warm-up routines depends on levels of fitness, time of the year, and the individual's idiosyncrasy
- The intensity of warm-up mainly depends on the dancers' levels of fitness
- A comprehensive warm-up routine takes approximately 20 minutes
- Sweating does not always indicate optimal warm-up
- Resting periods between the end of warm-up and the start of dance should not be greater than 10–15 minutes; these times also depend on the clothing and the environmental temperatures
- Dance studios should be heated to approximately 21 °C
- Dancers should be suitably dressed to avoid body heat losses
- Exercises should be selected to suit the individual needs
- Complexity of exercises should be varied to avoid boredom
- Warm-up should take place in a different venue to that of actual dance
- Warm-up exercises should progress from simple to complex, easy to difficult and from large to small muscle groups

THE STRUCTURE OF A WARM-UP SESSION

In order to produce the required changes, the warm-up must consist of a conservative 20 minutes of activity at various intensities, ranging to a more liberal approach set at 35–40 minutes. This length of time may be further extended—in elite sports it may be in excess of an hour—but no dancer should go for less than 20 minutes, if the full benefits of warm-up are to be gained. Table 6.2 shows some of the goals of warm-up, and the suggested length and the type of exercises to meet them successfully. It should always be remembered that stretching exercises in the warm-up routines should not be regarded as muscle flexibility and joint mobility activities. In general, a warm-up session may be divided into three stages.

Stage 1 (Preparatory). The duration of this stage is 5–10 minutes. Its main aim is to activate the cardiovascular system. Start with jogging, shift to jogging–running activities, and finish with gentle stretching of large muscle groups.

Stage 2 (Main). Lasts for 10–15 minutes. Main aims include stimulation of energy pathways, elevation of muscle temperature and injury prevention. Dancers should also start this stage with some jogging–running– playing activities and finish with stretching. However, jogging and other exercises are now of higher intensity than before, whereas muscles– tendons–connective tissue are stretched towards the full range. At the end of this stage, all muscle groups should have been effectively stretched, while sweating should reach moderate levels.

Stage 3 (Individual). Lasts for 5–10 minutes. During this stage the dancer concentrates on individual exercises which concern specific movements and/or muscle groups. Improvements of joint movements with more limited range due to, say, injury are the most common problems to be attended to at this stage. Dancers should also include movement patterns that are to be performed during class.

Table 6.2 Length, type and goals of warm-up

Goal	Length of warm-up	Type of warm-up
Activation of the cardiovascular system	At least 5 minutes @50–60% of HR max[a]	Activation of continuous nature. Any muscle group may be employed
Stimulation of energy pathways and Prevention of soft tissue injury	10–15 minutes	Continuous exercise performed between 60–70% of HR max[a]. Activities should engage as many muscle groups as possible.
Prevention of soft tissue injury	5–15 minutes	Mainly stretching exercises mobilizing the muscles to be used during actual dance.

[a] Maximal heart rate (HR max) = 220 − age

There is relatively little published information on warm-up in relation to dance. Anecdotal evidence points to the fact that the majority of dancers have a distorted perception of the meaning and the effects of warm-up. Usually, there is a set warm-up routine which individual dancers practise on 'special' occasions, often without taking into consideration aspects such as environmental temperature and clothing. These routines are principally based on stretching exercises during which the cardiovascular system has little or no involvement. However, whatever the actual perception and interpretation of the term, most dancers do try to warm-up before classes, rehearsals and stage performances, with modern dancers being more consistent with their warm-up procedures than ballet dancers (Fig. 6.3). Whether this difference is due to 'athletic' backgrounds often found in modern dancers is open to discussion. Further education and research are required on the effects of optimally conducted warm-up routines in dancers.

3.3 Cool-down

Cool-down is as critical for dance and long-term fitness as warm-up. Just as warm-up is a step between rest and successful dance, cool-down is a

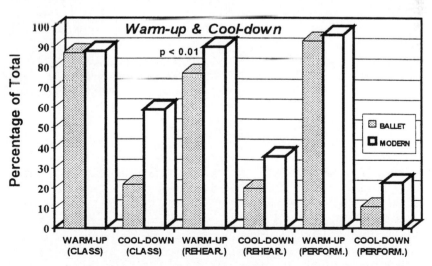

Fig. 6.3 Warm-up and cool-down exercises before and after classes, rehearsals and performances in professional dancers (expressed in % of 324 dancers)
Source: From: Koutedakis, Pacy, Carson and Dick Vol. 12, Medical Problems of Performing Artists (1997). Reproduced by permission of Hanley & Belfus, Inc.

step from dance to recovery. However, although some type of cool-down has been part of the athletes' training and competition routine for a long time, dancers have generally failed to take advantage of its benefits. This is clearly supported by the responses of 324 professional dancers presented in Fig. 6.3. While the majority reported some form of warm-up before classes, rehearsals and stage performances, relatively few of them spent time on winding-down. Again, modern dancers seem to be more consistent compared to ballet dancers. The values of cool-down for dancers are often lost in the excitement of after-dance euphoria and meetings with friends and admirers.

The term is usually understood as a set of procedures aiming to gradually slow down the 'biological motor'. Cool-down makes it possible to attain a physiological balance more quickly after exercise. Abrupt cessation of exercise—especially vigorous exercise—leads to a number of unwelcome physiological manifestations, such as pooling of blood, sluggish circulation, and slow removal of waste products. It may also contribute to muscle soreness and cramping.

More specifically, during exercise much of the venous return to the heart is accomplished by the milking action caused on limb veins by the alternate contraction and relaxation of the active muscle. Therefore, if physical activity is halted suddenly, a great deal of blood remains in the limbs and if it is not returned soon enough to the heart, cardiac function is impaired to the extent that transient dizziness or even faintness may occur. By contrast, light activity and stretching exercises after the end of the main physical effort continue the action of muscles on veins, thus helping the circulation and the removal of metabolic wastes (e.g. lactic acid). The more serious implications of sudden cessation of exercise include the high levels of the hormone *noradrenaline* present immediately after intensive exercise, making the heart more subject to irregular beats. Cool-down procedures help to remove excess noradrenaline (Sharkey 1997).

Cool-down procedures have also been used as synonymous to 'active recovery' through which a speedy reduction of metabolic by-products from the working muscles can be achieved. Indeed, it has been found that these procedures are more effective in, say, lactic acid removal following intensive physical effort compared to complete rest (Koutedakis and Sharp 1985). This finding becomes of greater significance when two or more stage performances have to be undertaken in relatively short periods of time. In general, optimal warm-down routines may be associated with a number of physiological changes (Fox and Mathews 1981; Noble 1986), including:

- The control mechanisms for heart rate, stroke volume, blood pressure, and respiration do not have to undergo rapid and erratic changes

- Elevated circulatory function to perfuse muscle
- Fast removal of lactic acid from muscle and blood ensured
- Body acidity returns more quickly to balance
- Smooth readaptation of the thermoregulating system to resting conditions
- Prevention of overloading of the cooling system when it is hot, and reduction of chilling in cold weather
- Minimization of post-exercise soreness and stiffness, especially in not very fit individuals
- Boost to the rate at which muscle recovers after workouts and classes

Regarding muscle recovery following workouts and classes, research has shown that stretching exercises—which are normally used during cool-down—stimulate the transport of *amino acids* (the building blocks of protein) into muscle cells, accelerate protein synthesis inside cells and inhibit protein breakdown (Vandenburgh and Kaufman 1983). Cool-down is also important for attaining an emotional balance after the possible disappointment of a poor performance. In situations where the next appearance follows soon afterwards, it is even possible to prepare for it during the cool-down from the previous appearance. At the same time, these procedures can be utilized to mentally analyse the causes of faults or failures, always with the help of a teacher. Failures in performance are best addressed during cool-down periods, given that they follow soon after action.

In designing a cool-down programme, the same principles and stages described in the previous section concerning warm-up may be adopted, but in the reverse order. It also takes approximately the same time to complete a cool-down routine compared to warm-up.

4   FATIGUE

4.1   Introduction

All dancers, and everybody else, feel fatigue. This may be defined *as the inability to generate or maintain an appropriate muscle force (as in a lift or a jump)*, or *as the inability to maintain a particular rate of physical work, as in especially fast, or long, or repeated dance or practice sequences*. One way of viewing fatigue is that it is a natural means of forcing the recipient to slow down from the activity in order not to regress to injury or illness. Prepubescent children, for example, generate much less of the fatiguing metabolic end product lactic acid in their muscle, which may be viewed as acting as a natural safety measure against serious overload. Consequently, in dance training situations it is possible for an ignorant teacher to make them overwork, which may result in a degree of overheating and dehydration, leading perhaps to headache and nausea. The same will not so readily happen to an equivalent group of young adults, as the pain and discomfort of lactic acid build-up will force them, at least temporarily, to stop the session before they become too hot or dehydrated. Nevertheless, fatigue itself may affect co-ordination, and possibly lead to injury.

The dancer's training involves two main aims; first to improve or maintain dance technique. Normally this is approached specifically. The second aim, although not always a specifically programmed one, is to reduce fatigue.

4.2   Main Reasons for Fatigue

Physical fatigue in the dancer, as in any other athlete, occurs for a number of different reasons, most of them concerned with chemical events inside each muscle cell. These events relate to the sources of energy, as described in Part I, and they depend mainly on the intensity and duration of the muscular effort being made, as well as the state of training of the particular dancer. Thus, the main reasons for physical fatigue are:

- Depletion of *Phosphocreatine*
- Build-up of *Lactic Acid*
- Decrease in Blood *Glucose*
- Depletion of Muscle Glycogen

DEPLETION OF PHOSPHOCREATINE (PC) IN THE MUSCLE CELL

This may occur in a short routine of the highest intensity, as in a series of jumps or fouettés. It will be remembered that in terms of power output, the PC system can, for a few seconds, produce about twice the power of the longer anaerobic system (glycolysis), which in turn can produce about four times the power of ordinary aerobic muscle effort. Muscle has about 4–8 seconds-worth of PC, whose fall-off is easily seen, for example, in the 100-metre sprint. If this is carefully timed every 10 metres, it is seen that virtually all the runners begin to slow down from about 60–80 metres onwards—because they have run out of PC. The winner is he or she who decelerates least, that is whose PC lasts just that fraction longer.

A short very intense dance routine may well involve an exhaustion of PC, where fatigue may not be felt as a positive feeling of tiredness, but simply as an inability to gain as much elevation in the leaps, or rotational speed in the fouettés. Nevertheless, this is a definite form of muscle fatigue. There is no specific end-product penalty following PC exhaustion, apart from the decline in power. The PC does recharge itself within a few minutes, up to a gradually declining maximum if it is repeatedly exhausted.

BUILD-UP OF LACTIC ACID IN MUSCLE AND BLOOD

This would occur in fairly short vigorous routines of up to a minute—or a repeated series of shorter routines, as in jazz dance, or in the show Riverdance, or in some modern classical dance. The second major muscular energy source, already described in Part I, is the metabolic cycle of *anaerobic glycolysis*. In this energy cycle the glucose or glycogen in the muscle is degraded, without any oxygen, through the 'glucose-splitting' cycle whose end product is *pyruvic acid*. You may remember that pyruvic acid, which still contains over 90% of the energy of the glucose molecule, can then go on to release it via *Krebs cycle*. However, if the power need is greater than all of Krebs can supply, then the huge mass of glycolysis comes into play, to produce less power than PC, but still four times more than Krebs. In sport, a very good example is the 400 metres—one lap of the track, lasting between 45 and 55 seconds, whose main energy source is anaerobic glycolysis. Other examples are any maximal physical efforts, lasting between 20 and 50 seconds—a fast dance routine, fast skipping, or a very hard rally at squash.

After this, fatigue is most certainly felt, and not just as an inability to keep going. Genuine discomfort and soreness or even transient pain is felt in the fatigued muscles. In the main, this is due to the large amount of pyruvic acid produced—far too much to be removed by *mitochondria* via Krebs cycle. The muscle cell, trying to escape fatigue, gains temporary respite by turning it into lactic acid. But this also quickly builds up, and forces a marked slowdown—due to the fact that lactic acid has no escape, and acts as an acid, that is it releases a very active chemical particle called an ion, a *hydrogen ion*, usually written as $[H^+]$. This interferes with the cross-bridges of the very molecules of contraction, the actin and myosin, and it also interferes with the function of the enzymes of glycolysis itself, and of Krebs cycle. And it diffuses out of the muscle cells and activates adjacent pain-fibres. In part this is a protective process, to stop you exhausting muscle to the point of no return—when it would go into rigor (as in rigor mortis: when the muscle really does run out of energy!). However, the dancer or the athlete is not normally appreciative of these fine philosophical points—they simply feel pain and fatigue, and have to markedly slow down, or even stop.

With frequent repetitive use (i.e. training!), muscle builds up a defence against lactic acid, by increasing its internal *buffering* mechanisms. However, much of the lactic acid spills out of the muscle cell. Some may go back into nearby, less fatigued, muscle cells and be changed back into pyruvic acid and delivered on to Krebs cycle. But most of it will go into the capillaries, and thus enter the bloodstream. Once there, a reasonable proportion (depending on the state of fitness of the dancer) will be buffered by blood 'bicarbonate'. A sodium atom from the bicarbonate bonds with the lactate part of the lactic acid to form harmless sodium lactate. The $[H^+]$ combines with the rest of the bicarbonate molecule to form carbonic acid, a very weak acid, that soon breaks down into carbon dioxide and water. The water simply stays in the blood, and the carbon dioxide is breathed out by the lungs. Indeed, the extra carbon dioxide from lactic acid stimulates the respiratory centre even more—which is partly why dancers and athletes breathe so hard after a bout of intensive (anaerobic) exercise. This is spoken of as the *oxygen debt*, but an important part of the breathing after a hard bout of anaerobic work is to get rid of the extra carbon dioxide, as well as taking in oxygen.

The fitter the dancer, the more bicarbonate he or she will have, and the longer they will be able to work anaerobically. Also, the fitter the dancer, the more quickly they can remove lactic acid from the blood, and perhaps the greater amount of lactic acid they can tolerate without feeling fatigued.

DECREASE IN BLOOD GLUCOSE LEVELS

This is a general feeling of tiredness which may come on after a few hours of work even of moderate intensity, usually when the dancer has missed a mealtime. Normally blood *glucose* is at a level of around 5 units (mmol/litre). After a couple of hours of sustained moderate work, the levels may have dropped about 25%, which is a lot in biological terms. Glucose is virtually the only fuel that there is for the brain, and for the retina (which may be thought of as an extension of the brain into your eye). When glucose drops, it induces feelings of tiredness and irritability, as well as a degree of muscular tremor and reduced co-ordination. This is often associated with yawning, the, 'hunger yawn' (which is different from the 'nervous yawn').

The cure for this is to stop and eat at least a snack—a muesli bar, or a sandwich, with some sweet tea or coffee. The prevention is not to let the glucose drop, by trying to eat regularly, even if the meals are just snacks. Often, of course, if one has been working physically hard, one does not feel hungry for a larger meal, or it may not be available, or it may be too near curtain up. Here, the energy drinks are useful.

DEPLETION OF GLYCOGEN IN MUSCLE

This is a more general feeling of fatigue and lack of energy, which occurs following many hours of work, or even one or two or more days of physical work, such as class, rehearsals and a demanding long performance, especially on matinee days. On tour, it is often harder to eat properly, resulting in glycogen depletion, which may also accompany the perceived need to stay slim. But remember, what is being discussed here is day-to-day fuelling of the working muscles.

If one doesn't eat over a few hours, blood glucose depletes, as just mentioned. But if one eats too little/works too hard over a longer period, then the muscles' own store of glucose, in its storage form glycogen, may be used up. The muscle can still function, of course, by using fat. But fat needs more oxygen to release the same amount of energy as glycogen; also, fat is used at a much slower rate. Muscle *can* function for days or weeks with very little glycogen, but it will work much more slowly, and performance suffers.

GLYCOGEN REPLACEMENT

A marathon runner, working entirely aerobically, will deplete muscle glycogen in about two hours. But anaerobic work, such as features to a considerable extent in dance, causes glycogen to be used nearly 12 times as fast. Thus in a long mixed day, a dancer can deplete the muscle glycogen by well over half in the working muscles. The way to restore it is to eat a reasonably substantial evening meal, providing about two thirds of its calories from carbohydrate or starchy foods—bread, pasta, potatoes, rice, cereals, as well as some cakes and jams. Note that bread, especially white bread, has a higher glycaemic index than sugar; that is, it delivers glucose into the bloodstream more quickly.

Costill and Miller (1980) asked two groups to exercise very hard for two hours on each of three consecutive days. They let one group eat what they wanted, but asked the other group to eat the meals they provided—which contained over two thirds of their calories as *carbohydrates*. Both groups ate the same total number of calories.

They also took a *biopsy* sample from the working muscle of all the runners before and after each day's run. In the group who simply ate their normal diet (which was low in carbohydrate, at only 40%, the rest being fat and protein), the levels of muscle glycogen fell markedly each day, and did not recover much overnight. But in the group on the much higher carbohydrate feeding, with 70% of their calories coming from carbohydrate, the glycogen levels also fell each day but were restored almost to normal (Fig. 6.4).

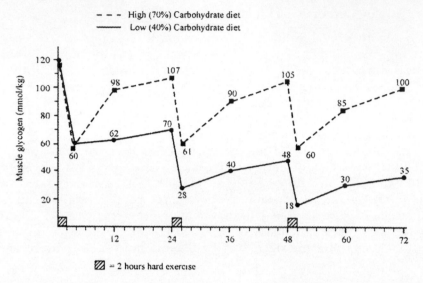

Fig. 6.4 The effects of diets with different carbohydrate content on levels of muscle glycogen. Note the much higher muscle glycogen levels in the 'high carbohydrate' group
Source: Redrawn from Costill and Miller Vol. 1, International Journal of Sports Medicine (1980). Reproduced by permission of Georg Thieme Verlag

Before this, many athletes had believed that they should eat large steaks and fried meals as the best food for exercise. But Costill and Miller (1980) reasoned that as the optimal muscle fuel is carbohydrate, that is what should form a major part of the diet of physically active people. And they demonstrated that in the experiment just quoted, which has now been amply confirmed by others. There is more information on glycogen replacement, and on nutrition in general, in Part I.

4.3   Other Reasons for Fatigue

DEHYDRATION

Taking on too little fluid may also induce muscle fatigue, partly by cutting down the effectiveness of body cooling, which affects both muscle and brain. A male dancer can sweat at a rate of up to 1.5–2 litres of fluid an hour, working hard on a hot and humid day, and a woman dancer will sweat about 20–30% less. The fluid of sweat is taken from the blood, which in turn replenishes itself from the *interstitial fluid* which bathes all body cells, including muscle cells. When the interstitial fluid diminishes, it draws fluid from within the cells themselves, including brain and muscle, and this may upset their function, leading to weakness and reduced co-ordination. The proportions of the three 'fluid compartments'—the blood, the interstitial fluid, and the intra-cellular fluid—are shown in Table 6.3.

Losing about 3% of your body weight as sweat will just begin to register as a drop in physical performance; losing about 5% will begin to induce inco-ordination; 3% of 70 kg is around 2 kg, and of 55 kg is just over a kilogram and a half. Thus if you weigh yourself at the beginning and end of a long hard session, you will get a pretty good idea of how much fluid has been lost. Indeed, after a long rehearsal or performance, you might be surprised how much fluid weight you have lost. But you certainly should not wait until the end of such a session before drinking. Little and often is the key. A small coffee cup full of water every 15–20 minutes is about all that can be absorbed if you are working hard. In other words, you can sweat faster than you can absorb. But drinking judiciously during the work will minimize *dehydration* effects.

Strong coffee and spirits both act as diuretics, that is they cause a relative over-production of urine. Which is just what you don't want if you are a bit dehydrated. A beer or two are fine in this respect, as are a glass or two of wine, especially if accompanied at some point with tap or bottled water. The salts in sweat do not normally have to be replaced other than by the normal level of salts or minerals in food.

One consequence of a degree of dehydration is that the heart will beat at some 10 to 25 beats higher than normal for a given work rate. Another problem is that the body temperature may rise a degree or so higher than the normal 2 °C or 3 °C rise with upwards of 40 minutes of exercise. The increased temperature or relative *hyperthermia* induces its own feeling of fatigue. So, when appropriate, one should break work down into a series of smaller sessions, with reasonable rests between.

THE BRAIN

Another longer-term fatigue effect, which may also follow too many uninterrupted days of hard physical work, especially if associated with

Table 6.3 Volumes, in litres, of fluid in the average male or female dancer

	Blood plasma	Interstitial fluid	Intra-cellular fluid
Man	4	12	40
Woman	3	9	30

too low a carbohydrate intake, and perhaps also a lack of rest and sleep, is a subtle change in blood chemistry, with effects on the brain. When muscle is near to overwork, and fuel (food) intake is marginal, muscle may begin to use a little more protein as fuel than before. It always uses some protein, for perhaps 5% of its energy needs. However, it may begin to use more of the *amino-acid* protein building blocks as fuel, especially three known as *valine, leucine* and *isoleucine*. But these three also enter the brain by a special entry-site carrier molecule. This is a bit like a revolving door, and they compete for this entrance with another amino acid, tryptophan. Oxford biochemist Eric Newsholme and his colleagues (1992) noted that when muscle is overtired, or relatively starved, it takes up more valine and its two companions, so lessening the blood content. However, without its three competitors, *tryptophan* enters the brain in greater quantities. And tryptophan is the precursor of the brain-active chemical *serotonin* (or 5-hydroxy-tryptamine), which is an important cause of tiredness and central (i.e. brain) fatigue. It increases the mental effort needed to keep up a rate of work.

As proposed by Jones and Bigland-Ritchie (1986), possibly this mechanism, or possibly other lesser known effects (perhaps via a drop in glucose supply to the brain?), seems to cause a drop in muscle tension or strength, due to a fatiguing effect on the motor centre itself—the site in the brain where the impulses for voluntary movement are generated. Failure of the brain's motor centre can be assessed by superimposing direct electrical stimulation of nerves on maximal voluntary contractions. It was reasoned that if the electrical stimulus can increase the force above the voluntary maximum, then this could be evidence that the brain itself is fatiguing, in terms of its passing fewer motor impulses down the nerves to the muscles. The main causes of fatigue in sport, where it has been extensively analysed, are shown in Table 6.4.

JOINT FATIGUE

Another, and unlikely seeming, cause of fatigue is the joints themselves. This was confirmed in the 1970s by the great *electromyographer* Basmajian. He seated a group of subjects with weights attached to their wrists. The weights were tied on, so that no muscular effort was required to hold them in place. He then placed electrodes over the muscles of the shoulders and upper and lower arms to record, by the process of electromyography, any electrical activity in the muscles, which would indicate that they were actively bearing some of the weight. However, he noted that there was no electrical activity—therefore the muscles were quite relaxed, and not working. Nevertheless, a short time later, the subjects began to complain of fatigue. Since the fatigue could not have been muscular,

Table 6.4 The main causes of fatigue in various athletic events, from 100 metres to the marathon, lasting from about 10 seconds to just over two hours

Event	Duration	% Aerobic energy	Possible main fatigue causes
100 m	10 sec	4	CP depletion
200 m	20 sec	10	CP depletion
400 m	44 sec	25	Lactic acid accumulation
800 m	1 min 45 s	50	Lactic acid accumulation
1500 m	3 min 30 s	65	Lactic acid accumulation
5000 m	13 min	87	Glycogen depletion
10 000 m	27 min	97	Glycogen depletion
Marathon	2 hrs 7 m	100	Glycogen depletion, Dehydration Hyperthermia Serotonin build-up

Basmajian concluded that it was the joints themselves which were fatiguing, and signalling so to the brain. When a dancer or athlete is fatigued, it is usually from a mixture of causes, but a contribution may well be coming from the joints themselves. Mountain runners often complain of fatigue in their hips, which does not feel muscular, and does indeed appear to be coming from the hip joint, and some dancers have said the same.

There is little one can do to alleviate this, and it is not known what training makes any difference. Nevertheless, it is presumed that training does damp down joint fatigue, possibly by strengthening the joint ligaments. So perhaps flexibility and strength work may be important in this context.

OVERTRAINING AND OVERWORK

The topic of overtraining/overwork and its effects will be extensively discussed in the following part of the present text. Briefly, fatigue, in general, may also be part of the '*over-training syndrome*', or of the '*post-viral-fatigue-syndrome*', or indeed of the so-called '*myalgic encephalitis*' or ME, which is a genuine and seriously debilitating fatigue syndrome. Fatigue experienced as constant tiredness may be part of the eating disorder *anorexia nervosa*, it may be at least partly due to a low muscle glycogen level, and it is often part of the early symptoms of upper respiratory disease such as colds, as well as influenza itself. *Glandular fever* (infectious mononucleosis) is a condition of young adults in which fatigue and tiredness are major symptoms.

An early warning of these conditions is often found in a morning pulse rate which is raised about ten beats a minute over normal. Most athletes and some dancers keep a training diary, in which they also record their morning pulse rate. This should be taken within a short time of waking, but before getting up, and before any tea or coffee (or a cigarette!). Sit up, and swing your legs onto the floor, and sit there for about half a minute. Count your pulse at your wrist or neck for a full minute, and record it. If you do this daily, you will get to know your own normal variation, and something markedly outwith this, say a rise of ten beats per minute over normal, could indicate that you are incubating a viral (or bacterial) condition. And if that is the case, you should go easier on the physical work, until something either develops, or your immune system stops it from surfacing clinically, as shown by your heart rate returning to normal.

4.4   Effects of Fatigue

CRAMP

One of the most dramatic manifestations of fatigue is cramp, which is the acute involuntary contraction of whole or part of one or several muscles. Several factors are associated with cramp, such as intense exercise, over-heating, overcooling, or even the time just before sleep or after sex (both associated with cramp in the feet). The one common factor seems to be holding the muscle in a shortened position, but a true single cause has yet to be identified. It would appear that a small area of muscle goes into a self-triggered spastic contraction, and the pain of this leads to further local contraction; in other words a vicious cycle of widening contraction is set up as a spinal reflex.

However, whatever the cause, the immediate remedy is to voluntarily contract the muscle with the antagonistic or opposite action to its cramped fellow. For example, if you have a calf cramp, then activate the opposing muscle (the foot flexors) by *dorsi-flexing* your foot (i.e. bringing your toes nearer your shin). If you have a hamstring cramp, actively straighten your leg (by using the quads, which are the hamstring antago-nists). For a biceps cramp, straighten your arm with the antagonistic triceps. Do this actively if possible, that is without helping it; but if you can't do this, then vigorously help the process by pulling your foot up with your hands, or straightening your leg against a resistance, or straightening one arm with the other. The important thing is to lengthen the cramped muscle.

The rationale behind this is that when, for example, you straighten your arm fairly quickly from a flexed position, you send a shower of nerve impulses down to the triceps muscle, which contracts to straighten or extend your arm; but the same action is associated with an inhibition on impulse traffic going down the nerves to the biceps and brachialis muscles, which relaxes them and allows the arm to strengthen unimpeded. This is known as *reciprocal inhibition*. It would be dangerous to have both the prime mover (the triceps) and the antagonists (biceps and brachialis) acting hard at the same time—muscle would tear, or bone might even break. Hence the wise programming of reciprocal inhibition. Therefore, if you activate the antagonist, you induce inhibition of nerve impulses to the cramped muscle; and as cramp appears to be maintained, if not actually started, by activation of a muscle's motor nerve, then this should have the desired effect of relaxing the cramped muscle by invoking a sort of nerve block.

One location where this does not seem to work quite as well is in cramp of the abdomen. Straightening your back is helpful, but not as effective as the equivalent in other sites. Perhaps the abdominal muscles are not regarded by the brain as antagonists to the extensors of the spine.

It is said that a degree of *acupressure*, by pressing hard on the upper lip, may reduce calf cramp, but the current author has not yet tried it. It works to suppress a sneeze, so it might be worth a try! Incidentally, there is little truth in the idea that a cold drink will induce abdominal cramp, an idea which possibly came from the condition of 'colic' in horses. Indeed, cool (around 8–12 °C) drinks may be absorbed faster than warm drinks, as they pass through the stomach more quickly.

'STITCH'

'Stitch' is another puzzling phenomenon related to fatigue. Perhaps it is more accurate to say that some stitch, at least, is related to fatigue in the unfit. There are several kinds of stitch. First is the pain felt on the right shoulder, which is very probably caused by the liver reducing its size too rapidly as it donates several hundred millilitres of blood to the general circulation, as part of the 'vascular shunt' of blood away from the abdomen at the start of exercise. Such pain, distant from the point of origin, is called 'referred pain', and it is due to the original embryonic site of formation of the liver. The brain still thinks your liver is near your neck.

A second stitch is that felt at the lower borders of the ribcage on either side. This is usually the crurae or strong muscle attachments of the diaphragm indicating fatigue.

Third is stitch felt more generally in the abdomen. This is usually due to exercising too soon after eating a meal. Food doesn't cause too much trouble if it is in the stomach (perhaps some nausea and sickness—but not stitch). But if it has reached the intestine, it then pulls on the mesentery, the membrane which helps anchor some abdominal organs in position, and this 'mesenteric stitch' signals discomfort.

Dancers and athletes undergo a variety of contortions to alleviate stitch, but all they seem to do is pass the time until the stitch wears off, and there is no 'scientific' way of alleviating it. As far as is known, stitch is not in any way harmful. However, types one and two mentioned above are common in subjects trying to exercise at a rate or for a duration that is greater than their norm, that is these tend to occur in the relatively unfit. The mesenteric stitch may occur in anyone who dances or exercises too soon after too much food. In sport, competitors usually have a fairly light meal about two and a half to three hours before their competition, and they will drink up to about half a pint of fluid about three-quarters to an hour before, and that would seem a reasonable regimen for dancers to follow.

4.5   Management of Fatigue

The biological purpose of fatigue is to stop the subject from continuing to exercise at the particular intensity or volume, in order to stop real harm to the relevant tissues. Hence, the natural feeling of a fatigued dancer is to rest. Rest in this context implies more than simply stopping activity, although that is important. Good dancers and athletes know how much fatigue they can tolerate. The problem arises with dancers and professional athletes in that both may very well have to perform or compete when fatigued, because it is how they earn their living. Management of fatigue after hard performance or rehearsal should have a few core components:

- Some degree of *cool-down* (see previous section) should be gone through. This low-intensity exercise routine need last no more than 5–10 minutes, but it is important to maintain a reasonable circulation of blood through tired muscle for this short time after it has stopped being active. The maintenance of a heightened circulation brings a supply of blood glucose, and will remove heat as well as lactic acid and other metabolites.
- *Physical rest* after the cool-down is obviously the single most vital component of fatigue management, as in sitting or lying in warmth and comfort.
- The rest may be aided by soaking in a *warm bath*, aided by gentle flexion and extension of limbs and back. If possible, a small massage, before or after, will help the relaxation process. Even a degree of massaging oneself is helpful.

- Appropriate *nutrition* is vital. Replace the fluid lost in sweat—drink water in its various forms until your urine is fairly clear and plentiful. Eat adequately—something savoury to replace the salts, and a fair amount of carbohydrate in the form of starchy food to replace the lowered muscle glycogen. The muscles' glycogen depots are particularly responsive to absorbing glucose within an hour or so after finishing exercise. You may not feel at all like eating so soon, but it is important to get some carbohydrate into the system, even in the form of any of the energy drinks or sweet tea, or a muesli bar or equivalent.
- Some dancers add in a valuable component of *mental relaxation*, in the form of relaxation tapes, meditation, yoga, or other techniques. A glass or two of wine or an equivalent may have a similar effect for others, as may sex with one's partner. This all helps maximize the quality of sleep.

5 CONCLUSIONS

While *fitness* has been the key element behind both survival and progress in all species, *training* is the result of a conscious and planned attempt by humans to become physically better. The latter is primarily based on the fact that, unlike machines that begin to wear out from the moment they are first used, human bodies improve with use. If exercise is done on a regular basis, the body begins to adapt by making adjustments, also known as *training effects*. Specificity, reversibility, overload, and individuality are the main principles of physical training. Periodization, resting, warm-up and cool-down are also important training components. However, current data, although limited, indicate that dancers undertake insufficient warm-up and cool-down exercises. One of the consequences of such malpractice is to prolong fatigue. This may be summarized as the results of the depletion of some substances in muscle, such as phosphocreatine, or of glycogen, or the accumulation of others, such as lactic acid. Rest, fluid, food and sleep are the four vital components in the management of muscle fatigue.

6 FURTHER READING

Bouchard C, Shephard R, Stephens T (eds) (1994) *Physical activity, fitness, and health*. Champaign, IL: Human Kinetics
De Vries HA, Housh TJ (1994) *Physiology of exercise* (5th edition). Madison, WI: Brown and Benchmark

Jones D, Round J (1990) *Skeletal muscle in health and disease*. Manchester, UK: Manchester University Press
Paffenbarger RS, Olsen E (1996) *Lifefit*. Champaign, IL: Human Kinetics
Sharkey B (1997) Physiology of fitness (4th edition). Champaign, IL: Human Kinetics
Wilmore JH, Costill DL (1994) *Physiology of sport and exercise*. Champaign, IL: Human Kinetics

ACKNOWLEDGEMENT

Craig Sharp would like to acknowledge help with references from Matthew Wyon MSc of the Roehampton Institute, University of Surrey, and Yiannis Koutedakis thanks Bev Parker of the Wolverhampton University for his expert help with the drawings in this book.

References to Part II

Abraham S (1996) Eating and weight controlling behaviours of young ballet dancers. *Psychopathology*, **29**(4): 218–22

Ackland TR, Bloomfield J (1995) Applied anatomy. In: Bloomfield J, Fricker PA, Fitch KD (eds), *Science and medicine in sport*. Oxford, UK: Blackwell: pp. 2–31

Alter MJ (1996) *Science of flexibility*. Champaign, IL: Human Kinetics

Åstrand PO, Rodahl K (1986) *Textbook of work physiology: physiological bases of exercise* (3rd edition). New York: McGraw-Hill

Bale P, Colley E, Mayhew JL, Piper FC, Ware JS (1994) Anthropometric and somatotype variables related to strength in American football players. *Journal of Sports Medicine and Physical Fitness* **34**(4): 383–9

Bar-Or O (1987) The Wingate anaerobic test: an update on methodology, reliability and validity. *Sports Medicine* **4**: 381–94

Bejjani FJ (1987) Occupational biomechanics of athletes and dancers: a comparative approach. *Clinical Podiatric Medicine & Surgery*, **4**(3): 671–711

Bell GJ, Syrotiuk DG, Attwood K, Quinney HA (1993) Maintenance of strength gains while performing endurance training in oarswomen. *Canadian Journal of Applied Physiology*, **18**: 104–15

Black A, Ribeiro JP, Bochese MA (1984) Effects of previous exercise on the ventilatory determination of the aerobic threshold. *European Journal of Applied Physiology*, **52**: 315–19

Bouchard C, Shephard R (1994) Physical activity, fitness, and health: The model and key concepts. In: Bouchard C, Shephard R, Stephens T (eds), *Physical activity, fitness, and health*. Champaign, IL: Human Kinetics pp. 14–15

Brinson P, Dick F (eds) (1996) Fit to dance? The report of the national inquiry into dancers' health and injury. London, Calouste Gulbenkian Foundation

Brozek J, Grande F, Anderson JT, Keys A (1963) Densiometric analysis of body composition: revision of some quantitative assumptions. *Annals of the NY Academy of Sciences*, **110**: 113–40

Buroker K., Schwane JA (1989) Does postexercise static stretching alleviate delayed muscle soreness? *Physician and Sportsmedicine*, **17**(6): 65–9

Carter C, Wilkinson J (1964) Persistent joint laxity and congenital dislocation of the hip. *Bone Joint Surgery*, **45**B: 40–5

Chandler TJ, Kibler WB, Uhl TL *et al.* (1990) Flexibility comparisons of junior elite tennis players to other athletes. *American Journal of Sports Medicine* **18**(2): 134–6

Chatfield SJ, Byrnes WC, Foster VL (1992) Effects of intermediate modern-dance training on select physiologic performance parameters. *Kinesiology and Medicine for Dance*, **14**(2): 13–26

Chmelar RD, Schultz BB, Ruhling RO *et al.* (1988) A physiological profile comparing levels and styles of female dancers. *Physician and Sportsmedicine*, **16**(7); 87–96

Claessens AL, Hlatky S, Lefevre J, Holdhaus H (1994) The role of anthropometric characteristics in modern pentathlon performance in female athletes. *Journal of Sports Science*, **12**(4): 391–401

Claessens ALM, Beunen GP, Nuyts MM *et al.* (1987) Body structure, somatotype, maturation and motor performance of girls in ballet schooling. *Journal of Sports Medicine and Physical Fitness*, **27**(3): 310–17

Clarkson PM, Freedson PS, Keller B, Carney D, Skrinar M (1985) Maximal oxygen uptake, nutritional patterns, and body composition of adolescent female ballet dancers. *Research Quarterly for Exercise and Sport*, **56**: 180–4

Cohen JL, Potosnak L, Frank O, Baker H (1985) A nutritional and haematological assessment of elite ballet dancers. *Physician and Sportsmedicine*, **13**: 43–54

Cohen JL, Segal KR, Witriol I, McArdle WD (1982) Cardio–respiratory responses to ballet exercise and the maximal oxygen intake of elite ballet dancers. *Medicine & Science in Sports & Exercise*, **14**: 212–17

Cohen JL, Segal KR, McArdle WD (1982) Heart rate response to ballet stage performance. *Physician and Sportsmedicine*, **10**: 120–33

Corbin CB, Noble L (1980) Flexibility: A major component of physical fitness. *Journal of Physical Education and Recreation*, **6**: 23–60

Costill DL, Miller JM (1980) Nutrition for endurance exercise: carbohydrate and fluid balance. *International Journal of Sports Medicine*, **1**: 2–14

Coyle EF (1991) Timing and method of increased carbohydrate intake to cope with heavy training, competition and recovery. *Journal of Sports Science*, **9**(Special Issue): 29–52

Dahlström M, Esbjörnsson Liljedahl M, Gierup J *et al.* (1997) High proportion of type I fibres in thigh muscle of young dancers. *Acta Physiological Scandinavia*, **160**: 49–55

Dahlström M, Inasio J, Jansson E, Kaijser L (1996) Physical fitness and physical effort in dancers: a comparison of four major dance styles. *Impulse*, **4**: 193–209

de Vries HA, Housh TJ (1994) *Physiology of exercise* (5th edition). Madison, Wisconsin, USA: Brown and Benchmark

DeLorme T, Watkins A (1948) Techniques of progressive resistance exercise. *Archives in Physical Rehabilitation and Medicine*, **29**: 263–6

Decoster LC, Vailas JC, Lindsay RH, Williams GR (1998) Prevalence and features of joint hypermobility among adolescent athletes. *Archives of Pediatrics & Adolescent Medicine*, **151**: 989–92

Dowson A, Evans A, Randolph C *et al.* (1997) The effect of an exercise programme on fitness levels and health in female ballet students. Paper presented at the 7th Annual Meeting of the International Association for Dance Medicine and Science, Tring, England

Durnin JVGA, Rahaman MM (1967) The assessment of the amount of fat in the human body from measurements of skinfold thickness. *British Journal of Nutrition*, **21**: 681–9

Etnyre B, Abraham LD (1988) Antagonist muscle activity during stretching: a paradox re-assessed. *Medicine and Science in Sports and Exercise*, **29**(3): 285–9

Etnyre B, Lee EJ (1988) Chronic and acute flexibility of men and women using three different stretching techniques. *Research Quarterly for Exercise and Sport*, **59**(5): 222–8

Ferris MF (1988) Warm-up, flexibility and exercise. *Scottish Journal of Physical Education*, **16**(1): 8–11

Fox EL, Mathews DK (1981) *The physiological basis of physical education and athletics* (3rd edition). Philadelphia, PA: Saunders College Publishing

Franks BD (1983) Physical warm-up. In: Williams MH (ed.), *Ergogenic aids in sport*. Champaign, IL: Human Kinetics pp. 340–75

Galanti MLA, Holland GJ, Shafranski P *et al.* (1993) Physiological effect of training for jazz dance performance. *Journal of Strength and Conditioning Research*, **7**(4): 206–10

Groer S, Fallon F (1993) Supplemental conditioning among ballet dancers: preliminary findings. *Medical Problems of Performing Artists*, **12**: 25–8

Hamilton WG, Hamilton LH, Marshall P, Molnar ME (1992) A profile of the musculoskeletal characteristics of elite professional ballet dancers. *American Journal of Sports Medicine*, **20**(3): 267–73

Harrey J, Tanner S (1991) Low back-pain in young athletes: a practical approach. *Sports Medicine*, **12**(3): 394–406

Hebbelinck M (1988) Flexibility. In: Dirix *et al.* (eds), *The Olympic book of sports medicine* Oxford, UK: Blackwell Scientific Publications: pp. 212–17

Hergenroeder AC, Brown B, Klish WJ (1993) Anthropometric measurements and estimating body composition in ballet dancers. *Medicine and Science in Sports & Exercise*, **25**(1): 145–50

Hergenroeder AC, Fiorotto ML, Klish WJ (1991) Body composition in ballet dancers measured by total body electrical conductivity. *Medicine and Science in Sports & Exercise*, **23**: 528–33

Holland, G (1968) The physiology of flexibility: a review. *Kinesiology Review*, **1**: 49–62

Jones D, Round J (1990) *Muscle in health and disease*. Manchester, UK: Manchester University Press

Jones D, Bigland-Ritchie B (1986) Electrical and contractile changes in muscle fatigue. In: Saltin B (ed.), *Biochemistry of exercise VI*, International Series Sports Science, **16**: 377–92

Katch FI (1993) The body profile analysis system (BPAS) to estimate ideal body size and shape: application to ballet dancers and gymnasts. *World Review of Nutrition and Dietetics*, **71**: 69–83

Karvonen J (1992) Importance of warm-up and cool down on exercise performance. Karvonen J, Lemon RWR, Iliev I, (eds), *Medicine in sports training and coaching*. London: Karger pp. 190–214

Kelitman N, Titelbaum S, Feiveson P (1938) The effect of body temperature on reaction time. *American Journal of Physiology*, **121**: 495–501

Kirkendall DT, Calabrese LH (1983) Physiological aspects of dance. *Clinics in Sports Medicine*, **2**(3): 525–37

Klissouras V (1971) Heritability of adaptive variation. *Journal of Applied Physiology*, **31**: 338

Knapik JJ, Bauman CL, Jones BH *et al.* (1991) Preseason strength and flexibility imbalances associated with athletic injuries in female collegiate athletes. *American Journal of Sports Medicine,* **19**: 76–81

Komi PV, Häkkinen K (1988) Strength and power. In: Dirix A, Knuttgen HG, Tittel K, (eds), *The encyclopaedia of sports medicine: the Olympic book of sports medicine,* Vol. 1 Oxford, UK: Blackwell: pp. 181–93

Koutedakis Y (1994) The physiology of fitness. In: *The runner's guide,* London: Collins Willow

Koutedakis Y, Agrawal A, Sharp NCC (1998) Isokinetic characteristics of knee flexors and extensors in male dancers, Olympic oarsmen, Olympic bob–sleighers and non–athletes. *Journal of Dance Medicine and Science,* **2**(2): 63–7

Koutedakis Y, Boreham C, Kabitsis C, Sharp NCC (1992) Seasonal deterioration of selected physiological variables in elite male skiers. *International Journal of Sports Medicine,* **13**: 548–51

Koutedakis Y, Cross V. Sharp NCC (1996) The effects of strength training in male ballet dancers. *Impulse,* **4**: 210–19

Koutedakis Y, Frischnecht R, Murphy M (1997) Knee flexion to extension peak torque ratios and low-back injuries in highly active individuals. *International Journal of Sports Medicine,* **18**: 290–5

Koutedakis Y, Khalouha M, Pacy PJ *et al.* (1997b) Thigh peak torques and lower-body injuries in dancers. *Journal of Dance Medicine & Science,* **1**: 12–15

Koutedakis Y, Pacy PJ, Carson RJ, Dick F (1997a) Health and fitness in professional dancers. *Medical Problems of Performing Artists,* **12**: 23–7

Koutedakis Y, Pacy P, Sharp NCC, Dick F (1996) Is fitness necessary for dancers? *Dance Research* **14**: 105–18

Koutedakis Y, Sharp NCC (1985) Lactic acid removal and heart rate frequencies during recovery after strenuous rowing exercise. *British Journal of Sports Medicine,* **19**: 199–202

Koutedakis Y, Sharp NCC (1990) Fitness assessment of elite competitors. *Rheumatology Now,* **1**: 18–20

Koutedakis Y, Soulas D, Sharp C *et al.* (1999) The effects of 3–5 weeks of holiday on dance–related physiological parameters. *International Journal of Sports Medicine,* in press

Kraemer WJ, Fleck SJ, Evens WJ (1996) Strength and power training: Physiological mechanisms of adaptation. *Exercise Sport Science Review,* **24**: 363–97

Kraemer WJ, Patton J, Gordon SE *et al.* (1995) Compatibility of high intensity strength and endurance training on hormonal and skeletal muscle adaptations. *Journal of Applied Physiology,* **78**, 976–89

Krivickas LS, Feinberg JH (1996) Lower extremity injuries in college athletes; relation between ligamentous laxity and lower extremity muscle tightness. *Archive of Physical Medicine and Rehabilitation,* **77**: 1139–43

Kujala UM, Orava S, Jarvinen M (1997) Hamstring injuries: current trends in treatment and prevention. *Sports Medicine,* **23**: 397–404

Kuno M, Fukunaga T, Hirano Y, Myashita M (1996) Anthropometric variables and muscle properties of Japanese female ballet dancers. *International Journal of Sports Medicine,* **17**(2): 100–5

Lamb DR (1984) *Physiology of exercise* (2nd edition) New York: Macmillan

McAtee RE (1993) *Facilitated stretching.* Champaign, IL: Human Kinetics

McKenzie DC, McLuckie SL, Stirling DR (1994) The protective effects of continuous and interval exercise in athletes with exercise–induced asthma. *Medicine and Science in Sports and Exercise*, **26**(8): 951–6

McNaught BR, Callander R (1990) *Illustrated physiology*. Edinburgh, UK: Churchill Livingstone

Margaria R, Aghemo P, Rovelli E (1996) Measurement of muscular power (anaerobic) in man. *Journal of Applied Physiology*, **21**(5): 1662–4

Micheli LJ, Gillespie WJ, Walaszek A (1984) Physiological profiles of female professional ballerinas. *Clinics in Sports Medicine*, **3**(1): 199–209

Morris FL, Payne WR (1996) Seasonal variations in the body composition of lightweight rowers. *British Journal of Sports Medicine*, **30**(4): 301–4

Newsholme E, Leech T, Duester G (1994) *Keep on running: the science of training and performance*. Chichester, UK: Wiley, p. 350

Newsholme E, Blomstrand E, Ekblom B (1992) Physical and mental fatigue: metabolic mechanisms and importance of plasma amino acids. *British Medical Bulletin*, **48**: 3; 477–95

Nilsson C, Wykman A, Leanderson (1993) Spinal sagittal mobility and joint laxity in young ballet dancers. *Knee Surgery, Sports Traumatology, and Arthroscopy*, **1**: 206–8

Noble BJ (1986) *Physiology of exercise and sport*. St Louis, MO: Times Mirror/ Mosby College Publishing

Norris CM (1994) Flexibility: principles and practice. London: A&C Black

Pacy PJ, Khalouha M, Koutedakis Y (1996) Body composition, weight control and nutrition in dancers *Dance Research*, **14**: 93–105

Paffenbarger RS, Olsen E (1996) *Lifefit*. Champaign, IL: Human Kinetics, p. 50

Pekkarinen H, Litmanen H, Mahlamaki S (1989) Physiological profiles of young boys training in ballet. *British Journal of Sports Medicine*, **23**(4): 245–9

Peterson MS (1986) A comparison of nutrient needs between dancers and other athletes. In: Shell CG, (ed.), *The dancer as athlete*. Champaign, IL: Human Kinetics, 117–21

Ploutz LL, Tesch PA, Biro RL, Dudley G (1994) Effect of resistance training on muscle use during exercise. *Journal of Applied Physiology*, **76**: 1675–81

Reid DC (1988) Prevention of hip and knee injuries in ballet dancers. *Sports Medicine*, **6**(5): 295–307

Rimmer JH, Jay D, Plowman SA (1994) Physiological characteristics of trained dancers and intensity level of ballet class and rehearsal. *Impulse*, **2**(2): 97–105

Rodenburg JB, Steenbeek D, Schiereck P, Bar PR (1994) Warm-up, stretching and massage diminish harmful effects of eccentric exercise. *International Journal Sports Medicine*, **15**(7): 414–19

Romney NC, Nethery VM (1993) The effects of swimming and dryland warm-ups on 100-yard freestyle performance in collegiate swimmers. *Journal of Swimming Research*, **9**: 5–9

Rosenbaum D, Hennig EM (1995) The influence of stretching and warm-up exercises on Achilles tendon reflex activity. *Journal of Sports Sciences*, **13**(6): 481–90

Safran MR, Garrett WE, Seaber AV, Glisson RR, Ribbeck BM (1988) The role of warm-up in muscular injury prevention. *American Journal of Sports Medicine*, **16**(2): 123–9

Sawyer-Morse MK, Smolik T, Mobley C, Saegert M (1989) Nutrition beliefs, practices, and perceptions of young dancers. *Journal of Adolescent Health Care*, **10**: 200–2

Schantz PG, Åstrand PO (1984) Physiological characteristics of classical ballet. *Medicine & Science in Sports Exercise*, **16**: 472–6

Schott J, McCully K, Rutherford OM (1995) The role of metabolites in strength training: Short versus long isometric contractions. *European Journal of Applied Physiology*, **71**: 337–41

Schwane JA, Watrous BG, Johnson SR, Armstrong RB (1983) Is lactic acid related to delayed-onset muscle soreness? *Physician & Sportsmedicine*, **11**: 124–31

Sen C, Grucza R, Pekkarinen H, Hanninen O (1992) Anaerobic power response to simulated warm-up procedures for skiers. *Biology of Sport*, **9**(3): 103–8

Sharkey B (1997) *Physiology of fitness* (4th edition). Champaign, IL: Human Kinetics

Sharp NCC, Karasowitz EG, Harper EM, Shields RS (1966) Canine survival on treatment with hyperbaric oxygen following hepatic artery ligation. *Surgery*, **59**: 255–63

Simoneau JA, Lortie G, Boulay MR *et al.* (1986) Inheritance of human skeletal muscle and anaerobic capacity adaptation to high intensity intermittent training. *International Journal of Sports Medicine*, **7**(3): 167–71

Siri WE (1956) The gross composition of the body. In: *Advances in biological and medical physics*. New York: Academic Press, **4**: 239–80

Sohl P, Bowling A (1990) Injuries to dancers: prevalence, treatment and prevention. *Sports Medicine*, **9**: 317–22

Stalder MA, Noble BJ, Wilkinson JG (1990) The effects of supplemental weight training for ballet dancers. *Journal Applied Sport Science Research*, **4**: 95–102

Stanley DC, Kraemer WJ, Howard RL *et al.* (1994) The effects of hot water immersion on muscle strength. *Journal of Strength and Conditioning Research*, **8**(3): 134–8

To WW, Wong MW, Chan KM (1997) Association between body composition and menstrual dysfunction in collegiate dance students. *Journal of Obstetrics & Gynaecology Research*, **23**(6): 529–35

Torii M, Yamasaki M, Sasaki T (1996) Effect of prewarming in the cold season on thermoregulatory responses during exercise. *British Journal of Sports Medicine*, **30**(2):102–11

Vandenburgh HH, Kaufman S (1983) Stretch and skeletal growth: what is the physical to biochemical linkage? In: *Frontiers of exercise biology*. Champaign, IL: Human Kinetics

van Marken Lichtenbelt WD, Fogelholm M, Ottenheijm R, Westerterp KR (1995) Physical activity, body composition and bone density in ballet dancers. *British Journal of Nutrition*, **74**: 439–51

van Mechelen W (1992) Running injuries. A review of the epidemiological literature. *Sports Medicine*, **14**(5): 320–35

Westblad P, Tsai-Fellander L, Johansson C (1995) Eccentric and concentric knee extensor muscle performance in professional ballet dancers. *Clinical Journal of Sport Medicine*, **5**(1):48–52

Williford HN, East JB, Smith FH, Burry LA (1986) Evaluation of warm-up improvement in flexibility. *American Journal of Sports Medicine*, **14**(4): 316–19

Wolman RL, Clark P, McNally E *et al.* (1990) Menstrual state and exercise as determinants of spinal trabecular bone density in female athletes. *British Medical Journal*, **301**: 516–18
Young A, Dinan S (1994) Fitness for older people. *British Medical Journal*, **309**: 331–4

Part III
THE HEALTHY DANCER

Introduction

According to the World Health Organization, *health is a state of complete physical, mental and social well-being*. This complex of factors, that represents the spectrum of vitality, goes beyond the traditional view of health which, for thousands of years, was perceived as *merely the absence of disease or infirmity*. However, the practice of placing illness (or injury) on one side of a rather narrow line and health on the other is still alive and kicking. Most dancers, for instance, see health simply as the absence of any serious skeletal, joint and/or muscle injuries which prevent them from doing their classes, rehearsals and, of course, performances.

In response to this traditional point of view, most of the available literature in dance medicine and science has almost exclusively referred to injuries and their treatment. The result has been the creation of a treatment-oriented culture within the dance world which, by definition, pays little attention to the prevention of injuries, and/or to other components of health and fitness such as overtraining (or burnout), body weight control and exercise-induced asthma. Therefore, the main aims of this chapter are to (1) introduce a selection of relevant health components to dancers and their teachers, (2) compare medical and health problems seen in dancers with those seen in sport, and (3) assess the present state of the art of dance medicine and science. It is hoped that the reader will appreciate that dancers are indeed 'performing athletes', and that dance, like sport, involves a number of health risks which may develop into disabling conditions if no or inappropriate action is taken. The reader will also understand that dance medicine and science are in a healthy state and growing. However, for better or worse, 'tradition' may inhibit the pace of development in areas which are not universally thought of in a dance context.

Chapter 7

Overtraining—Burnout

Yiannis Koutedakis

1 SUMMARY

Data on overtraining (or burnout) in dancers and the causes of it are currently limited. However, there is no doubt that the condition does exist, and that it may well account for the increased number of early retirements, injuries, minor but frequent illnesses, and reduced performances, both in the class and on stage. Most of the relevant information comes from sport. According to this, the stress of increased volumes of physical work—in conjunction with social, economic, academic and fitness problems—can overload the mechanisms of adaptation to exercise and can cause undesirable hormonal, immunological and neural changes. Acute or short-term overtraining must be distinguished from chronic or long-term overtraining that can lead to more severe and prolonged side-effects. It should be emphasized that many and complex changes are caused by severe exercise, and that these represent adaptive responses to exercise and training and are part of normal physiology. To prevent or reverse overtraining, there needs to be tailoring of physical (dance) quality and quantity, diet, good hydration, physical rest and sleep according to the individual needs and levels of fitness.

2 INTRODUCTION

The positive relationships between practice or physical training and performance in the field (or on the stage) have been documented since the time of classical Greece. What has only recently been appreciated is the concept of a threshold of physical activity beyond which further increases may result in a deterioration of both health and performance.

In the last 15–20 years, the idea that *the more you put in the more you get out*, together with the ever increasing demands for better performances, have forced preparation for dance to become virtually a year-round endeavour. However, as many dancers have learned to their cost, the path to successful performances is strewn with risks as well as benefits. These risks include the fact that very high quantities and/or intensities of physical stress (i.e. dance) may overload the physiological mechanisms of adaptation, and make dancers experience feelings of constant fatigue, lethargy, frequent respiratory tract infections, and reduced physical performance. Indeed, more than 2000 years ago, the father of modern medicine, Hippocrates of Cos (c. 469–399 BC), wrote, 'the physical conditioning is at risk when exercise is at very high levels'.

Both health and physical performance may be further affected if excessive exercise training is employed during the vulnerable pre-adolescent stages. Supporting this observation, Aristotle (*Politics*, Book VIII) wrote that 'the disadvantages of excessive (systematic) training in early years are amply proved by the list of Olympic victors, not more than two or three of whom won a prize both as boys and as men. The discipline to which they were subjected in childhood undermined their powers of endurance'.

The exact point where 'training' becomes 'overtraining' is difficult to define. It is known, however, that the frequency and intensity of exercise undertaken in a given time are among the factors that determine the adaptations to training. Disproportional increases in either frequency or intensity of physical work may overload the mechanisms of adaptation, creating havoc in the muscle tissue, upsetting the body's immunity and harassing the delicate balance of the hormonal system.

3   DEFINITION OF TERMS

The terms 'overtraining' (also referred to as 'overtraining syndrome', or 'burnout', or 'overwork'), 'staleness', 'chronic fatigue' (or 'chronic fatigue syndrome') and 'post-viral fatigue' are interchangeably used to describe the condition where active individuals:

- Complain of reduced physical performances, for no apparent medical or other obvious reasons (Wilmore and Costill 1988)
- Suffer from constant fatigue (Lehman, Lormes, Optitz-Gress *et al.* 1997)
- Show behavioural and emotional changes (Kuipers and Keizer 1988)

Although the above terms are used by many as synonyms to describe more or less the same condition—that is, poor physical performances, coupled with chronic and unexplained fatigue and certain behavioural changes—the condition itself may have different origins, or be triggered by different chains of events. Historically, chronic fatigue as a presenting complaint in the absence of other identifiable organic illness was seldom reported before the second half of the nineteenth century, when it spread in an almost epidemic-like manner. An interesting feature was, however, that this epidemic was largely limited to women of the middle and upper classes (Shorter 1993), celebrated for their rather loose connection with tasks requiring physical effort. By the time of the First World War, chronic fatigue was a common complaint in the industrialized world. The term 'chronic fatigue syndrome' was introduced in the 1930s when the (same) main symptoms remained persistent for at least six consecutive months. Depending on the country, chronic fatigue is further known as 'neuromyasthenia' (USA), or 'myalgic encephalomyelitis'—ME (UK). Whatever the term employed, chronic fatigue has become an increasingly common complaint in most countries. In the 1980s, at least 20% of British adults said that they had 'always felt tired' in the previous month (Cox, Blaxter, Buckle *et al*. 1987).

Although the causes of the classical chronic fatigue are still unclear, the main triggering element of overtraining is not. In this circumstance, fatigue and the consequent underperformance in physical tasks are somehow linked to increased volumes and levels of exercise training. In other words, overtraining describes a condition indicating an imbalance between habitual exertion and recovery, with severe and prolonged fatigue resulting. Unlike the chronic fatigue syndrome, 'overtraining' is a relatively new entry in the medical vocabulary, with the confirmed cases spreading worldwide in line with the popularity (and demands) of sport and dance.

Post-viral fatigue is close to overtraining, as it is also characterized by identifiable source(s): (1) a virus infection having preceded the condition, and/or (2) inadequate recovery from infection, before returning to demanding training and exercise schedules.

4 FACTORS CONTRIBUTING TO OVERTRAINING

Clinically, overtraining is a complex condition of indeterminate cause with a range of symptoms and signs varying from person to person. This interpersonal variability can also affect the factors that may contribute to the development of the condition. These factors may include:

- Increased physical work and training
- Lack of optimal recovery
- Personality characteristics (e.g. overachievers)
- Fitness levels
- Type of activity (i.e. 'individual' vs 'team' activities)
- External factors (e.g. media attention, financial difficulties)

In general, overtraining tends to occur in dancers during periods of increased commitments in class or on stage and with proportionally less time for *recovery*. In fact, it has been suggested that optimal recovery should be an integral part of any programme designed to improve fitness and physical performance (Keast and Morton 1992). But, why might lack of optimal recovery from exercise lead to overtraining?

Following intense dance, for example, microdamage to body structures (mainly in muscle) needs to be repaired to prevent further, more serious damage in subsequent workouts. At the same time, more contractile proteins must be laid down so that the muscles can produce greater forces, more energy-production enzymes must be synthesized for muscles to work harder without becoming fatigued, and more oxygen has to be supplied to the energy-production sites via a sufficiently developed capillary network. However, for the muscle to succeed in these 'repair' and 'growth' (adaptation) processes, an appropriate length of time is required where little or no physical activity takes place. This seems to last about 24 hours after exercise, when muscle protein synthesis reaches its highest rates. Fig. 7.1 shows the relationship between exercise load and recovery during which positive changes (i.e. adaptations) in key physical performance parameters—such as strength, power and endurance—occur. Inadequate recovery may negatively affect the mechanism of adaptation and, therefore, levels of fitness and health.

Although ordinary individuals are not immune from imbalances

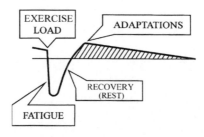

Fig. 7.1 Following recovery, the tissues adapt to tolerate higher exercise loads, that is the dancer is in a higher state of fitness

between physical activity and recovery from it, athletes, as well as dancers at different levels of competence, have produced most of the reported cases of overtraining. This is partly associated with the long-held belief that there is a linear relationship between volumes of work and performance in the field or on the stage, hence the well known saying *no pain, no gain*. However, this is true only up to a certain point, beyond which further increase in training and exercise volumes brings about reductions in physical performance (Fig. 7.2). Steinacker (1993) has cautioned that if active individuals undertake very high volumes of exercise and training (more than 1000 hours per year), even work at moderate levels may be perceived to be hard and excessive.

Individuals most prone to reach the stage of overtraining or burnout are the very highly motivated, the overachievers, those who set ultra-high standards for themselves. They tend to train conscientiously through injury and illness as long as performances do not suffer. In committed dancers, feelings of guilt quickly emerge if a day or two passes without a certain number of hours of practice in the studio, as they

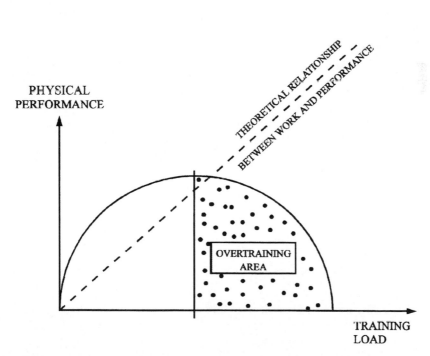

Fig. 7.2 A model showing relationships between exercise training, performance and overtraining

mistakenly believe that lack of practice, even for short periods of time, may negatively affect their dance performance. Indeed, preliminary data have indicated that 3–5 weeks of rest (summer holidays) after the end of a professional season have actually led to increases in most dance-related performance parameters, such leg strength (Koutedakis, Soulas, Sharp *et al.* 1999). Once again, this finding stresses two important factors: (1) that rest should not be treated as negative influence, and (2) that fatigue—and perhaps overtraining before the rest period—may prevent dancers from showing their true potential.

Relatively low levels of *physical fitness* as well as the 'type' of the activity in question may also play an important role in the development of overtraining. For the same workload, fitter persons are working relatively more easily than their unfit counterparts (Hendrickson and Verde 1994). Also, *individual* activities (e.g. running, cycling, swimming and dance) are likely to produce more cases of overtraining than team events such as basketball and volleyball.

External factors (or stresses) such as *family* and *personal relationships, media attention, conditions at work,* and *financial difficulties,* may further contribute to cases of overtraining. Unfortunately, the response to any setback in physical performance is often to increase the volume and intensity of exercise training in a misguided attempt to recover lost ground. As Fig. 7.3 illustrates, failure to break the circle of poor perform-

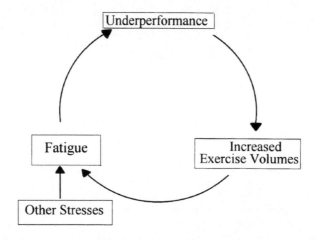

Fig. 7.3 The response to setbacks in physical performance is often to increase the training volume and intensity. This causes fatigue and, together with the influence of other external stresses, may further detract from performance

ance, increased excrcise volume, external stresses and fatigue may cause much unhappiness and even blight career prospects.

5 DIAGNOSIS OF OVERTRAINING

Given that no simple or specific tests have been developed to date, diagnosis has traditionally been reserved for the elite athlete or the professional dancer because of their arduous work schedules. Affected individuals are directed towards medical help by their coaches or dance teachers, because of feelings of constant fatigue and unexplained underperformance. When no underlying disease can be found from medical history, clinical examination or routine haematology and biochemistry, overtraining may be tentatively diagnosed. Diagnoses should normally be supported by: (1) the coach/teacher, team or company physician and the individual involved reporting a reliable history of at least 2–3 weeks of reduced rates of recovery following exercise training, with no overt cause apart from increased workloads or competition/performance frequency; and (2) a cluster of particular symptoms and signs such as loss of motivation for physical work, loss of appetite and body weight, and increased susceptibility to infections. Some psychological tests may offer an additional tool in verifying overtraining.

6 SYMPTOMS

In physically active individuals such as dancers, fatigue is part of the expected response to daily exercise routines. Consequently they may accept it as normal or their complaints may fall on unsympathetic ears and prevent them from communicating this element of supposed weakness. However, dancers are different from other patients complaining of fatigue in that they have an objective measure of the symptom, their physical performance. When feelings of constant fatigue and poor class and stage performance are simultaneously present, then other symptoms have to be considered. These are rather non-specific and subjective and may vary from dancer to dancer. Symptomatology may include (Budgett 1990):

- Excessive sweating
- Inability to recover optimally following intensive dancing
- Loss of desire and enthusiasm for dance (feelings of helplessness)
- Breakdown of technique
- Poor concentration

- Loss of appetite, and loss of body weight
- Disturbed sleep often with nightmares or vivid dreams
- Increased need to visit the toilet at night
- Increased susceptibility to injuries
- Increased anxiety and irritability
- Signs of depression

7 SIGNS

As in the case of symptoms, there are no consistent signs on clinical examination or laboratory testing associated with overtraining. For present purposes, the reported signs have been grouped according to those indicating *acute overtraining* (lasting for up to one month), and those related to *chronic overtraining* (lasting for many weeks or months).

7.1 Acute Overtraining

Acute overtraining (also known as 'short-term overtraining' or 'physical overstrain') is the result of an imbalance between exercise and recovery over a period of just a few days or weeks. It occurs when sudden increases in exercise-training load are introduced in order to meet emergency needs such as new productions, last-minute changes due to injuries, and so on. Very often this demanding work has to be completed in the presence of a number of external stressors (e.g. academic, social, economic). However, the effects of this type of overtraining quickly disappear, when the reasons for causing it are removed. The most common signs include (Dressendorfer 1985; Jeukendrup and Hesselink 1994; Wilmore and Costill 1988):

- Increased normal resting heart rates by 5–10 beats per minute
- Increased resting blood pressure
- Raised resting lactic acid concentrations
- Decreased maximal lactic acid levels following intensive physical exercise
- Following specific dance routines, heart rate recovery to resting levels may take 2–3 times longer than normal
- Decreased ability by the body to utilize oxygen during maximal exercise
- Muscle damage

Muscle damage is perhaps the most common outcome of acute overtraining, indicating that the body is not ready to accommodate large volumes of work (normally due to lack of fitness), or that the muscular work exceeds the capabilities of the muscles in question, or both. For example, exercise enthusiasts participating in marathon racing often feel the results of acute overtraining soon after the end of their race, by experiencing severe muscular pain and fatigue lasting for several days, or even weeks. Acute overtraining at the muscle level may be related to one or more of the following:

- Increased acidity
- Mechanical damage to the muscle cell
- 'Metabolic failure' (i.e. extreme reductions in *phosphocreatine*—PC
- *Free-radical* damage to muscle regulatory proteins; the longer and harder the exercise, the higher the free-radical levels in the muscle

7.2 Chronic Overtraining

Chronic overtraining (or 'long-term overtraining' or 'overtraining syndrome') is the result of imbalances between exercise and recovery over a period of weeks or months. It occurs in individuals who: (1) are highly motivated; (2) have relatively inadequate levels of fitness; and/or (3) are primarily involved in 'individual' activities (e.g. swimming, running, dance). When the condition is fully developed, the following signs may appear in addition to some of the signs mentioned in the previous section (Koutedakis, Frischnecht, Vrobova *et al.* 1995; Sharp 1993; Sharp and Koutedakis 1992; Parry-Billings, Budgett, Koutedakis *et al.* 1992):

- Menstrual irregularities, even cessation of menstruation
- Increased susceptibility to infections, especially of the skin and upper respiratory tract
- Increased rates of allergies
- Minor scratches may heal slowly
- Loss of maximal voluntary muscle strength

Barron and Noakes (1985) suggested that the overtraining syndrome is due to hypothalamic-pituitary dysfunction, as may be the case in very active women who frequently develop menstrual irregularities. However, menstrual irregularities may also be secondary to reduced body-fat stores in such women, and therefore to lower energy reserves (Dueck, Manore and Matt 1996).

As will be described in the next section, the second, third and fourth signs above clearly indicate a lowering of the body's resistance to infection, that is *immune system* malfunction. It is now widely recognized that excessive exercise can have detrimental effects on many aspects of immune function. The last of the listed signs seems to be more related to impairment of 'central' (i.e. brain) rather than 'peripheral' (i.e. muscle) mechanisms, and it will also be discussed separately.

8   OVERTRAINING AND THE IMMUNE SYSTEM

It is widely known that moderate exercise with optimal resting intervals causes either no changes to, or enhances the functions of the immune system. However, exhausting exercise and/or busy dance timetables tend to produce adverse changes in these functions, particularly if strenuous physical activity is accompanied by other environmental and professional stressors. If exercise is pursued to the level of overtraining, the immune system may be chronically affected. This can have substantial negative implications for many aspects of immune function, including lowered resistance to acute infections, HIV infections, and even cancer (Berglund and Hemmingsson 1990; Shephard and Shek 1994).

The first scientific papers showing relationships between intense exercise training and the susceptibility to illness appeared early in the twentieth century. In 1918, Cowles noted that virtually all cases of pneumonia at a boys' school occurred in pupils engaged in sport, and that simple respiratory infections could escalate to pneumonia after physical effort which resulted in increased muscular fatigue. With the advances in medicine and pharmacology, this relationship between exercise and susceptibility to illness was dismissed as coincidental, until the 1970s when fitness was established as being among the basic ingredients for healthy life. The massive participation in exercise and sport, and the expansion of exercise science that followed, reconfirmed the original negative relationship between high volumes of exercise and immune function. For instance, it has been found that ultramarathon runners may exhibit increased symptoms of upper respiratory infections (Peters and Bateman 1983), and that athletes who run more than 100 km a week are twice as likely to exhibit infectious illness than individuals who average less than 32 km per week (Nieman, Johanssen, Lee and Arabatzis 1990). Preliminary data on dancers have indicated that even short, but very intensive bouts of exercise, can negatively affect important aspects of the chemical defence mechanism of innate immunity (Koutedakis and Perera 1998). Such changes may then impair the dancers' natural immunity and increase susceptibility to infection for a short period after exercise.

There is no universal agreement as to what might be the actual mechanism which links increased physical exercise and the reported incidence of infections in athletes. However, Parry-Billings, Budgett, Koutedakis *et al.* (1992) provided evidence in support of the hypothesis that the susceptibility to infections following periods of increased exercise training may be due to lower plasma *glutamine* levels found in overtrained individuals.

Glutamine is a non-essential amino acid produced in the muscle. It is required for the biosynthesis of the rapidly dividing cells of the immune system, while it is also used as a fuel to generate a substantial part of the energy required by this system (Newsholme, Crabtree and Ardawi 1985). It becomes obvious therefore, that an optimal supply of this amino acid is an important tool against illness, whereas low levels may lead to frequent infections and a worsening cycle of poor physical performances. Athletes suffering from chronic overtraining appear to maintain low plasma glutamine levels for months or years.

During exercise, plasma glutamine concentrations may increase, decrease or remain unchanged depending on the type, duration and intensity of exercise. Lowered plasma glutamine has been observed following prolonged physical efforts leading to glycogen depletion. The lowest concentration of plasma glutamine is seen about 2 hours after such efforts, and it takes more than 7 hours to return to pre-exercise resting levels. Therefore, prolonged exercise (and thus less recovery time) may be associated with a lower capacity to synthesize glutamine. Commercially available glutamine supplements may be utilized as a short-term solution of the overtraining problem, as recent data suggest a link between this supplement and lower infection rates following prolonged exercise (Castell, Poortmans and Newsholme 1996; Castell and Newsholme 1997).

9 OVERTRAINING AND LOSS OF MUSCLE STRENGTH

In individuals suffering from chronic overtraining, loss of maximal voluntary muscle strength is amongst the confirming signs. It could be said therefore, that the reduced physical performance reported for such individuals might be the result of a loss of the ability voluntarily to produce high values of muscle strength.

The development of large muscle forces (i.e. strength and power) is a complex mechanism that depends on multiple steps leading from the central nervous system (i.e. motor cortex in brain), via the nerves, to the actual activation of muscle. However, muscle strength may be affected even though muscle function is not impaired, as evidenced by a normal ability to respond to external electrical stimulation. This has led to the development of the 'central-fatigue' hypothesis to explain reduced outputs during voluntary muscular exercise in overtrained individuals. This hypothesis is also in line with reported data which show an impairment of the brain's central motor-drive in chronic fatigue syndrome sufferers (Stokes, Cooper and Edwards 1988).

Koutedakis and colleagues (1995) tested this hypothesis by examining whether overtrained elite athletes were able to recruit all their motor units during a 12-second *isometric* maximal voluntary contraction (MVC). During the last 6 seconds of the contraction, an electrical stimulation was superimposed on the exercising muscle by a computerized muscle stimulator. Fig. 7.4 gives us an example of the main findings of

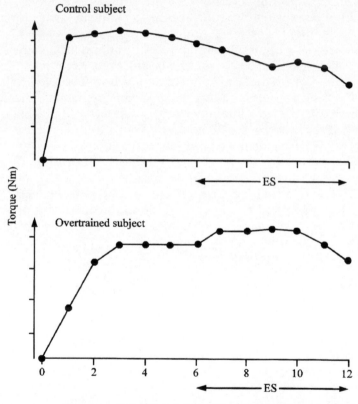

Fig. 7.4 The effect of electrical stimulation (ES) superimposed on an isometric maximal voluntary contraction of the quadriceps muscle from a healthy control (top) and an overtrained (bottom) subject

Source: From Koutedakis, Frischnecht, Vrbova and Sharp Vol. 19, International Journal of Sports Medicine (1995). Reproduced by permission of Georg Thieme Verlag

this study. The electrical stimulation superimposed upon a healthy control subject did not increase the performance of the quadriceps during the isometric maximal contractions. This subject seems, therefore, to be voluntarily able to fully activate his muscles. However, in the overtrained subject, the added electrical stimulation increased the quadriceps torque, revealing an inability to voluntary activate all his muscle fibres. It was concluded that these data fit with the idea of an impaired central drive in the brain as an explanation for muscular weakness in overtrained individuals.

10 SEASONAL VARIATIONS IN OVERTRAINING

It has been mentioned in this section that overtraining in dancers may be developed in two seemingly similar forms: (1) *acute overtraining* lasting from a few days to a month; and (2) *chronic overtraining* lasting for several weeks or months. The former can occur during periods of sudden increase of physical activity both in the class and on stage, and may emerge at any time. Acute overtraining may be diagnosed at the start, middle or end of the season, and—in line with relevant information from sport—demonstrate no particular seasonal pattern. But what about chronic overtraining?

As with many aspects related to science and medicine in dance, there is a lack of information on possible patterns followed by occurrence of overtraining, in relation to professional dance seasons. Yet knowledge of such variation is very useful in an attempt to prevent or minimize its occurrence.

In sport, many investigators have described the effects of seasons or periods of competition, training, detraining, and reduced training on aspects of physical fitness (Koutedakis, 1995). Depending on performance level, type of sport, and the fitness parameter in question, the reported swings may be as high as 18% from one season to another. Seasonal variations also exist in medical conditions, which may interrupt or prevent normal training and competition. Athletes are more likely to develop an injury and/or become overtrained during their competition and pre-competition cycles, compared to preparation phases (Koutedakis and Sharp 1998).

The same authors also found that neither the type of physical activity nor the sex of participants affected the seasonal variation of injuries and overtraining. Indeed, given that the ability to perform in sport is determined more by training and biological potential than by gender, it is the duration, frequency and intensity of exercise training which affect performance in both males and females. Marked increases in duration, frequency or intensity of physical work may overload adaptation mechanisms, thus leading to increased rates of injury and overtraining, mainly through overuse and fatigue respectively.

Similar overtraining patterns to those found in sport may also apply in dance. The fact that dancers are more likely to become overtrained towards the end of their professional season is supported by some preliminary data on female ballet dancers (Koutedakis, Soulas, Sharp *et al.* 1999). It has been reported that 3–5 weeks of rest after the end of a professional season is associated with increases in most dance-related fitness parameters, such as flexibility and leg power and strength. It is possible that fatigue, and perhaps, overtraining before the resting period, prevented dancers from showing their true fitness potential. However, reduced ability to reach fitness potential not only affects dance performance, but also brings dancers closer to a potential injury (Koutedakis, Khaloula, Pacy *et al.* 1997).

11   DIET AND OVERTRAINING

Poor diet could potentially be one of the dancers' worst enemies. According to the relatively limited data on the effects of diet on overtraining, calorie deficiency (Aakvaag 1985) as well as vitamin and iron deficiency (Beek 1984) have been identified as precipitating factors. For example, lack of muscle fuel (i.e. glycogen) may lead to rapid fatigue, and may predispose to prolonged fatigue and overtraining. Also, some vitamins, especially the *antioxidant* vitamins C, D and E, may possibly have a role to play in the function of the immune system.

Full hydration should always be among the dancer's priorities since dehydration is an important cause of fatigue and underperformance. It is advisable for a diary to be kept of food and drink, which will serve the dual purpose of highlighting any deficiencies and educating the dancer.

12   PREVENTION OF OVERTRAINING

Unfortunately, there is no objective test or method that can be reliably used to detect those dancers who may become overtrained during periods of increased and/or prolonged commitments in the class and on stage. It should be remembered, though, that the longer the history of fatigue before any measure is taken (e.g. cessation or reduction of exercise), the longer it takes to recover, while drop in performance is often a late signal to avoid a prolonged period of fatigue and its deleterious effects.

With this in mind, dancers should primarily try to avoid the physical and psychological stresses mentioned earlier in this chapter. Where possible, enriching their lives with other mental and physical interests than dance alone is perhaps the best strategy to prevent overtraining in the long term. Dancers should never attempt to increase physical loads suddenly, and a steady increase of up to 5% per week is the optimal work- and training-dose for most active individuals. Furthermore, dancers should introduce, if possible, weekly cycles of activity, where 'heavy' weeks of work are followed by the occasional 'easier' week.

Once a case of overtraining has been diagnosed and dealt with, there is a danger of relapse at around 3 months (Budgett 1990). Therefore, it is advisable that a reduced or 'controlled' amount of dance-related stresses (e.g. classes, rehearsals, etc.) should be maintained for up to 4 months. Even if there are no overtraining problems, it is still recommended for dancers to have at least a month's break from hard work each year, to allow full recovery in terms of repairing all the tissue microtraumas and to mentally and physically prepare the body for the new season.

13 MANAGEMENT OF OVERTRAINING

Dancers and other athletes have a different perception of life compared to what is regarded as 'normal'. In particular, signs of a possible illness or injury do not worry them as long as they feel positive about the future and dance commitments are met. It is only when the latter suffer that help is sought, by which time the dancer may be in a crisis from which he or she sees little or no escape. This is their most vulnerable time as they may become difficult individuals to deal with. They can become aggressive, they are unused to being ill (as opposed to injured) and desperately in need of a treatable cause to their malaise. When the cause is found, treatment itself must be quick, painless and preferably administered within a dance studio. However, it does not always work like that.

The concept *'no pain no gain'* should be played down in the dancers' phraseology, as there is normally little gain to be made by working through fatigue, illness or injury. Although extremely rare, working through viral infections may sometimes cause serious problems that include damaged *myocardium*, resulting in possible cardiac arrhythmia. Research has clearly demonstrated that periods of physical rest (or periods of reduced physical activity) may result in a drop in the incidence

of infectious illness, and may, therefore, contribute to physical performance improvements in active, but tired individuals. This rest period
should be 3–5 weeks long for optimal recovery from spells of overtraining (Koutedakis, Budgett and Faulmann 1990), during which 'mono-
tonous' types of exercise training should be avoided (Kuipers and Keizer
1988). However, dancers should be aware that it is possible to produce
premature and unexplained personal best performances 'out of the blue'
before apparent complete recovery. If that happens, it gives the wrong
recovery signals, work restarts in full swing, and a reoccurrence of
overtraining is likely to manifest itself.

Apart from rest, other regeneration techniques may also be used. These
techniques include reduction of all stresses through counselling and
sleep, in conjunction with the use of saunas, massage, aromatherapy,
hydrotherapy and, of course, dietary advice.

14 CONCLUSIONS

There is no objective early test that can reliably detect those dancers
who will go overboard and become overtrained during periods of
increased exercise training. Although very difficult to implement,
'undertraining' (or reduced training) is better than overtraining, and
this seems to be the best way to avoid prolonged fatigue and everything it entails. To prevent or reverse overtraining, there needs to be
tailoring of dance quality and quantity, diet, good hydration, physical
rest and sleep according to the individual needs and levels of fitness.
An exciting area of dance medicine and science research will be to
define the anatomic parameters and the exercise doses that cause
overtraining, and to devise fitness examinations and training programmes that will allow maximal performance with minimal overload
risk. The development of specific psychological tests, or further valida-
tion of existing ones, should also be incorporated in future dance
medicine and science research.

15 FURTHER READING

Ciba Foundation (1993) *Chronic fatigue syndrome*. Chichester, UK: Wiley.
Koutedakis Y, Sharp NCC (1998) Seasonal variations of injury and overtraining in
    elite athletes. *Clinical Journal of Sports Medicine*, **8**(2): 131–7
Koutedakis Y, Soulas D, Sharp C *et al.* (1999) The effects of 3–5 weeks of holiday
    on dance-related physiological parameters. *International Journal of Sports Medi-
    cine*, in press

Kuipers H, Keizer HA (1988) Overtraining in elite athletes: Review and directions for the future. *Sports Medicine*, **6**: 79–94
Sharp C, Koutedakis Y (1992) Sport and the overtraining syndrome: immunological aspects. *British Medical Bulletin*, **48**(3): 518–533
Watson RR, Eisinger M (eds) (1992) *Exercise and disease*. Boca Raton, FL: CRC Press
Wilmore JH, Costill DL (1988) *Training for sport and activity* (3rd edition). Dubuque, IA: Wm. C. Brown, pp. 195–200

REFERENCES

Aakvaag A (1985) Hormonal response to prolonged physical strain, effect of calorie deficiency and sleep deprivation. In: Fotherby B, Pal C (eds), *Exercise endocrinology*. Berlin: de Gruyter: pp. 25–64
Barron GL, Noakes TD (1985) Hypothalamic dysfunction in overtrained athletes. *Journal of Clinical Endocrinology and Metabolism*, **60**(4): 803–6
Beek vander EJ (1984) Effects of marginal vitamin intake on physical performance in man. *International Journal of Sports Medicine*, **5**(Suppl): 28–31
Berglund HP, Hemmingsson P (1990) Infectious disease in elite cross-country skiers: a one-year incidence study. *Clinical Sports Medicine*, **2**: 19–23
Budgett R (1990) Overtraining syndrome. *British Journal of Sports Medicine*, **24**: 231–6
Castell LM, Newsholme EA (1997) The effects of oral glutamine supplementation on athletes after prolonged, exhaustive exercise. *Nutrition*, **13**(7–8): 738–42
Castell LM, Poortmans JR, Newsholme EA (1996) Does glutamine have a role in reducing infections in athletes? *European Journal of Applied Physiology*, **73**(5): 488–90
Cox B, Blaxter M, Buckle A et al. (1987) *The health and lifestyle survey*. London: Health Promotion Research Trust: pp. 61–2
Cowles WN (1918) Fatigue as a contributory cause of pneumonia. *Boston Medical & Surgery Journal*, **179**: 555
Dressendorfer RH (1985) Increased morning heart rate in runners: a valid side of overtraining? *Physician and Sportsmedicine*, **11**: 93–100
Dueck CA, Manore MM, Matt KS (1996) Role of energy balance in athletic menstrual dysfunction. *International Journal of Sports Nutrition*, **6**(2): 165–90
Hendrickson DC, Verde TJ (1994) Inadequate recovery from vigorous exercise. *Physician & Sportsmedicine*, **22**(5): 56–8, 61, 62, 64
Jeukendrup AE, Hesselink MKC (1994) Overtraining—what do lactate curves tell us? *British Journal of Sports Medicine*, **28**(4): 239–40
Keast D, Morton AR (1992) Long-term exercise and immune functions. In: Watson RR, Eisinger M (eds), *Exercise and disease*. Boca Raton, FL: CRC Press: pp. 121–48
Koutedakis Y (1995) Seasonal variations in fitness parameters in competitive athletes. *Sports Medicine*, **19**: 373–92
Koutedakis Y, Budgett R, Faulmann L (1990) Rest in underperforming elite competitors. *British Journal of Sports Medicine*, **24**: 248–52
Koutedakis Y, Frischnecht R, Vrbova G, Sharp C (1995) Maximal voluntary quadriceps strength patterns in Olympic overtrained athletes. *Medicine & Science in Sports & Exercise*, **27**(4): 566–72

Koutedakis Y, Khaloula M, Pacy PJ *et al.* (1997) Thigh peak torques and lower-body injuries in dancers. *Journal of Dance Medicine & Science,* **1**(1): 12–15

Koutedakis Y, Perera S (1998) The effects of intensive exercise on salivary lysozyme in trained individuals. *Kinesiology,* in press

Koutedakis Y, Sharp NCC (1998) Seasonal variations of injury and overtraining in elite athletes. *Clinical Journal of Sports Medicine,* **8**(1): 18–21

Koutedakis Y, Soulas D, Sharp C *et al.* (1999) The effects of 3–5 weeks of holiday on dance-related physiological parameters. *International Journal of Sports Medicine,* in press

Kuipers H, Keizer HA (1988) Overtraining in elite athletes: Review and directions for the future. *Sports Medicine,* **6**: 79–94

Lehmann MJ, Lormes W, Optitz-Gress A *et al.* (1997) Training and overtraining: an overview and experimental results in endurance sports. *Journal of Sports Medicine & Physical Fitness,* **37**(1): 7–17

Newsholme EA, Crabtree B, Ardawi MSM (1985) Glutamine metabolism in lymphocytes: its biochemical, physiological and clinical importance. *Journal of Experimental Physiology,* **70**: 473–89

Nieman DC, Johanssen LM, Lee JW, Arabatzis K (1990) Infectious episodes in runners before and after the Los Angeles marathon. *Journal of Sports Medicine & Physical Fitness,* **30**(3): 316–28

Parry-Billings M, Budgett R, Koutedakis Y *et al.* (1992) Plasma amino acid concentrations in the overtraining syndrome: possible effects on the immune system. *Medicine and Science in Sports and Exercise,* **24**(12): 1353–8

Peters EM, Bateman ED (1983) Ultramarathon running and upper respiratory tract infections. *South African Medical Journal,* **64**: 582–4

Steinacker JM (1993) Physiological aspects of training in rowing. *International Journal of Sports Medicine,* **14**: S3–S10

Sharp C (1993) Immunological aspects of exercise, fitness and competition sport. In Macleod DAD, Haughan RJ, Williams C *et al.* (eds), *Intermittent high intensity exercise; preparation, stresses and damage limitation.* London, UK: E and FN Spon

Sharp NCC, Koutedakis Y (1992) Sports and the overtraining syndrome: immunological aspects. *British Medical Bulletin,* **48**(3): 518–33

Shephard RJ, Shek PN (1994) Potential impact of physical activity and sport on the immune system—a brief review. *British Journal of Sports Medicine,* **28**(4): 247–55

Shorter E (1993) Chronic fatigue in historic perspective. In: *Chronic fatigue syndrome* (Ciba Foundation Symposium 173). Chichester, UK: Wiley: pp. 6–16

Stokes MJ, Cooper RG, Edwards RHT (1988) Normal muscle strength and fatigability in patients with effort syndrome. *British Medical Journal,* **297**: 1014–17

Wilmore JH, Costill DL (1988) *Training for sport and activity* (3rd edition). Dubuque, IA: Wm. C. Brown: pp. 195–200

Chapter 8

Asthma and Dance

Ray Carson

1 SUMMARY

Asthma is a lung disease that involves reversible narrowing of the airways. It can be caused by a variety of agents, such as *allergens*, or by exercise. It is now known that asthma is an inflammatory disease of the walls of the airways. The incidence and severity of asthma is increasing in the population, but the reasons for this are not yet known. Exercise-induced asthma has a higher incidence among active individuals. However, mild to moderate asthma does not necessarily affect physical performance. Carefully designed exercise programmes and the use of warm-up routines before a performance can reduce the risk and severity of exercise-induced asthma. A range of drugs is available which can effectively treat the symptoms of asthma. The correct use of medicaments can enable asthmatic dancers to perform to their full potential.

2 INTRODUCTION

Asthma is on the increase in developed countries. Both the incidence of asthma and its severity have escalated in recent years. In a survey carried out in 1991/92 in the UK nearly 10% of the population sample had or had had asthma, with an even higher figure among children (Dept. of Health 1995a). Asthma now causes over 1600 deaths per year, and the total number of deaths has increased over the last two decades. The underlying reasons for these increases are not known, but some theories will be discussed later. As well as the personal costs of this disease, there is also an increasing cost to society—the total cost of prescriptions was £350 million in 1993 (Dept. of Health 1995a).

3 DEFINITION OF ASTHMA

Asthma may be defined as *a clinical syndrome characterized by widespread airway obstruction, which is reversible either spontaneously or with treatment* (Montefort and Holgate 1991). The important point is that the airway or bronchial tube narrowing must be shown to be reversible in a true case of asthma. However, a wheezy or persistent cough is sometimes wrongly perceived as asthma, particularly in children.

It has been known for some time that asthma is predominantly an allergic disease. *Atopic* (or susceptible) individuals often show several symptoms of allergy, such as eczema, hay fever and rhinitis (runny nose), as well as asthma. However, it is also known that asthma is a chronic inflammatory disease. In susceptible individuals, the walls of the airways become inflamed, causing constriction and making them *hyperreactive*. This is the most common form of asthma known as *extrinsic* asthma, but there is also *intrinsic* asthma, where the cause is unknown; *exercise-induced* asthma, where exercise causes asthma symptoms; and *occupational* asthma associated with irritants (Fig. 8.1).

4 DIAGNOSIS

4.1 Extrinsic Asthma

This usually begins in early childhood in susceptible individuals. The usual symptoms are wheezing, shortness of breath and a persistent cough. Often there are other symptoms of allergy such as hay fever and

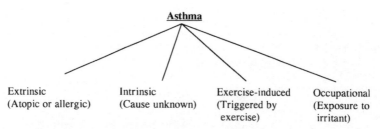

Fig. 8.1 Known types of asthma

cczema. A simple lung function test of measuring the *peak expiratory flow rate* (PEFR) may confirm a reduction in peak flow due to airway narrowing. A *spirometer*, such as a Vitalograph, can be also used to measure the effective lung capacity, known as the *vital capacity* (VC), and also the *volume of air exhaled in the first second of a forced expiration* (FEV$_1$). The VC is usually not affected in mild asthma, but the FEV$_1$ may be reduced compared to 'normal' values (Fig. 8.2). The reduction in the volume exhaled in the first second indicates airway narrowing. It should be emphasized again that the airway obstruction should be shown to be reversible for a definitive diagnosis of asthma. Often a few puffs from a Ventolin® inhaler are given to the patient and the test repeated after 10 minutes, to see if expiration increases. It is also usual for the patient to be referred for skin tests to establish which substances, if any, they may be allergic to. Grass pollen, the faecal pellets of the house dust mite and animal fur are some of the main culprits.

Fortunately, extrinsic asthma that begins in childhood often abates in adulthood. Over half of children with mild asthma will 'grow out' of it by the time they are 21 years of age (Rees and Price 1995). The mechanism by which this occurs is not understood at all. The important point is that a history of childhood asthma should not necessarily impede an adult dancer, as by the time a dancer reaches adult performing age they would probably be free of symptoms.

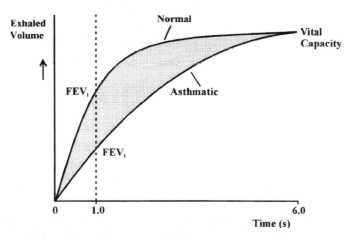

FEV$_1$: (Forced expiratory volume in the first second) is the volume of air that can be exhaled during the first second of a maximal expiration

Fig. 8.2 Example of Vitalograph recordings. The shaded area indicates typical differences between asthmatic and normal individuals

4.2   Intrinsic Asthma

Intrinsic asthma usually has a late onset, often in middle age. There may be no associated allergy and the cause is often unknown. The symptoms are the same, but the severity of the condition is often greater than that of the extrinsic type.

4.3   Exercise-induced Asthma

Exercise-induced asthma can occur in anyone at any time. It is more common in children, and some adults are more susceptible than others. The usual symptoms are wheezing, shortness of breath, tightness in the chest and coughing, following vigorous exercise. If these only occur after exercise then this suggests exercise-induced asthma, rather than the other types. A controlled exercise test can be performed in a Chest Clinic to confirm the diagnosis.

4.4   Occupational Asthma

Occupational asthma usually presents as the usual symptoms when exposed to a causative agent at the workplace. There may be a pattern of feeling unwell at work with an improvement at weekends or during holidays (not uncommon!). It should be stressed that it involves long-term exposure to a causative agent such as a solvent. It may be possible to identify the agent quite simply. Some good detective work in a Spanish port recently identified that the cause of regular increases in asthma incidence and severity throughout the city was due to dust from grain ships loading and unloading. Over 5% of cases of adult asthma may be linked to an occupational cause, and more than 200 possible agents have been identified. It should be stressed that prolonged exposure to such agents is necessary for symptoms to develop. Agents that are relevant to dancers, during rehearsal, performance and class, might include wood dust, cotton dust, solvents used in glues, hair sprays, and fungal spores.

5   DISEASE MECHANISMS

Exercise-induced asthma may be of most relevance to dancers. The mechanisms involved here have not been resolved and are still hotly debated. The main theory is that during exercise the lungs are physically vibrated, which causes mast cells in the walls of the airways to disrupt, releasing their inflammatory mediators and causing transient broncho-constriction (Hough and Dec 1994). An alternative theory is that during exercise heat is lost from the lungs, which may cause temporary *vasocon-striction* of blood vessels supplying the walls of the airways. Then after the exercise a reflex increase in blood flow may cause swelling of the airway walls and airway obstruction (McFadden and Gilbert 1994). A third theory is that water lost by evaporation during exercise may cause the walls of the airways to absorb fluid from the blood, leading to swelling and airway obstruction (Weiler 1996). Cold air stimulates irri-tant receptors in the walls of the airways. Normally inhaled air is warmed and moistened by passing through the nasal cavities, but during exercise, mouth breathing occurs to get air into the lungs more quickly. In a cold studio, this inhaled cold air has direct access to the airways and stimulates the irritant receptors, causing reflex bronchoconstriction.

In general, asthma has been the subject of intense and quite well-funded medical research for the past 30 years. A great deal is now known about the mechanisms involved at the cellular and molecular level but there are still many unknowns. The interested reader with some know-ledge of biology is referred to some recent, comprehensive review articles (Barnes 1996; Rees and Price 1995).

Normally, the internal surface of the airways is protected by a contin-uous lining of *epithelial* cells covered in a layer of mucus (Fig. 8.3). This usually prevents the penetration of allergens into the walls of the air-ways. Recently, it has been shown that in asthmatics, damage to the *epithelium* allows the penetration of allergens into the walls of the airways (Djukanovic, Roche, Wilson *et al.* 1990). This damage also exposes nerve endings, which makes the airway super-sensitive or 'hyperreactive' to noxious stimuli. It has been suggested that pollutant gases, such as nitrogen dioxide, ozone and sulphur dioxide could dissolve in the fluid lining the airways and damage the epithelium. Also, these gases are known to trigger *bronchoconstriction* at quite low concentrations by acting on irritant receptors in the airways (Dept. of Health 1991, 1992, 1993). In other words, asthma is characterized by a number of chemical proce-dures, as well as 'neural' aspects.

5.1 Chemical Process

The first time an antigen or trigger substance penetrates the wall of an airway it is picked up by a cell of the immune system called an *antigen presenting cell*. This cell 'presents' the antigen to a *Th$_2$-helper T cell* that recognizes it as being 'foreign'. The Th$_2$ cell stimulates *B cells* to produce an *antibody* called *immunoglobulin E* (IgE), which coats the walls of cells

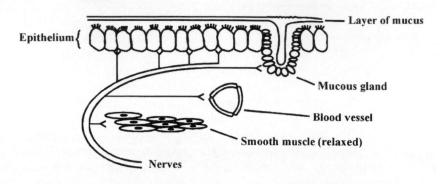

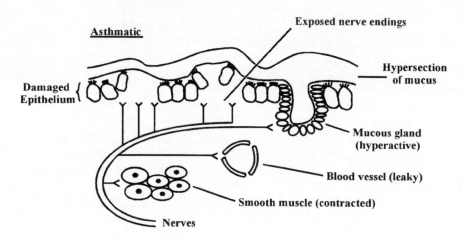

Fig. 8.3 Longitudinal sections through small airways in normal and asthmatic individuals

such as *mast cells* and *eosinophils*. From now on, any subsequent exposure to the allergen is detected by these sensitized IgE coated cells, which are then activated. The mast cells contain granules of stored *inflammatory mediators*, such as histamine. When activated, the membrane surrounding the cell is disrupted causing the release of the stored inflammatory mediators as well as the production of more of them. Inflammatory mediators are a range of reactive molecules, such as *prostaglandins*, which contract smooth muscle, cause tissue damage, make capillaries more 'leaky' and stimulate nerve endings. The nerve stimulation causes reflex constriction of the airways and activates the mucous glands, producing excess mucus secretion that further obstructs the airways. It is now well established that this 'chronic inflammatory process' is the main mechanism involved in asthma (Barnes 1996). The main causal allergens identified are the faecal pellets of house dust mites, grass pollen, tree pollen, fungal spores and animal fur.

5.2 Neural Aspect

The main nerve supply to the smooth muscle in the walls of the airways belongs to either the *sympathetic* or the *parasympathetic nervous system*. Activation of the sympathetic nervous system causes relaxation of the smooth muscle and dilation of the airways, via the release of *noradrenaline*. The sympathetic system may be activated by nervousness, or before vigorous exercise, producing the so-called 'fight or flight response', and prepares the lungs for exercise. Longer-term stress and anxiety tend to activate the opposing parasympathetic nervous system, causing constriction of the airways. It is quite possible for anxiety or panic to induce or exacerbate an asthma attack.

6 EFFECTS ON PERFORMANCE

It is important to emphasize the point that being asthmatic, having a history of asthma or being diagnosed as asthmatic does not necessarily affect performance. Some Olympic gold-medal-winning athletes are asthmatic (Enright 1996). For a professional dancer, developing exercise-induced asthma does not mean that it is time to hang up the shoes.

In order to understand how asthma might affect performance, we will have to delve into some lung physiology at this point. Each person's lung capacity is determined genetically and is related to their height, gender, age and ethnic origin. The role of the lungs in exercise is obviously to supply enough oxygen for the exercising muscles and to excrete the waste carbon dioxide produced. Most physiologists agree that lung capacity is not a common limiting factor in exercise performance (Harries 1994). The limiting factor is the heart and blood vessels, as they set the rate of delivery of oxygen to the muscles via the blood. Thus the rate of delivery of oxygen is dependent on the blood flow, which in turn depends on the heart. The heart can only beat so fast, and each person has a maximum heart rate, which is roughly equal to 220 minus their age in years. In contrast, the lungs have a huge reserve that we rarely fully use even during maximal exercise. At rest we use about one tenth of the lungs' capacity. To illustrate this, it is possible to measure the volume inspired and expired, and the flow rate generated during a breath, using a device called a *pneumotachograph*. A typical recording is shown in Fig. 8.4, and I hope that this emphasizes that—even at maximal exercise—not all of the 'envelope' of lung capacity and flow rate is normally utilized.

Asthma has to be quite severe before it will affect submaximal performance. In mild asthma the vital capacity is usually not affected. However, in chronic asthma, the continuous inflammation causes a gradual reduction in lung capacity, because the walls of the airways thicken, the lung tissue becomes less elastic, and air is trapped in smaller airways by mucus plugs. Peak flow is affected in all forms of asthma, as

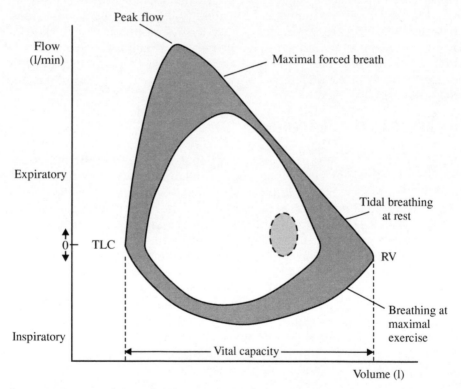

TLC: Total lung capacity (full inspiration)
RV: Residual volume (full expiration)

Fig. 8.4 Flow-volume loops. The flow-volume loop at maximal exercise does not normally occupy the entire available envelope, so some lung capacity is still reserved (shaded area)

any narrowing of the airways will cause a reduction in the maximal flow rate possible through them. An analogy is to compare a narrow hosepipe with a fire hose. The fire hose has a much greater diameter and can deliver a much greater volume of water per minute than could a garden hosepipe. The flow rate through a tube is proportional to the radius of the tube to the power of 4. Therefore if the radius of a tube is halved this causes a 16-fold reduction in flow rate. By far the most numerous airways in the lungs are the small airways, which have a diameter of less than 2 millimetres. Because they are numerous and narrow they contribute the greatest resistance to airflow in the lung. Unfortunately, asthma tends to affect these very airways at an early stage, producing the clinical symptoms known as wheezing. Although a person suffering an asthma attack appears to be fighting to get air in, the real problem is the difficulty of breathing out through the narrowed airways.

Obviously severe asthma will substantially limit exercise capacity, but mild asthma may not affect moderate levels of exercise too greatly. Some dance may involve moderate aerobic exercise over prolonged periods of time, although at other times it may be very strenuous. There do not appear to be any specific studies of asthma in dancers. A recent study of figure skaters found that about one third of the group studied had exercise-induced asthma (Mannix, Farber, Palange *et al.* 1996), but this did not appear to affect their performance. This relatively high incidence may have been due to exposure to cold air above the ice rink. A recent review estimated that up to 14% of athletes exhibit exercise-induced asthma (Enright 1996). A study of children with mild to moderate asthma found that they showed no significant difference in exercise performance compared to healthy controls (Santurz, Baraldi, Filippone and Zacchello 1997). Interestingly, the main determinant of their exercise tolerance was found to be the level of physical conditioning.

It has been known for some time that exercise-induced asthma can affect peak performance of elite athletes (Voy 1986). The condition may not be immediately apparent, and symptoms such as poor performance, fatigue and shortness of breath may be blamed on an upper respiratory tract infection or poor fitness levels.

7 PREVENTION

Prevention is always better than cure. There are ways of preventing or minimizing the symptoms of asthma, in which education and sensible precautions have a role to play.

7.1 Minimize Exposure to Specific Allergens

In extrinsic asthma, often a triggering allergen, or allergens, has been identified by skin tests. If this is the case, then every precaution should be taken to avoid or minimize exposure to the specific allergens. This is not as easy as it sounds. For example, most people would find it difficult to give away a pet dog or cat, if they found they were allergic to the fur. It is impossible to avoid exposure to grass or tree pollen, without a mask, in the summer. Microscopic house dust mites are present in every home, no matter how clean the owner may be. They live in soft furnishings, mattresses, carpets and curtains, and unfortunately they thrive in modern, centrally heated, double-glazed homes. Their faecal pellets are so small that they are difficult to filter out effectively. The mite-proof bedding which is commercially available may be of some benefit. Also, the specially developed anti-mite sprays can be used on bedding to some effect (Rees and Price 1995). Regular cleaning to prevent dust collecting would be beneficial, and special medical vacuum cleaners with a fine filter are available.

7.2 Minimize Lung Vibrations and Cold Environments

Lung vibrations in conjunction with cold, dry air are known to be amongst the causative agents in exercise-induced asthma. Avoiding these conditions would be beneficial. For example, going for a run on hard pavements or roads on a frosty morning is about the worst thing possible to do. Running on soft surfaces such as grass would be better and the use of good running shoes or trainers is essential. As an alternative to running, cycling involves less vibration and can be conducted indoors on an exercise bicycle in warm, moist air. It has been known for some time that swimming can be beneficial for asthmatics and is probably the least likely form of exercise to cause exercise-induced asthma (Bar-Or and Inbar 1992). One reason for this could be the inhalation of warm, moist air, although some asthmatics may react to chlorine in the water, and immersing the face in cold water triggers the diving reflex which can cause *bronchoconstriction*. On the whole, swimming can be a valuable part of preparation and training programmes for the asthmatic.

Dance performance is often energetic, and will obviously involve vibration of the lungs, which could cause exercise-induced asthma. It may be impossible to avoid this, but there are possible ways of minimizing the severity of the bronchoconstriction caused. Good shoes and dance surfaces can reduce the transmission to the lungs of impacts on landing. For the asthmatic dancer the use of warm-up routines may significantly decrease post-exercise bronchoconstriction. A study by McKenzie, McLuckie and Stirling (1994) showed that a warm-up of 15 minutes at fairly high intensities significantly reduced post-exercise bronchoconstriction in moderately trained athletes. It is thought that moderate exercises may actually cause *bronchodilation*, as an adaptation of the lungs that improves their efficiency. Exercise training appears to reduce the harmful bronchial obstruction response and increases the beneficial bronchodilator response. In a study of 14 elite athletes with asthma, Todaro (1996) found evidence for bronchodilation after exercise. However, intensive endurance training has been found to cause exercise-induced asthma. Helenius, Tikkanen and Haahtela (1997) suggested that long-distance runners had a greater risk of developing exercise-induced asthma than speed and power athletes. The suggested reasons for this were prolonged hyperventilation and thus increased exposure to allergens and irritants.

7.3 Always Warm-up

It has been known for some time that athletes with exercise-induced asthma have a refractory period after exercise, during which further exercise causes little bronchoconstriction (Weiler, 1996). This refractory period can last 1–4 hours, but it may not occur in all individuals. The asthmatic dancer may be able to make use of this by exercising (i.e. warming-up) at a level that does not induce bronchoconstriction for about 20 minutes before a performance. The mechanism responsible for this is not fully understood. However, breathing exercises, yoga, meditation and hypnosis can be useful in preventing exercise-induced asthma. The use of aerobic dance has even been suggested as therapy for mildly asthmatic patients (Wolf and Lampl 1988).

7.4 Avoid Smoking

All types of smoke are irritant to the airways, therefore asthmatics should avoid prolonged exposure to smoky environments (Rees and Price 1995). It cannot be emphasized enough that smoking, both active and passive, is highly detrimental to asthmatics and should be strongly discouraged. There is ample evidence that smoking increases the rate of decline in lung function with age in people with atopy (Connellan, Carson, Holland *et al.* 1981a,b), and in healthy individuals (Scott, Douglas, Sullivan and Carson 1985). There is also evidence that dancers have a high incidence of smoking.

8   TREATMENT

Fortunately, most types of asthma can be effectively treated and managed for the majority of the time. Some very effective drugs have been developed which are efficient at relieving the symptoms of asthma. These include the β-agonist drugs, steroid drugs, cromones, xanthines and anticholinergic drugs:

- The mainstays of the pharmacological treatment are the *β-agonist* drugs. Their name comes from the fact that these drugs act on special sites, termed *β-receptors*, on the surface of smooth muscle cells in the walls of the airways. Binding of drug molecules to these receptors interferes with the contraction mechanism in the smooth muscle cells, leading to relaxation. Therefore the administration of β-agonists causes bronchodilation and counteracts the bronchoconstriction of asthma. The most widely used drug of this type in Britain is salbutamol, which has a variety of trade names, such as Ventolin®. Other similar drugs in use are terbutaline, albuterol and fenoterol. One of the disadvantages of these drugs is that they have a short half-life (2–3 hours), and so regular doses are required (Page, Curtis, Sutter *et al.* 1997). However, longer acting β-agonists are now available, such as salmetorol, aformoterol and bambuterol. All of these drugs are usually administered by inhalation, either by an aerosol inhaler ('puffer') or via a nebulizer. This route of administration directs the drugs to the required site of action and minimizes systemic side-effects. In severe asthma they can be given orally as tablets or during an asthma attack intravenously for a rapid effect.
- Steroid drugs are currently the second most common type of treatment, often given in combination with β-agonists. Now that it is well established that asthma is an inflammatory disease, the use of steroids to 'dampen down' the underlying inflammation is a sensible approach. It could be argued that it is better to use steroids to treat the disease itself rather than β-agonists which really only treat the symptoms. Some researchers argue that the widespread use of β-agonists has contributed to the increase in severity of asthma (Page and Costello 1992). The theory behind this is that bronchoconstriction is a defence reaction which prevents an allergen from penetrating deeper into the lungs. By artificially dilating the airways with β-agonists, this could allow an inhaled allergen or irritant to reach the smaller airways, causing more widespread inflammation. Steroid drugs reduce inflammation by blocking an enzymatic biochemical pathway, which normally gives rise to inflammatory mediators. The most common steroids prescribed are beclomethasone (trade name

Becotide™), budesonide, fluticasone and prednisolone. For severe asthma, these drugs can be given orally, but they then have widespread side-effects. For mild to moderate asthma, steroids can be administered via an inhaler. It should be emphasized that they should be taken regularly and that the benefits may not be immediately apparent.

- A family of drugs which are very effective for preventing exercise-induced asthma are the cromones, such as sodium cromoglycate (trade name Intal) nedocromil sodium and ketotifen. They can be inhaled as a powder and must be taken before exercising, as they are preventive, and are not a treatment. However, used correctly they have virtually no side-effects and can completely obliterate exercise-induced asthma, and have allowed asthmatic athletes to win Olympic gold medals. A recent study showed the efficacy of an inhaled dose of 4 mg of nedocromil sodium in reducing exercise-induced bronchoconstriction in athletes (Valero, Garrido, Malet *et al.* 1996). The mechanism of action of cromones is not completely known, but one effect is that they stabilize the membranes of mast cells, preventing them from degranulating and releasing the inflammatory mediators, which cause the bronchoconstriction.

- Another useful family of drugs is the methyl xanthines, such as theophylline. These are given orally in severe asthma and cause bronchodilation by relaxing bronchial muscle. The problem with theophylline is that it has serious side-effects, such as speeding up the heart rate, while the plasma levels should be monitored regularly.

- Anticholinergic drugs are another useful family of drugs for some types of asthma. They are toxic compounds, but when given by inhalation very little of the drug is absorbed into the circulation to cause side-effects. They are useful when the asthma is caused by irritation of the airways or is associated with stress and panic attacks.

As well as drugs, dietary factors may be involved. Some vitamins, such as vitamin C and vitamin E, have an 'antioxidant' role in the body, and they mop up so-called *free radicals*. Free radicals are highly reactive molecules that are produced during the inflammatory process and cause cell damage. There is evidence for the involvement of free radicals in asthma (Barnes 1996; Dept. of Health 1995b), and therefore these vitamins might be expected to be beneficial. A recent study found evidence that a (quite large) dose of 2.0 g of vitamin C gave some protection from exercise-induced asthma (Cohen, Newman and Nahum 1997).

9 CONCLUSIONS

Asthma does not necessarily affect exercise performance, if it is mild to moderate in severity. Dancers are at greater risk of developing exercise-induced asthma, which can be minimized by fitness training exercises such as swimming or aqua-aerobics. Also, the use of warm-up exercises prior to performance can reduce the chance of exercise-induced asthma occurring. Effective drugs are available, which can alleviate the symptoms of asthma and can allow the asthmatic dancer to excel.

10 FURTHER READING

Dept. of Health (1995a) *Asthma. An epidemiological overview*. London: HMSO: pp. 2–20

Dept. of Health (1995b) *Asthma and outdoor air pollution*. London: HMSO: pp. 3–55

Enright T (1996) Exercise-induced asthma and the asthmatic athlete. *Wisconsin Medical Journal*, **95** (6): 375–8

Rees J, Price J (1995) *ABC of asthma*. London: BMJ (3rd edition)

Voy RO (1986) The US Olympic Committee experience with exercise-induced bronchospasm. *Medical Science Sports and Exercise*, **18**: 328–30

Wolf SI, Lampl KL (1988) Pulmonary rehabilitation: the use of aerobic dance as a therapeutic exercise for asthmatic patients. *Annals of Allergy*, **61** (5): 357–60

REFERENCES

Barnes PJ (1996) Pathophysiology of asthma. *British Journal of Clinical Pharmacology*, **42**: 3–10

Bar-Or O, Inbar O (1992) Swimming and asthma. Benefits and deleterious effects. *Sports Medicine*, **14** (6): 397–405

Cohen HA, Newman I, Nahum H (1997) Blocking effect of vitamin C in exercise-induced asthma. *Archives of Pediatric Adolescent Medicine*, **151** (4): 367–70

Connellan SJ, Carson R, Holland F, Joyce H, Pride NB (1981a) Role of atopy in determining susceptibility of smokers to chronic airway narrowing. *Thorax*, **36**: 716–17

Connellan SJ, Carson R, Holland F, Joyce H, Pride NB (1981b) Role of bronchial hyperreactivity and atopy in enhancing decline of lung function in male smokers. *European Journal of Respiratory Diseases*, **62** Suppl. 113: 130–1

Dept. of Health (1991) *First Report: ozone*. London: HMSO

Dept. of Health (1992) *Second Report: sulphur dioxide, acid aerosols and particulates* London: HMSO

Dept. of Health (1993) *Third Report: oxides of nitrogen. Advisory group on the medical aspects of air pollution episodes*. London: HMSO

Dept. of Health (1995a) *Asthma. An epidemiological overview*. London: HMSO: pp. 2–20

Dept. of Health (1995b) *Asthma and outdoor air pollution*. London: HMSO: pp. 3–55

Djukanovic R, Roche WR, Wilson JW, Beasley CRW, Twentyman OP, Howarth

PH, Holgate ST (1990) Mucosal inflammation in asthma. *American Review of Respiratory Diseases*, **142**: 434–57

Enright T (1996) Exercise-induced asthma and the asthmatic athlete. *Wisconsin Medical Journal*, **95** (6): 375–8

Harries M (1994) Pulmonary limitations to performance in sport. *British Medical Journal*, **309**: 113–15

Helenius IJ, Tikkanen HO, Haahtela T (1997) Association between type of training and risk of asthma in elite athletes. *Thorax*, **52** (2): 157–60

Hough DO, Dec KL (1994) Exercise-induced asthma and anaphylaxis. *Sports Medicine*, **18** (3): 162–72

McFadden Jr ER, Gilbert IA (1994) Exercise-induced asthma. *New England Journal of Medicine*, **330**: 1362–77

McKenzie DC, McLuckie SL, Stirling DR (1994) The protective effects of continuous and interval exercise in athletes with exercise-induced asthma. *Medical Science Sports and Exercise*, **26** (8): 951–6

Mannix ET, Farber MO, Palange P, Galasetti P, Manfredi F (1996) Exercise-induced asthma in figure skaters. *Chest*, **109** (2): 312–15

Montefort S, Holgate ST (1991) Asthma as an immunological disease. *Medicine International*, **89**: 3699–702

Page C, Costello J (1992) Controversies in respiratory medicine: regular inhaled beta-agonists—clear clinical benefit or a hazard to health? (2). Why beta-agonists should not be used regularly. *Respiratory Medicine*, **86** (6): 477–9

Page CP, Curtis MJ, Sutter MC, Walker MJA, Hoffman BB (1997) *Integrated pharmacology*. London: Mosby: pp. 233–40

Rees J, Price J (1995) *ABC of asthma*. London: BMJ (3rd edition)

Santurz P, Baraldi E, Filippone M, Zacchello F (1997) Exercise performance in children with asthma: is it different from that of healthy controls? *European Respiratory Journal*, **10** (6): 1254–60

Scott GE, Douglas RB, Sullivan KR, Carson R (1985) *Pulmonary function of firemen: a follow-up study*. London: Home Office

Todaro A (1996) Exercise-induced bronchodilation in asthmatic athletes. *Journal of Sports Medicine and Physical Fitness*, **36**(1): 60–6

Valero A, Garrido E, Malet A, Estrush A, Gispert J, Rubio E (1996) Exercise-induced asthma prophylaxis in athletes using inhaled nedocromil sodium. *Allergol Immunopathology (Madrid)*, **24** (2): 81–6

Voy RO (1986) The US Olympic Committee experience with exercise-induced bronchospasm. *Medical Science Sports and Exercise*, **18**: 328–30

Weiler JM (1996) Exercise-induced asthma: a practical guide to definitions, diagnosis, prevalence and treatment. *Allergy and Asthma Proceedings*, **17**: 315–25

Wolf SI, Lampl KL (1988) Pulmonary rehabilitation: the use of aerobic dance as a therapeutic exercise for asthmatic patients. *Annals of Allergy*, **61** (5): 357–60

Chapter 9

Body Weight Control

Paul Pacy

It is my firm belief that human society is divided into three distinct castes: Russian dancers, dancers, and very ordinary people   (Haskell 1979)

1 SUMMARY

This chapter explores a number of issues related to body weight and body weight control. The information provided includes general principles and basic concepts, as well as practical advice, and is designed to allow dancers to make informed choices concerning their optimal diet and lifestyle.

2 INTRODUCTION

It is hoped that the information in this chapter will prove valuable, not only to the professional dancer, but also to all individuals engaged in dance. However, before focusing on the various aspects involved in body weight control in dancers two general issues need addressing.

First, it is abundantly clear that the body weight of the average UK citizen, in common with that of all developed countries, is constantly on the increase. The frequency of obesity has risen by over 50% in both males and females since 1980 and now accounts for approximately 14% of males and 17% of females. This has been associated with a parallel decline in physical activity by the population at large. Higher standards of living and affluence have been accompanied by marked reductions in physical activity and energy expenditure, as individuals increasingly adopt a sedentary lifestyle. It has been estimated that the amount of television watching has doubled since the 1960s to about 28 hours per week. Several large fitness and health surveys conducted in the early 1990s make for depressing reading. For instance it has been revealed that in the month before one questionnaire survey, over 80% of the population had not walked continuously for 2 miles; 90% had not cycled, while only 20–30% had been involved in physical activity of any kind (Prentice and Jebb 1995).

A second issue is that professional dancers appear to have been subjected to much less rigorous scientific interest and scrutiny than is the case with their athletic counterparts. This relates to all aspects of dance, not merely nutrition.

There is an obvious contrast with sport, where many innovations (from training techniques to equipment changes) have been made in the last 20 years as a consequence of increasing scientific understanding. This 'revolution' has resulted in tremendous increases in athletic performance, as well as bringing substantial financial rewards. To match these, there has to be a desire within the dance community to ask why things are done as they are, and whether there is not some way of improving them. In addition, and perhaps even more importantly, there must be an ability to answer the questions posed, which is the whole basis of scientific debate. It is hoped that the general principles outlined in this chapter will contribute to relevant knowledge in body weight control in dancers.

3   ELEMENTS OF BODY WEIGHT—BODY FAT

Many individuals, particularly in the world of professional sport and dance, feel they need information about their body composition. Simply this means how much of one's body weight is fat—usually measured in percentage—and how much is non-fat. The *fat-free mass* mainly comprises muscle and bone, together with organs such as liver, heart, lungs, and so on.

This subdivision of weight into fat and fat-free mass is crude, but remains widely used. The same applies to the relevant measurements. As discussed in Part II (Chapter 5), although there are many ways to measure fat and fat-free mass (ranging from simple *skinfold thickness* measures to sophisticated and expensive techniques such as *magnetic resonance imaging*), none are perfect. It is also important to appreciate that body composition values are, at best, an approximation, so dancers should not be too concerned with small differences. Furthermore, in individuals such as dancers who tend to be very lean, body fat measures are prone to greater error than in sedentary non-lean individuals (Pacy, Cox, Khalouha *et al.* 1996).

The vast majority of the published body-fat data in dancers come from ballet, where typical values range from about 17% in females (Clarkson, Freedson, Keller *et al.* 1985), to about 11% in males (Hergenroeder, Fiorotto and Klish 1991). In general, female dancers, like other women, normally have a higher percentage of body fat than their male counterparts of the same height and weight; similarly males have higher non-fat values than females. Given that muscle is the main non-fat body component, and that it uses relatively high portions of energy during both rest and exercise, differences in body composition partly explain why males use more calories than females, weight for weight.

4 ARE THERE IDEAL BODY WEIGHTS?

Dancers frequently ask 'what is my ideal body weight?' The answer depends on many factors including what is meant by the term 'ideal'. For instance, the weight of an individual which is likely to minimize the long-term risk to health may well be very different from the weight that the dancer needs to attain for a particular role. In addition, there are queries about how the weight is actually made up (fat versus non-fat components), where the fat is deposited (central versus peripheral distribution), as well as what is the gender and age of the individual in question. Therefore, it becomes clear that the answer to 'what is my ideal body weight?' is not straightforward. Let's now briefly describe one of several ways in which weight is categorized.

4.1 Body Mass Index

If one is asked to describe what a 57 kg (9 stone) female or male looks like it soon becomes apparent that until the height of the individual is known any description is meaningless. If the 57 kg man were 1.98 m (6 ft 6 in.) then he would be very thin, while if he were only 1.30 m (4 ft 3 in.) he would be exceedingly fat. This example highlights the need to consider height when making any valid judgement about ideal body weight.

The most frequent weight:height relationship used for categorizing weight by nutritionists and doctors is the *body mass index* (BMI) which was first described by the Belgium astronomer/mathematician Quetelet in the late 1860s. The BMI (or 'Quetelet's index') represents the weight in kilograms (kg) divided by the height in metres squared (m^2). Thus, the BMI of a dancer who is 1.7 metres (5 ft 7 in.) and weighs 57 kg (9 st) is:

$$\frac{57}{1.7^2} = \frac{57}{1.7 \times 1.7} = \frac{57}{2.89} = 19.7 \text{ kg/m}^2$$

When the MBI is used, neither the sex nor the age of the individual influences its calculation. This means that, in the above example, it does not matter whether the dancer was male or female, young or old. However, it is not advisable to use BMI in children below 16.

How is BMI categorized and how does it relate to ideal body weight? Again there is no universal consensus, but the recent guidelines from Scotland (Table 9.1) are practical, particularly for those in the dance profession. Using the example of the dancer who is 1.7 m (5 ft 7 in.) tall, and using height and ideal BMI range (18–24.9) to estimate weight, the ideal body weight, for both males and females, ranges between:

$$1.7^2 \times 18 = 52 \text{ kg} \qquad \text{to} \qquad 1.7^2 \times 24.9 = 72 \text{ kg}$$

Embarking on a body weight control programme, it is advisable to set the lower value as a target to reach up to for individuals who are considered too lean with the upper value as a goal to come down to for those who are overweight. Targets must be attainable, which is more likely if the weight change required is kept to a minimum.

Table 9.1 The five most commonly used categories of body mass index (BMI)

BMI (kg/m^2)	Category
Less than 18	Lean
18–24.9	Normal
25–29.9	Grade 1 obesity
30–40	Grade 2 obesity
Greater than 40	Grade 3 obesity

5 FACTORS AFFECTING BODY WEIGHT

As already mentioned in Part I (Chapter 1), the body weight of an individual reflects the difference between the total amount of energy expended in a given time (day or year) and the total amount of energy absorbed in this time, which is related to food intake. Thus, factors that effect *total energy expenditure* (*TEE*) and *total energy intake* will influence body weight, and both will be considered briefly. However, it should be stressed that TEE represents the sum of several components, the three most important of which are:

- *Resting energy expenditure* (REE) which represents the energy expended lying quietly on a bed at a thermoneutral temperature, while awake and not having eaten for about 12 hours. This accounts for about 60–70% of TEE and although itself greatly influenced by body weight, it is nevertheless relatively constant from day to day
- *Postprandial thermogenesis* which represents the increase in energy expended each time one eats. This represents about 10% of TEE
- *Exercise-induced thermogenesis* or the increase in energy expended each time one undertakes exercise. This is variable, but represents between 15 to 20% of TEE

Factors that affect any of these three components will obviously have an impact upon TEE—and therefore body weight—and those influencing REE are the most powerful. These factors range from habitual exercise, hormones and drugs to genetic factors and the food consumed.

Physical activity influences REE as does energy (i.e. food) intake. In terms of REE, several experts have suggested that extended participation in aerobic exercise (long steady state activity such as cycling, or swimming) increases underlying metabolism. However, the amount of exercise required to do this is very large and beyond the capacity of most individuals, including dancers (Pacy, Cox, Khalouha, Elkin, Robinson and Garrow 1996). But what about the effect of exercise and appetite? Work undertaken about 40 years ago suggested that even modest amounts of exercise resulted in significantly lower energy intake compared to no exercise, or to very vigorous activity. Despite extensive experimental work, it has been proved difficult to confirm this, and many authorities are unconvinced of an appetite-suppressing effect of mild exercise.

Instead, drugs which suppress appetite (anorectic agents) have been introduced in the battle for weight loss. *Amphetamines* have long been recognized to do this but have many serious side-effects and should never be used. More recently, drugs such as fenfluramine and dexfenfluramine have been used to aid weight loss in the obese, but have lately been withdrawn from use owing to serious side-effects. In the last few years much work has focused on the substance *leptin* (derived from a Greek word for 'thin') which has been shown to control weight in animals by regulating appetite.

Certain *hormones*, especially *thyroxine*, from the thyroid gland, can also affect REE and, hence, body weight. More specifically, thyroxine stimulates energy expenditure. However, it also promotes appetite and thus energy intake, but to a lesser degree. Individuals with an overactive thyroid usually show weight loss, despite increased appetite and evidence of excess metabolism (sweating, tremor and hyperactivity).

Occasionally thyroxine tablets have been given to promote weight loss, but this practice is highly dangerous.

Apart from the scientifically researched factors that affect body weight, there is a number of myths that are associated with the ever-increasing efforts to comply with society's standards of leanness. One of them is *cigarette smoking*. Many dancers claim that smoking helps them control their weight. Is there any validity in this belief?

Smoking does increase energy expenditure, to a very small extent, but is unlikely to have a great impact on weight control. Certainly established smokers tend to have lower weights than non-smokers or recent ex-smokers. However, this might reflect the tendency of ex-smokers to increase their habit of 'snacking' and a possible appetite-suppressing effect of smoking. Lower weight in smokers might also reflect the detrimental effects smoking has on health. Indeed, the vast majority of health professionals are in no doubt that cigarette smoking, including passive smoking, is extremely dangerous for health and well-being. Despite this, a worrying trend for young people to smoke has recently been established. In 1996, 28% of boys aged 15 and 33% of girls were regular smokers. Ideally, the dance environment should be made smoke free.

6 THE ROLE OF NUTRITION

A 1990 International Congress on Sports Nutrition reported that: 'Diet significantly influences athletic performance. An adequate diet, in terms of quantity and quality before, during and after training and competition will maximize performance.' There is little doubt that such sentiments are equally true for dance. The obvious question is what forms an 'adequate' diet.

It cannot be emphasized strongly enough that while it is easy to ask important questions relating to diet, nutrition and dance, it is much harder to provide answers. There are many reasons for this, several of which are listed below:

- Dancers differ from each other in the amount of energy (calories) and nutrients they require
- The absorption of nutrients may differ between individuals and even within the same person at different times
- Most nutrients have more than one function in the body, so which should be taken to determine optimal intake? (e.g. the amount of vitamin C to prevent scurvy is different from that thought to help prevent colds)

- There is a lack of a universally accepted definition of optimal health in dance

Nutritionists have devised *dietary reference values* (DRVs), which represent attempts to assess the adequacy, or otherwise, of diets of both individuals and populations (for more information see Part I, Chapter 2). The use of the term reference is not accidental, but highlights the fact that such values must not, and should not, be interpreted as representing recommended or even desirable intakes, although this is frequently done. DRVs are guidelines and need to be used as such. In addition it needs to be remembered that DRVs apply to relatively healthy sedentary individuals.

The food we eat consists of two broad categories, namely *macronutrients* (carbohydrate, protein, fat and alcohol) and *micronutrients* (vitamins and trace elements). The energy component of the diet is contained in the macronutrients. Nevertheless, there are no deficiency signs or symptoms associated with lack of either fats (with the extremely rare exception of *essential fatty acids* and possible fat-soluble vitamin deficiencies) or carbohydrates (sugars or starches). Theoretically therefore, there are no requirements for these dietary components. However, given that fats and carbohydrates are major contributors to overall energy intake, and that weight loss is a direct consequence of inadequate intake of energy, these two macronutrients play the major role in body weight control.

Matters are different regarding proteins, vitamins and minerals which, if consumed in insufficient quantities, will ultimately lead to signs and symptoms of a specific nutrient deficiency. Again, it should be emphasized that all DRVs for proteins, vitamins and trace elements/minerals should be treated with caution and viewed as indications of nutrient requirements.

6.1 Food for Energy

'Why do we need food?' is another frequent question. However, as with most seemingly simple questions there is a potentially large number of correct answers, which in part reflects the questioner's interest. In purely biological terms we need food to provide us with the *energy* that our bodies need for life. It is very important to understand that we are not inanimate objects; even when we appear to be doing nothing, we are continuously in a state of change and the processes involved in change require energy. For instance, skin, which might appear inert, is being broken-down and reproduced constantly and rapidly. This is why we lose our hard-earned and often expensively derived holiday suntan after only a few weeks.

The same is true of nearly all tissues and organs of the body. This process of 'manufacture' and 'destruction' requires energy that under normal circumstances will be provided entirely from the energy content of food. When insufficient energy is provided by food then it is obtained from energy stored in the body as tissue (for practical purposes mainly fat) and is, of course, the reason people lose weight during periods of calorie restriction (i.e. starvation or strict dieting).

Overall, individuals are in one of three energy states (see Fig. 1.3, Part I). Firstly, an individual may be in energy balance when energy expenditure equals intake and weight remains constant. Secondly, individuals may be in negative energy balance when energy expenditure is greater than intake and weight will be lost. Finally, individuals may be in positive balance when energy intake exceeds expenditure and weight is gained.

It has already been pointed out in Part I that energy exists in several forms, and that there are different ways to quantify it. In practice this means that there are essentially two units that describe energy, namely calories (usually kilocalories) or Joules. What is important to remember is that the terms energy, calories and Joules are interchangeable, that is, they mean the same thing. For reference, 1 calorie is equivalent to 4.184 (usually rounded up to 4.2) Joules. The actual amount of energy required from the diet at any point depends on many additional factors and will be discussed next.

6.2   Energy Needs

The energy requirement of an individual represents the level of energy intake from food that will balance energy expenditure when the individual has a body size and composition, and level of physical activity, consistent with long-term good health.

World Health Organization (1985)

Such sentiments may be useful, but are very much of the 'soundbite' variety, as it is virtually impossible to define precisely what is meant by 'long-term good health'. However, inherent in such a statement is the acknowledgement that energy requirement is governed, among other factors, by body size (weight) and composition (the amount of fat and non-fat), and by physical activity. Thus, any attempts to provide answers about the energy requirement of an individual must take into account his/her weight, body composition and levels of physical activity. Age and sex are additional major factors that have to be considered in estimating energy requirements.

A large number of other factors may influence individual energy needs (see previous section 5), but each of them usually exerts a relatively small effect, and for practical purposes may be ignored. Based on research involving the assessment of professional contemporary female dancers, by means of 4-day weighed dietary histories, it seems likely that male and female dancers should consume, on average, around 45 and 40 kcal/kg body weight per day, respectively.

6.3   Predicting Energy Needs

There are many published predictive equations in use, although only a few will be described in this section. The majority of them attempt to estimate resting energy expenditure (REE) which is the most expensive component of the human daily energy requirement. It should be noted that the different equations tend to provide slightly different estimates of REE. Analysis of the equations shows that sex and weight are the most important factors, with age and height less so. The most widely used formula in the UK is that published by Schofield (1985), which appears in Table 9.2. Some predictive equations need the input of more sophisticated information, and an example of one of these, published by Ravussin and colleagues (1991) from USA, is given in Table 9.3. A further set of equations is given in the first part of this book (Chapter 1). Using the

Table 9.2   The Schofield formulae for the calculation of resting energy expenditure (REE). The units are kcal per day

Age (years)	Men	Women
18–30	REE = 15.1 × weight (kg) + 693	REE = 14.8 × weight (kg) + 488
31–60	REE = 11.5 × weight (kg) + 872	REE = 8.13 × weight (kg) + 846
Above 60	REE = 11.7 × weight (kg) + 588	REE = 9.08 × weight (kg) + 660

Table 9.3   More complicated formulae for the calculation of resting energy expenditure (REE), in kcal per day. Effective use of these formulae requires prior knowledge of fat-free body weight (fat free mass—FFM), fat weight, and the individual's age. The units are kcal per day

Female	REE = (13.9 × FFM [kg]) + (6.3 × fat [kg]) − (4.4 × Age [yr]) + 794
Male	REE = (13.9 × FFM [kg]) + (6.3 × fat [kg]) − (4.4 × Age [yr]) + 941

latter set, REE can be calculated either on a 24-hour basis or for any given length of time.

By using these equations, it becomes obvious that, on average, males expend more energy (i.e. calories) than women of the same body weight. Practically, this means that men have to consume more calories to maintain weight than do equally heavy women. In part this reflects the fact that men have more fat-free mass (i.e. muscle) per kilogram than do women.

7   EATING HABITS AND BODY WEIGHT CONTROL

7.1   What is the Best Diet for Me?

The majority of nutrition experts have advised that of the total energy intake at least 55% should be from carbohydrate, and 30% from fat, while the rest should be from protein. No recommendations are made for alcohol but it should be at the very most no more than 5% of daily energy intake.

The suggestion that dancers should regularly consume a diet with a fat content as low as 30% is somehow unrealistic. It is not clear why we appear unable to reduce the fat content of food to this sort of level, but it may reflect the fact that fat is a major component of taste and texture. Extreme low-fat diets are simply unpalatable. It is perhaps wiser to encourage dancers to alter the type of fat consumed rather than concentrating on reducing total levels to unsustainable long-term levels. Indeed, available data suggest that we should all try to reduce the amount of saturated fat (i.e. animal-derived fat) and increase the amount of mono-unsaturated fat (e.g. olive oil or rapeseed oil) and omega-3 fat (fish oil), and to a lesser extent polyunsaturated fats (vegetable oils).

This is happening already. Although the fat content of the average UK diet has been around 42% for the last two decades, the population does seem to have altered the polyunsaturated to saturated fat ratio of the diet, thus making meals generally 'healthier'. In general, it appears that the so-called *Mediterranean diet* (plenty of fresh fruit and vegetables, with olive oil and pasta) is beneficial to health and produces fewer body weight-related problems. It should be remembered that, contrary to popular myth, bread, potato, rice and pasta (termed staples) are not 'fattening'. Here are eight recently published guidelines for a healthy diet (Clayton 1997):

- Enjoy your food
- Eat a variety of different foods

- Eat the right amount to be at a healthy weight
- Eat plenty of foods rich in starch and fibre
- Eat plenty of fruit and vegetables
- Do not eat too many foods that contain a lot of fat
- Do not have sugary foods and drinks too often
- If you drink alcohol, drink sensibly

7.2 Are Vegetarians at Risk?

Are vegetarians at greater risk of nutritional deficiencies than meat-eaters? The answer to this is probably not. However, it is sensible to seek professional advice from a nutritionist/dietician before embarking along this road, particularly if one wants to do more than merely cut out dietary meat. Concern has long been voiced that vegetarians are theoretically at increased risk of not absorbing nutrients such as iron and calcium as these may be bound by the high fibre intake. In practice this does not seem to be a major problem, with the possible exception of iron, as much less iron from vegetables is absorbed compared to that from meat. It is worth remembering that vitamin C increases the absorption of non-animal iron, so drinking, for example, orange juice with a meal facilitates iron absorption.

For many years there has been concern that vegetable-derived protein is inferior to that from animals, as some of the essential amino acids are not present. However, with the normal mix of foods, any deficiencies can easily be rectified. In addition, work at Surrey University, examining the amounts of dietary protein required in our diet, has demonstrated that humans adapt to changes in protein intake (Millward and Pacy 1995). The more we regularly consume the more we need, and vice versa. It has not been possible to determine precisely the lowest amount of protein for maintaining optimal health, but it is less than even the strictest vegans would consume.

In marked contrast with the situation 10–20 years ago, being vegetarian does not any longer imply a boring and tasteless diet, while the range of foods that cater for vegetarians is ever increasing with tasty and nutritious results. The situation is different if a vegan diet is to be followed. There is little doubt that vegan vegetarians or those on macrobiotic diets are much more at risk of nutritional deficiencies, particularly in vitamin B12. These are by no means inevitable, but it is probably advisable to have blood examined every 6 months to look at the size of the red cells (Vitamin B12 deficiency is associated with an increased size of red blood cells). It is again advisable to seek professional assistance before embarking on such a nutritional regimen.

Apart from the moral comfort of being vegetarian, are there any physiological or health advantages compared to non-vegetarians? It is difficult to answer this question, but it may be worth pointing out that European vegetarians are generally lighter, and have lower blood pressure and lower blood fat levels than their meat-eating counterparts. This difference may then be linked to a number of medical issues, such as coronary heart disease. However, no obvious differences have been found between vegetarians and meat-eaters in terms of physical performance.

7.3   When is the Best Time to Eat and How Much?

This is a matter of individual preference. Many studies have been performed to see if there is any advantage in eating small amounts of food regularly (grazing) throughout the day versus eating large amounts once or twice a day (bolus). There appears to be no scientific consensus about this, or about the best time to eat. Provided daily energy intake equals expenditure, precisely when the intake occurs does not matter. However, the time of day when the major calorie intake is eaten will depend on many factors ranging from the practical consideration of the time of performance or practice to social reasons, such as the time at which members of the household eat.

Many overweight individuals claim to eat very little during the day and to consume most of their food at night, as a result of which they are unable to expend the calories. Most nutritionists do not believe this explanation. A more plausible one is that when one is hungry, expediency is paramount, which reduces the chance of making the most appropriate nutritional choices. Foods that are very easily consumed tend to be very rich but not filling, which promotes excess calorie intake.

The same is likely to occur with dancers. In addition, going for long periods of time without food and then eating a glucose-rich snack may well promote inappropriate insulin release which could result later in low blood sugar (*hypoglycaemia*). This would urge further food intake.

A potential problem with consuming a large meal, particularly carbohydrates, is that this may cause fluid to be drawn from the circulation into the intestines, resulting in a faint and bloated feeling. This is the so-called *dumping syndrome* and is prevented by taking small amounts of complex carbohydrate regularly. Spacing out intake throughout the day, which includes breakfast, minimizes this problem. It is sensible to eat some complex carbohydrate (such as bananas) 2 or 3 hours before activity so that by the time of the performance absorption is over, thereby minimizing potential problems of hypoglycaemia or dumping.

Consumption of non-calorie fluids should be continued throughout the day to prevent dehydration.

7.4 Is There Any Benefit in Taking Dietary Supplementation?

Dietary supplementation is widespread among student and professional dancers alike. In part, this may reflect the belief that supplements are advantageous to health, or perhaps it is because the dancers feel their diet lacks vital ingredients. Supplements may be divided into several broad categories:

- *Antioxidant* supplements designed to minimize the damage from the by-products of oxygen and oxygen use. These by-products are called *free radicals* and have the capability of destroying many body components. Free radicals have been implicated in many serious disease processes which include cancers, heart disease (free radical altered [oxidized] cholesterol enters blood vessel walls more readily) and even the ageing process itself. Epidemiological evidence suggests that high consumption of fruit and vegetables (which are the main antioxidant sources) is beneficial to health in general. However, Benson, Geiger, Eisesman and Wardlaw (1989) examined the use of such dietary supplementation on prevention of injury in dancers and failed to document any benefit.
- Supplements against common colds, which frequently affect dancers and athletes. A recent study from America (Mossad, Macknin, Medendorp and Mason 1996) has provided relatively good evidence that consuming zinc gluconate trihydrate (13.3 mg) lozenges reduces the duration of coughs, headaches and nasal and throat symptoms associated with the common cold by nearly 50%. Individuals had to start the medication within 24 hours of symptoms appearing and had to take a lozenge every 2 hours until symptoms disappeared. The main problem, however, with the zinc preparations is that they are associated with nausea and an unpleasant taste. If this form of zinc supplement can be purchased it would seem reasonable to take it when cold symptoms begin, to assess its effect and, dependent upon that, take it or not during subsequent colds. There appears to be much stronger evidence for zinc gluconate than for vitamin C in reducing the impact of the common cold.
- Performance-enhancing supplements such as *creatine, carnitine, caffeine* and *amino acids*. The evidence that is available, although not extensive, is exceedingly weak (less so for creatine) and not sufficient to advise individuals to purchase them.

- *Vitamins*. There may be a role for vitamin supplementation in dancers, although it is becoming increasingly apparent that a poor diet cannot be compensated simply by taking vitamins. Nutritionists are increasingly concerned that consumption of vitamins will lead individuals into a false sense of security with respect to diet and health, and as a consequence should not be recommended.
- Commercially available *sport drinks*. These are increasingly being promoted for use among individuals participating in vigorous activities. The majority contain a lot of sugar, so are calorific, costly and are increasingly being recognized as a cause of dental caries. Their use is not encouraged particularly as isotonic drinks can be made up by dancers themselves much more cheaply. A home-made sport drink is preferable as it is relatively cheap, and excessive calories can be controlled. The ingredients and the calorie content of three easily made drinks are as follows:

1. 50 grams of sugar dissolved in 1 litre of water will provide 200 kcals
2. 500 ml unsweetened orange juice mixed with 500 ml water contains 180 kcal
3. 200 ml orange squash diluted by water to 1 litre contains 215 kcal

7.5   What About Very Low-Calorie Diets and Weight Loss?

There are extremely few dancers who need to lose weight on health grounds, and certainly not by draconian reductions of calorie intake. Given the concerns about potential eating disorders, it is difficult to feel positive about weight reduction in dancers. However, because many dancers embark upon such actions for various reasons, two general issues with respect to weight loss will be briefly outlined.

Firstly is the level of diet. Very low-calorie diets (VLCD) typically supply less than the variable amounts of high biological value protein, and less than the recommended daily allowances of minerals and vitamins. It cannot be stressed enough that intakes of less than 800 kcal per day are likely to cause both short- and long-term health problems. It is likely to be detrimental to health if dancers attempt to carry on their daily routines unless they are consuming at least 1000 kcal per day.

If individuals find it impossible to lose weight when eating what they believe to be 1000 kcal, it is advisable that they try a milk diet. The milk diet was championed by Professor Garrow and is cheap and very nutritious, lacking only iron and B vitamins (which in the short term is of little significance). Dancers would be advised to drink 2.5 pints of full-fat milk per day (1000 kcal) plus non-calorie fluids like Diet Coke, Oxo, or Bovril, to provide a change of taste. The milk can be made up in coffee and tea or simply drunk neat. With this approach, it is likely that the weight loss will have a favourable fat to fat-free mass ratio of 3:1. This indicates that more fat can be lost than fat-free mass (i.e. mainly muscle), which brings us to the second general issue related to VLCD and body weight control.

The second issue relates to the nature of the tissue lost during dieting. It is not possible to lose fat alone as the tissue lost comprises a mixture of fat and fat-free mass. The ideal mix remains debatable, but it is probably 75% fat and 25% fat-free mass, which occurs when weight loss is slow. The faster the rate of weight loss the greater will be the loss of fat-free mass. Yiannis Koutedakis and I showed that when elite lightweight oarswomen lost weight rapidly it consisted of 50% fat and 50% fat-free mass. Thus, the key to effective weight loss is to do it slowly.

There is also a connection between the nature of the tissue lost during dieting and the level of diet. The energy deficit that results from the use of VLCDs is large and will favour the preferential loss of fat-free mass rather than fat as was the case with the lightweight oarswomen. A theoretical concern with this approach, particularly if used repeatedly, is that it results in changing body composition in favour of fat which, in practical terms for the dancer, means gaining a higher weight than their pre-diet weight when dieting ceases and usual eating patterns are resumed.

7.6 Are Eating Problems Common Among Dancers?

The answer is reluctantly yes, especially with young ballet dancers. This is supported by many authorities who have felt in recent years that the prerequisite leanness and sylph-like body shape of female ballet dancers is associated with significant and potentially serious eating disorders (Evers 1987; Le Grange, Tibbs and Noakes 1994; Abraham 1996). However, it is very difficult to get accurate figures on the size of this problem, but it may occur in up to 35% of professional and student ballet dancers.

This difficulty stems from the fact that there is no precise definition of, say, *anorexia*, while many individuals deny problems associated with eating disorders. Suzanne Abraham from Australia graphically illustrates these difficulties in recent publications. She examined the eating patterns of 60 young (mean age 17) female ballet dancers and concluded that only 1.7% had anorexia, 1.7% had bulimia, while overall 12% had some form of eating disorder. However, in contrast to these relatively benign figures was the finding that 34% had a BMI under 17, 13% admitted to abusing laxatives, 11.7% induced regular vomiting, 28% reported cycles of binge eating and starvation, 30% worried about becoming obese, and menstruation was absent in 58% of the 60-strong sample. Overall 73% of the dancers had experienced difficulties controlling their eating while 52% claimed to experience on-going problems with controlling their weight. This does seem a major problem among female ballet dancers, although it appears less so among other dancers.

Does it matter to the dancer if he or she has eating problems such as anorexia? The answer is most decidedly yes. This condition and the associated poor nutrition can interfere with the ability to perform, concentrate, and learn, and to heal what would otherwise be minor injuries. Benson and colleagues (1989) noted that dancers with abnormal menses, a feature of anorexia, were significantly more likely to have bone injuries than those who menstruated normally. The same authors also noted that very lean dancers (with a BMI of less than 19) were more prone to injury than their less lean counterparts. There are also long-term effects of such leanness and poor nutrition, namely the development of osteoporosis, which will be covered in the next chapter.

8 BODY WEIGHT AFTER RETIREMENT

Many dancers feel that once they retire from dancing they will rapidly gain weight. Is this a valid sentiment? Certainly there is evidence that individuals who weight cycle (constantly gaining and then losing weight) tend over the years to become heavier. However, information relating to dancers is very limited. Research workers from South Bank University (Lewis, Dickerson and Davies 1997) conducted a questionnaire-based investigation into this problem but unfortunately obtained a response rate of only 32%, raising serious doubts as to the applicability and validity of the findings. For this project only ballet dancers volunteered, who were almost exclusively white caucasian. However, on the subject of body weight after retiring, the authors reported that the BMI of female dancers rose from 18.5 to 20.4, and for men from 21.0 to 22.7. Only two dancers had a BMI greater than 25, and both were female, with values of

29.2 and 25.4. These results suggest that while retirement is associated with increased body weight, this is not detrimental to health for the majority of individuals.

9 CONCLUSIONS

Professional and student dancers tend to be lean, with lower than normal body fat. As a rough guide for weight maintenance, female dancers should consume about 40 kcal per kg body weight per day, and male dancers 45 kcal per kg body weight per day. In terms of health, virtually no dancer needs to lose weight and if they are required to do so on aesthetic grounds this must be done very slowly at a rate of no more than 2 lb per month in females and 4 lb in males. The leanness of dancers, allied to their frequency of eating disorders and prevalence of cigarette smoking, is almost certainly detrimental to long-term health, particularly among females. Healthy eating must be encouraged with little or, ideally, no reliance upon supplementation or undue emphasis on calorie restriction.

10 FURTHER READING

Abraham S (1996) Characteristics of eating disorders among young ballet dancers. *Psychopathology*, **29**: 223–9

Braisted JR, Mellin L, Gong EJ, Irwin CE (1985) The adolescent ballet dancer. Nutritional practices and characteristics associated with anorexia nervosa. *Journal of Adolescent Health Care*, **6**: 365–71

Brinson P, Dick F (eds) (1996) *Fit to dance?* London: Calouste Gulbenkian Foundation

Kirkendall DT, Calabrese LH (1983) Physiological aspects of dance. *Clinics in Sports Medicine*, **2**: 525–37

ACKNOWLEDGEMENTS

The author wishes to thank Professor Joe Millward, Malcolm Cox, Neil Gibson and Magita Khalouha for their help and support over the years. Their friendship is greatly appreciated. He also wishes to thank all at Dance UK for their invaluable assistance for which he is grateful. Finally, a big 'thanks' to all dancers who volunteered in his research projects.

REFERENCES

Abraham S (1996) Eating and weight controlling behaviours of young ballet dancers. *Psychopathology*, **29**: 218–22

Benson JE, Geiger CJ, Eiserman PA, Wardlaw GM (1989) Relationship between nutrient intake, body mass index, menstrual function, and ballet injury. *Journal of the American Dietetic Association*, **89**: 58–63

Clarkson PM, Freedson PS, Keller B, Carney D, Skrinar M (1985) Maximal oxygen uptake, nutritional patterns, and body composition of adolescent female ballet dancers. *Research Quarterly for Exercise and Sport*, **56**: 180–4

Clayton B (1997) Nutrition tasks: achievements and challenges for the future. *British Nutrition Foundation Nutrition Bulletin*, **22**: 32–46

Evers CL (1987) Dietary intake and symptoms of anorexia nervosa in female university dancers. *Journal of the American Dietetic Association*, **87**: 66–8

Haskell A (1979) *Balletomania*. London: Penguin Books: p. 21

Hergenroeder AC, Fiorotto ML, Klish WJ (1991) Body composition in ballet dancers measured by total body electrical conductivity. *Medicine & Science in Sports and Exercise*, **23**: 528–33

Le Grange D, Tibbs J, Noakes TD (1994) Implications of a diagnosis of anorexia nervosa in a ballet school. *International Journal of Eating Disorders*, **15**: 369–76

Lewis RL, Dickerson JWT, Davies GJ (1997) Lifestyle and injuries of professional ballet dancers: reflections in retirement. *Journal of the Royal Society of Health*, **117**: 23–31

Millward DJ, Pacy PJ (1995) Postprandial protein utilisation and protein quality assessment in man. *Clinical Science*, **88**: 597–606

Mossad SB, Macknin ML, Medendorp SV, Mason P (1996) Zinc gluconate lozenges for treating the common cold. A randomized, double-blind, placebo-controlled study. *Annals of Internal Medicine*, **125**: 81–8

Pacy PJ, Cox M, Khalouha M, Elkin S, Robinson A, Garrow JS (1996) Does moderate aerobic activity have a stimulatory effect on 24 hour resting energy expenditure: a direct calorimeter study. *International Journal of Food Sciences and Nutrition*, **47**: 299–305

Prentice AM, Jebb SA (1995) Obesity in Britain: gluttony or sloth? *British Medical Journal*, **311**: 437–9

Ravussin E, Zurlo F, Ferraro R, Bogardus C (1991) Energy expenditure in man: determinants and risk factors for body weight gain. *Progress in Obesity Research*: 175

Schofield C (1985) An annotated bibliography of source material for basal metabolic rate data. *Human Nutrition: Clinical Nutrition*, **39C** (Suppl. 1): 42–91

World Health Organization (1985) *Energy and protein requirements*. World Health Organization, Geneva. Technical Series Report 724

Chapter 10

Body Weight and Bone Density

Roger Wolman

1 SUMMARY

The aim of this chapter is to present the main aspects associated with a relatively new health risk, particularly in female dancers. Although *osteoporosis* does not directly affect performance on stage, its development can be traced back in the pre-pubertal years, and if one is not careful, its effects can make lives miserable at later stages. Menstrual abnormalities and low body weight, in association with high volumes of physical work, can negatively affect the mineral content of the skeleton and lead to increased incidents of stress fractures. Prevention of the disease should be based on the development of strong skeletons through proper diets and optimal body weights. However, this strategy might sometimes go against the general perception of the female dancer.

2 INTRODUCTION

Over the last 25 years there has been a female fashion fad for thinness. The low body weight of female dancers—although a current aesthetic requirement—can cause several well recognized medical problems. The female athlete 'triad' (Skolnick 1993) of disordered eating (leading to low body weight), *amenorrhoea* and *osteoporosis* is now well recognized and is seen just as commonly in dancers. However, the consequences of this triad may not become apparent until well after retirement from dancing. The present chapter will focus on the menstrual abnormalities that occur in association with low body weight and the related effects on the skeleton.

3 MENSTRUAL EFFECTS OF LOW BODY WEIGHT

Menstruation occurs as a result of a complex series of hormonal messages passed between several organs (Barnes and Chamberlain 1988). Hormonal signals pass from the *hypothalamus* to the *pituitary*, which are both areas of the brain, and then to the *ovaries*. The latter respond by releasing *oestrogen* and *progestogen* that stimulate the growth of the lining of the womb, the shedding of which produces the subsequent menstrual bleed. Although the hormonal signals that pass between these organs are well recognized the hormonal (or other) triggers that stimulate the hypothalamus to initiate this process are poorly understood.

Disorders or diseases involving any of the organs mentioned above may affect normal menstrual function and lead to irregular or even absent periods. There are therefore many causes of menstrual dysfunction (Warren 1996). Dieting and weight loss can affect normal *hypothalamic* function, which may cause menstrual dysfunction, in particular complete cessation of the periods. This is known as *amenorrhoea*. In this situation the hypothalamus fails to send the correct signals to the *pituitary*. The ovaries are then unable to function properly. This type of amenorrhoea occurs commonly in women with *anorexia nervosa*.

Menstrual dysfunction is also seen in active individuals participating in intensive aerobic exercise, such as marathon running. Amenorrhoea may occur and can be seen in up to 50% of athletes running over 60 miles per week (Feicht, Johnson, Martin *et al*. 1978). A similar incidence is seen in cyclists and lightweight rowers (Fig. 10.1) engaged in intensive training. This 'athletic' amenorrhoea is also associated with hypothalamic dysfunction although the exact mechanism is not fully understood. It is however related to several factors (Noakes and van Geld 1988):

- *The intensity of physical work*. At least in athletes, about 20% of them develop amenorrhoea when physical work amounts to 20 miles per week of running. The incidence increases as athletes increase their weekly running mileage.
- *Age*. Amenorrhoea is more common in those in the late teens and early twenties than in those in their late twenties. Activities that are affected as a

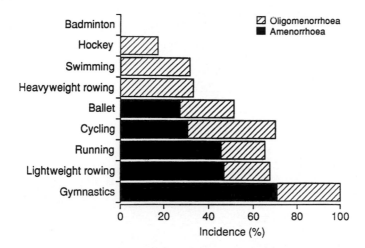

Fig. 10.1 The incidence of amenorrhoea and oligomenorrhoea in elite athletes and performers in the UK
Source: From Wolman and Harries (1989)

result include dance, swimming, and gymnastics where young hopefuls normally make an early start.

- *The degree of calorie restriction.* Amenorrhoea is more common in women involved in physical activities with low body weight requirements. For example, the incidence is much higher in women lightweight rowers, whose competition weight must be below 59 kg, compared to their heavyweight counterparts. Although both groups do similar types of training, the former often need to go on calorie-restricted diets.

Athletic amenorrhoea therefore occurs in those involved in intensive aerobic exercise (which places a large demand on the body's energy resources) who are also on relatively low calorie intakes in their diet (providing insufficient energy for the amount of exercise undertaken). This produces an energy imbalance (Fig. 10.2) which leads to weight loss and low body fat, both of which are related to the development of amenorrhoea. It may also affect the production and release of various specific *hormones*, some of which influence the function of the hypothalamus, and therefore may be responsible for the development of menstrual abnormalities. This is currently an area of intense research (Jenkins and Grossman 1993).

Athletic amenorrhoea bears many similarities to the amenorrhoea seen

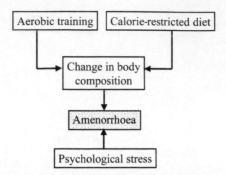

Fig. 10.2 The factors responsible for the development of amenorrhoea in dancers

in patients with *anorexia nervosa*. In fact, some research has suggested that the majority of the affected individuals also have an eating disorder (Gadpaille, Sanborn and Wagner 1987). It is important to recognize this connection when it comes to advice and treatment (see later in the section).

Both body weight and body fat measurements can provide a measure of the risk of developing amenorrhoea. Body weight may be assessed relatively to the height of the person. We use a measure called the Body Mass Index (BMI), which has been extensively discussed in the previous chapter. Briefly, this measure is defined as the (W)eight (in kg) divided by the (H)eight (in metres) squared, that is W/H^2. Amenorrhoea is more likely to occur when the BMI of the person falls below 18 (e.g. a dancer of height 5 ft 5 in. [1.65 m] and weight 7 stone 10 lb [49 kg] will have a BMI $= W/H^2 = 49/1.65 \times 1.65 = 18$).

Body fat is usually recorded as a percentage of the total body weight. As also stressed in the previous chapter, there is currently no simple and, at the same time, accurate method to assess body fat. Nevertheless the employment of body-fat callipers to measure skinfold thickness—at four or more specific sites on the body—has gained popularity. The sum of these can then be converted into a measure of body fat using a standardized conversion table. If it falls below about 17% of total body weight amenorrhoea is likely to occur (Frisch and McArthur 1974). It should however be emphasized that despite its simplicity and its very low cost, unqualified individuals should never use this method, as the possibility of reaching the wrong conclusions is very high.

3.1 Dancers

Most of the discussion so far has been based on athletes and not dancers. This is simply because the majority of the current research has involved the former. Work that has been conducted on dancers (especially classical) demonstrates that they also are vulnerable to the same effects. They too are commonly on low-calorie diets and also spend long periods of time training.

From the above it is possible to see why dancers are at risk of menstrual dysfunction. These include various degrees of infrequent periods (known as *oligomenorrhoea*) and absent periods (*amenorrhoea*). Surveys suggest that approximately a third of classical dancers have amenorrhoea, another third have oligomenorrhoea, and only a third normal periods. It is also well known that dancers tend to start their periods late with the onset of monthly periods occurring, on average, around the age of 15 to 16 years (Frisch, Wyshak and Vincent 1980). However in some dancers this may not occur until the late teens or even the early twenties.

There has been less research on contemporary dancers and therefore accurate figures on the incidence of menstrual abnormalities are not available. It is likely that the incidence is lower as the demand for weight reduction is less.

3.2 The Menarche

The *menarche* is defined as the age at which the first menstrual period occurs. This is usually around the age of 11 to 14 years and is influenced by several factors including body weight and body fat, both of which increase prior to the menarche. Intensive exercise and calorie restriction in this age group will delay the menarche, probably through delaying the increase in body weight and fat that is required (Warren and Brooks-Gunn 1989). This is commonly seen in athletes and dancers who start training in childhood. *Primary amenorrhoea* is said to occur when the menarche is delayed beyond the age of 16 years and is frequently seen in dancers.

Research has shown that delayed menarche in dancers affects, *inter alia*, the development of the bones in the back and increases the risk of developing a *scoliosis* (Warren, Brooks-Gunn, Hamilton *et al.* 1986), a condition that causes a twisting of the spine. Clearly this needs to be avoided, as scoliosis will affect the long-term prospects for the dancer and increases the risk of back problems in later life. As we will see later on, *stress fractures* are more common in dancers who have a delayed menarche.

4   BONE DENSITY AND OSTEOPOROSIS

Bone consists predominantly of a combination of protein and calcium that gives it strength. The term *bone density* refers to the calcium concentration within the bone. This is constantly changing, albeit at a very slow rate. Bone density is generally lower in women than men and varies with age (Peel and Eastell 1995). It increases during the teens to reach its peak around the late twenties or early thirties. This is called the *'peak bone mass'* (Fig. 10.3). It declines thereafter as part of the normal ageing process but in women there is an accelerated phase of bone loss around the time of the menopause. As bone density decreases the bone itself becomes weaker and eventually there is a risk of *fractures* occurring with very little trauma. This is known as *osteoporosis* and is more common in elderly females.

There are many factors that affect the risk of developing osteoporosis (Kelly, Sambrook and Eisman 1990). These include factors that appear in

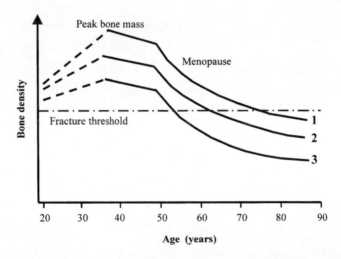

Fig. 10.3   The change in bone density with age. An average woman would follow line 2, crossing the bone-fracture threshold in her mid-sixties. A dancer with prolonged amenorrhoea in her twenties will have a reduced peak bone mass and eventually be at risk of fracturing at a much earlier age (line 3). A woman who increases her peak bone mass is likely to reduce her long-term risk of getting fractures (line 1)

childhood and/or early adult life and affect *peak bone mass*, as well as factors that occur at a later age affecting mainly the rate of loss of calcium from the bone. If someone acquires a high peak bone mass in their early thirties they will be able to withstand greater losses in bone density in later life before becoming osteoporotic. Dancers and other high-risk individuals must appreciate, therefore, that events which take place in childhood and early adult life will affect the chances of developing osteoporosis many years later.

4.1 Measurement

For those who might be at risk of developing osteoporosis we now have very accurate, specialized methods for measuring bone density (Compston, Cooper and Kanis 1995). The most popular involves using a DEXA (Dual Energy X-ray Absorptiometry) scanner (Fig. 10.4). During this technique the patients lie still on a comfortable couch for about 10–20 minutes, while the scanner passes above them. It is extremely safe as it uses a pencil-thin beam of X-rays, which exposes the patient to minimal

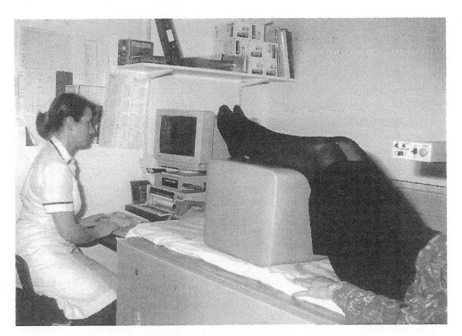

Fig. 10.4 A female patient having a DEXA scan

radiation but provides an extremely accurate measure of calcium concentration in different bones of the skeleton.

4.2   Factors Affecting Bone Density

Several well-known factors influence bone density (Riggs and Melton 1986) including physical activity, oestrogen levels in women (see below) and nutritional status. Other less important factors include smoking and alcohol, both of which can have an adverse effect on the skeleton. *Genetic* factors are also important, as osteoporosis tends to run in families (Sambrook, Kelly, Morrison and Eisman 1994).

There are several important nutritional factors too, but calcium and vitamin D seem to be the most crucial (Heaney 1993). Over 99% of the body's calcium is stored in the bone where it is needed to maintain the strength of the skeleton, but which also acts as a reservoir for this mineral. If there is a nutritional deficiency of calcium, then calcium will leak out from the skeleton to be used elsewhere. This can be prevented to a large extent by maintaining the dietary intake to meet these needs. The recommended daily intake of calcium is between 800 and 1000 mg, with larger requirements during pregnancy and following the menopause. Dairy products provide the best natural source of calcium. For example a pint of skimmed milk contains about 800 mg. There is also a high concentration of calcium in dark green, leafy vegetables such as spinach and broccoli.

Vitamin D enhances the absorption of calcium from the diet and improves its utilization in the body. There are usually adequate amounts of this vitamin in the diet, and it is especially effective in those exposed to natural sunlight.

'Mechanical stress' is another factor that affects bone density. This stress represents the forces generated during the various forms of physical activity. The bones of the skeleton respond to direct mechanical stresses placed upon them by laying down more calcium and becoming stronger. This is supported by the fact that the bone density of athletes is generally greater than that of sedentary people (Dalen, Laftman, Ohlsen and Stromberg 1985; Lane, Bloch, Jones *et al.* 1986). The bone density of the legs is greater in runners, while in tennis players the bone density of the racket arm is greater. In contrast the bone density of swimmers is not much different from non-athletes because swimming is a non-weight-bearing sport. This is telling us that when direct stresses on the bones are removed, bone density decreases.

The same effects can be further found in people on prolonged bed-rest due to, for instance, a bad injury. During such prolonged rest calcium leaks out of the bone quite rapidly, and the density falls (Lockwood, Lammert, Vogel and Hulley 1973). Interestingly, the same outcomes have been seen in astronauts whose bone density falls while they are in the gravity-free environment of space. Therefore, physical activity is important for maintaining the strength of the skeleton and the current trend for a sedentary lifestyle is one of the reasons why osteoporosis is getting more common.

5   EFFECTS OF LOW BODY WEIGHT ON THE SKELETON

These can be divided into a direct effect of body weight on the skeleton and an indirect effect through hormonal changes.

5.1   Direct Effect (Stress Loading)

The weight of a person will affect the stress loads placed upon the skeleton in a normal daily weight-bearing activity such as walking. Overweight people have greater bone density than those who are underweight. This may be a factor that increases the risk of getting thin bones in dancers. However, dancers perform large amounts of weight-bearing physical activity that tends to increase the stress loading and improve their bone density. This is especially true for jumping activity that has been shown to increase bone density in the hips (Bassey and Ramsdale 1994).

5.2   Indirect Effect (Hormonal)

There are many different hormones produced by the body that control and influence the metabolic activity of the bones. One of these is *oestrogen* whose production by the ovary is adversely affected by low body weight (see above). The body's output of oestrogen increases at puberty and is sustained until the time of the *menopause* (usually late forties or early fifties) when it falls dramatically. This hormone is essential both for normal menstrual function and several aspects of skeletal integrity including bone density, prevention of stress fractures and skeletal maturation.

Bone Density

Oestrogen helps to maintain bone density. Following the menopause oestrogen output falls significantly and there is an associated decline in bone density that may eventually lead to osteoporosis (one third of women by the age of 65 years).

Between puberty and the menopause, oestrogen production follows a monthly cycle that is responsible for the menstrual pattern. However, there are certain medical disorders that can lead to diminished oestrogen production and, therefore, amenorrhoea. When this occurs, irrespective of the cause, bone density falls (Aitken, Hart, Anderson *et al.* 1973; Rigotti, Nussbaum, Herzog and Neer 1984), affecting some parts of the skeleton more than others with the spine and the hip regions being at particular risk.

Physically active women who are amenorrhoeic, secondary to training and weight loss, have reduced bone density (Drinkwater, Nilson, Chesnut *et al.* 1984; Marcus, Cann, Madvig *et al.* 1985). The severity will depend on several aspects (Wolman 1990) including:

- *The length of time that they have been amenorrhoeic.* Although the most severe fall in bone density occurs in the first year the losses continue thereafter. Initially these losses are reversible once menstruation restarts. However, with prolonged amenorrhoea, beyond about 2 years, the losses become irreversible even when menstruation returns to normal.
- *The age of onset of the menarche.* Women who had a late menarche have a low bone density. This demonstrates that events in childhood and adolescence, which interfere with puberty, may influence the risk of osteoporosis many years later. This is particularly relevant to dancers, many of whom have a delayed menarche.
- *The degree of weight loss and other nutritional deficiencies.* The more severe the weight loss, the greater will be the impact on bone density. Dancers may also be on diets that are inadequate in specific nutrients, such as calcium and vitamin D.
- *Genetic factors.* There are genetic influences on bone density, but the exact genes responsible have not yet been worked out. People with certain types of genes may be at greater risk of getting osteoporosis and therefore it is often helpful to know something about the person's family history.

STRESS FRACTURES

Stress fractures are also known as fatigue fractures and occur as a result of repetitive stresses placed upon bone that is not given enough time to recover in between exercise sessions. The bone fatigues and eventually a small fracture occurs along its surface. This is extremely painful. They occur at different sites in different sports depending on the site of the stress. In dancers stress fractures most commonly occur around the shins and in the feet. Occasionally they occur in the back. The only treatment is complete rest from activity that allows the fracture to heal. This usually takes 6–10 weeks but occasionally it can be considerably longer.

Stress fractures are more common in dancers who are *amenorrhoeic* (Carbon, Sambrook, Deakin *et al.* 1990). The low oestrogen level causes thinning of the bone, putting it at greater risk. It may also impair the healing process in the bone once a fracture has occurred. Any treatment that helps to prevent the occurrence of stress fractures should be strongly considered.

DELAYED SKELETAL MATURATION

In early adolescence, around the time of puberty, there is a rapid growth spurt. This growth takes place at the ends of the long bones (e.g. the thighbone and the shinbone) where there are growth plates, known as the *epiphyses*. These are separated from the main bone and this is where the growth takes place. Once this is completed, the growth plates fuse with the rest of the bone. In women this process is strongly under the influence of the hormone *oestrogen*.

In young dancers, delayed puberty and oestrogen production is often followed by a delay in skeletal maturation and, in particular, a delay in the closure of the growth plates. The epiphysis is a site of potential weakness and it can become injured with an excessive application of mechanical stresses (e.g. intensive exercise). Injuries occasionally occur at the top end of the femur (i.e. thighbone) where it forms part of the hip joint (this disorder is known as a slipped upper femoral epiphysis). This is well recognized as a cause of severe hip pain in younger age groups (Wolman, Harries and Fyfe 1989; Warren, Shane, Lee *et al.* 1990). This injury may also affect the opportunity for further growth of the bone and can lead to *arthritis* in later life.

Delayed skeleton maturation also increases the risk of certain types of tendon injuries. More specifically, the site where tendons attach to bone is weaker in adolescents than in adults and is a common site for injury in youngsters. In dancers this includes the patellar *tendon* at the knee (Osgood–Schlatters Disease) and the Achilles tendon at the ankle (Severs Disease). Once the growth spurt is completed and the bones have fused these injuries tend to resolve.

6   REDUCED BONE DENSITY

In most *amenorrhoeic* dancers *bone density* will be 10–20% below the average for someone of their age, but occasionally it can be considerably lower and may even be as low as seen in someone in their seventies.

As a woman in her twenties usually has a higher bone density than one in her fifties, she will have to lose a greater amount of calcium from the bone before she develops *osteoporosis*. However as the bone loss in an amenorrhoeic dancer is occurring at an age when bone density should be going through a process of consolidation, this does not bode well for the future (Johnston and Longcope 1990). Many such dancers go on to develop *osteoporosis* in their fifties, which is about 15 years earlier than we normally see it.

In the more severe cases, osteoporosis and the associated fractures occur at an even younger age and may occasionally occur in the twenties. I have now treated several dancers in this age group with fractures one would expect to see only in the elderly (Wilson and Wolman 1994). This is clearly a very worrying problem and needs to be treated aggressively.

7   MANAGEMENT OF LOW BONE DENSITY AND OSTEOPOROSIS

Methods that prevent the development of osteoporosis are a more effective way of dealing with this condition than treating it once it is already established. The preservation of bone density can be enhanced by general factors such as diet (especially calcium and Vitamin D) and by not smoking (Compston 1990). Weight-bearing physical exercise is also important, but this is usually adequate amongst dancers.

7.1   Prevention and Treatment

Prevention of osteoporosis depends on identifying those at risk. Unfortunately it is a silent disease, not causing symptoms until a fracture has occurred. By this time the opportunity for prevention has been missed. We therefore need other ways of detecting those at risk. The menstrual status is the most important indicator in young adult female dancers, followed by optimal body weight. As mentioned previously, those with low body weight, even with regular periods, are still in danger of developing osteoporosis.

DEXA scanning provides a very effective way of screening for osteoporosis (Fig. 10.4). However, as this technique is not widely available, it

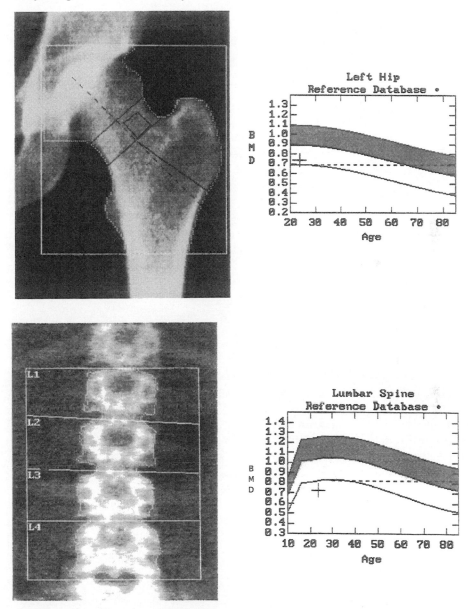

Fig. 10.5 The results of a DEXA scan on a 22-year-old dancer who had been amenorrhoeic for 3 years. Measurements for the bone mineral density on a (BMD) have been taken from the left hip (a) and spine (b) and then plotted on a graph (+) as shown. Note that especially in the spine the bone density is considerably below the average (the shaded area between the two lines) for her age. She is now receiving treatment

is important to limit its use to those at risk. Any dancer who has been amenorrhoeic for 6 months should be scanned (Fig. 10.5). Those with irregular periods for over a year and those with very low body weight should also be scanned.

Once those at risk have been identified, they should be offered advice to prevent any further bone loss. They also need to see a dietician who can determine whether they have any nutritional deficiencies. Treatment, which should aim at re-establishing natural menstruation as soon as possible, will depend on the underlying cause. Deficient calorie intake relative to the high level of physical activity is often the key causative factor. Successful treatment will therefore depend on increasing the calorie intake in the diet and possibly making adjustments to the training regime. However the dancer, because of the fear of gaining weight, may be unable to do this. The assistance of a counsellor or psychologist trained in the management of eating disorders may be needed to help the dancer at this stage.

If natural menstruation fails to occur with the regime outlined above, the dancer should be offered oestrogen replacement medication, as the dangers of remaining amenorrhoeic are unacceptable. This can be given either as the oral contraceptive or as hormone replacement therapy. Once treatment has been started, the DEXA scan should be repeated 6–12 months later to assess possible improvements in bone density. It is important to recognize that some women are unable to tolerate this medication due to side-effects of breast tenderness and pre-menstrual tension.

In those dancers who already have a low bone density the treatment is more difficult. Current treatments for osteoporosis aim at preventing any further bone loss because, at present, there are no treatments capable of significantly increasing bone density. The use of biphosphonates and calcitonin constitutes well-established treatment in post-menopausal women and the elderly, but not in young adults. There is therefore some concern about prescribing these medications to younger age groups.

8   CONCLUSIONS

The association of disordered eating, weight loss, amenorrhoea and osteoporosis is now well recognized in dancers. The dangers of developing osteoporosis should not be underestimated, while significant weight loss can cause major long-term medical problems. By improving the diet of the dancer and preventing significant weight loss, amenorrhoea and osteoporosis can be prevented. This requires education of dancers and the people working with them, so that they can appreciate the dangers and seek medical advice at an early stage. The support of a dietician is extremely helpful as they can define possible nutritional deficiencies. A counsellor/psychologist is also necessary in some cases to support the dancer when she is having difficulty coming to terms with dietary adjustments and possible weight gain.

9 FURTHER READING

Costa MD, Guthrie SR (eds) (1994) *Women and sport*. Champaign, IL: Human Kinetics

Warren MP, Brooks-Gunn J (1989) Delayed menarche in athletes: the role of low energy intake and eating disorders and their relation to bone density. In: Laron Z, Rogol AD (eds), *Hormones and sport*. New York: Sereno Symposia Publications from Raven Press, **55**: 41–55

Wilson J, Wolman R (1994) Osteoporosis and fracture complications in an amenorrhoeic athlete. *British Journal of Rheumatology*, **33**: 480–1

Wolman RL, Harries MG (1989) Menstrual abnormalities in elite athletes. *Clinical Sports Medicine*, **1**: 95–100

Wolman RL (1990) Bone mineral density in elite female athletes. *Annals of Rheumatic Diseases*, **49**: 1013–6

REFERENCES

Aitken JM, Hart DM, Anderson JB, Lindsay R, Smith DA, Speirs CF (1973) Osteoporosis after oopherectomy for non-malignant disease in pre-menopausal women. *British Medical Journal*, **2**: 325–8

Barnes J, Chamberlain G (1988) *Lecture notes on gynaecology* (6th edition). Oxford, UK: Blackwell Scientific: pp. 30–35

Bassey EJ, Ramsdale SJ (1994) Increase in femoral bone density in young women following high-impact exercise. *Osteoporosis International*, **4**: 72–5

Carbon R, Sambrook P, Deakin V *et al.* (1990) Bone density of elite female athletes with stress fractures. *Medical Journal of Australia*, **153**: 373–6

Compston JE (1990) Osteoporosis. *Clinical Endocrinology*, **33**: 653–82

Compston JE, Cooper C, Kanis JA (1995) Bone density in clinical practice. *British Medical Journal*, **310**: 1507–10

Dalen N, Laftman P, Ohlsen H, Stromberg L (1985) The effect of athletic activity on bone mass in human diaphysial bone. *Orthopaedics*, **8**: 1139–41

Drinkwater BL, Nilson K, Chesnut CH *et al.* (1984) Bone mineral content in amenorrhoeic and eumenorrhoeic athletes. *New England Journal Medicine*, **311**: 277–81

Feicht CB, Johnson TS, Martin BJ *et al.* (1978) Secondary amenorrhoea in athletes. *Lancet*, **2**: 1145–6

Frisch RE, McArthur JW (1974) Menstrual cycles: Fatness as a determinant of minimum weight for height necessary for their maintenance or onset. *Science*, **185**: 949–51

Frisch RE, Wyshak G, Vincent L (1980) Delayed menarche and amenorrhoea in ballet dancers. *New England Journal Medicine*, **303**: 17–19

Gadpaille WJ, Sanborn CF, Wagner WW (1987) Athletic amenorrhoea, major affective disorders, and eating disorders. *American Journal of Psychiatry*, **144**: 939–42

Heaney RP (1993) Thinking straight about calcium. *New England Journal Medicine*, **328**: 503–5

Jenkins PJ, Grossman A (1993) The control of the gonadotrophin releasing hormone pulse generator in relation to opioid and nutritional cues. *Human Reproduction*, **8**: 154–61

Johnston CC, Longcope C (1990) Pre-menopausal bone loss—a risk factor for osteoporosis. *New England Journal Medicine*, **323**: 1271–2

Kelly PJ, Sambrook PN, Eisman JA (1990) The interaction of genetic and environmental influences on peak bone density. *Osteoporosis International*, **1**: 56–60

Lane NE, Bloch DA, Jones HH *et al.* (1986) Long distance running, bone density, and osteoarthritis. *Journal of American Medical Association*, **225**: 1147–51

Lockwood DR, Lammert JE, Vogel JM, Hulley SB (1973) Bone mineral loss during bed rest. *Excerpta Medica ICS*, **270**: 261–5

Marcus R, Cann C, Madvig P *et al.* (1985) Menstrual function and bone mass in elite women distance runners. *Annals of Internal Medicine*, **102**: 158–63

Noakes TD, van Geld M (1988) Menstrual dysfunction in female athletes. *South African Medical Journal*, **73**: 350–5

Peel N, Eastell R (1995) ABC of rheumatology: osteoporosis. *British Medical Journal*, **310**: 989–2

Riggs BL, Melton LJ (1986) Involutional osteoporosis. *New England Journal of Medicine*, **314**: 1676–86

Rigotti NA, Nussbaum SR, Herzog DB, Neer RM (1984) Osteoporosis in women with anorexia nervosa. *New England Journal of Medicine*, **311**: 1601–6

Sambrook PN, Kelly PJ, Morrison NA, Eisman JA (1994) Genetics of osteoporosis. *British Journal of Rheumatology*, **33**: 1007–11

Skolnick AA (1993) 'Female athlete triad' risk for women. *Journal of American Medical Association*, **270**: 921–3

Warren MP, Brooks-Gunn J, Hamilton LH *et al.* (1986) Scoliosis and fractures in young ballet dancers. *New England Journal of Medicine*, **314**: 1348–53

Warren MP, Brooks-Gunn J, (1989) Delayed menarche in athletes: the role of low energy intake and eating disorders and their relation to bone density. In: Laron Z, Rogol AD (eds), *Hormones and sport*. New York: Sereno Symposia Publications from Raven Press, **55**: 41–55

Warren MP, Shane E, Lee MJ *et al.* (1990) Femoral head collapse associated with anorexia nervosa in a 20 year old ballet dancer. *Clinical Orthopaedics and Related Research*, 171–6

Warren MP (1996) Evaluation of secondary amenorrhoea. *Journal of Clinical Endocrinology and Metabolism*, **81**: 437–42

Wilson J, Wolman R (1994) Osteoporosis and fracture complications in an amenorrhoeic athlete. *British Journal of Rheumatology*, **33**: 480–1

Wolman RL, Harries MG (1989) Menstrual abnormalities in elite athletes. *Clinical Sports Medicine*, **1**: 95–100

Wolman RL, Harries MG, Fyfe I (1989) Slipped Upper Femoral Epiphysis in an amenorrhoeic athlete. *British Medical Journal*, **299**: 720

Wolman RL, (1990) Bone mineral density in elite female athletes. *Annals of Rheumatic Diseases*, **49**:1013–6

Chapter 11

Anatomical and Physiological Gender Differences

N.C. Craig Sharp

1 SUMMARY

This chapter focuses on those anatomical and physiological aspects which influence physical performance in dance, or sport, with a brief introduction to sexual dimorphism, or how we become two sexes. The important point to grasp in any description of such physical differences is that, although on average one sex may have one attribute more highly developed than the other, there is a very broad overlap. Thus, the average height of British men and women is 5 ft 9 in. (1.7 m) and 5 ft 4 in. (1.6 m) respectively, yet very many women are taller than the male average, and vice versa. Much of the difference between people relates to the genetic hand which they are dealt at conception. Rarely can existing training methods or techniques, or, indeed, medical interventions, bring dancers ahead of their better genetically endowed counterparts.

2 INTRODUCTION

Unlike sport, dance is one of the few activities where women have always been regarded as an equal or even more important part of the end product, that is performance. Thus, while women were not allowed even to watch the ancient Olympic Games (the only exception being the Priestess of the Goddess Hera) they were heavily involved together with men in the various festivals, where dance used to have an important and sacred role. In some cultures (e.g. Indian, Arabic) female dancers enjoy particular respect, and their performances have always been received as 'Heaven's gift to mankind'.

Although with a somewhat different emphasis and meaning to that of the older societies, Western countries tend to treat male and female dance similarly. Men and women are trained together in the dance studios using more or less the same methods and techniques. They also perform together, and this is true for most of the different forms of dance. But, are there any differences between the two genders? What about *genetics*? Can humans in general—and dancers in particular—alter their physical performance prospects? The answer is yes, but always in the context of one's genetic programme—which in physical terms is mediated through anatomy and physiology.

3 GENDER FORMATION

3.1 Internal Genitalia

Gender aspects as a whole in dance, as in sport and exercise, embrace genetic, hormonal, anatomical, physiological, psychological, and socio-logical factors. The term 'sexual dimorphism' refers to the two sexes that we grow into, triggered initially by genetic and then hormonal factors operating on the foetus.

Gender is coded by a specific pair of the 23 pairs of human *chromo-somes*, termed the 'sex chromosomes'. They are designated as XX codes for women and XY for men. It is important to note that all mammals are basically female unless specifically masculinized (vice versa with birds, in whom the males have the pair of identical sex chromosomes). In humans the sexing process is initiated in the sixth week of foetal life. If the chromosomes are XX, then female development automatically follows the pre-destined programme; that is the outer layers of the two small clumps of cells which form the undifferentiated sex glands or gonads, begin their development into ovaries. A double set of tubules known as the *Mullerian ducts* then simply grow to form the *fallopian tubes*, uterus and upper vagina.

However, following coded instructions from the male Y-chromosome, the medulla or middle of the undifferentiated gonads is stimulated into becoming the male sex glands or *testes*. Within days, these start to secrete two *hormones*. The 'male' *testosterone* promotes growth of another tubular system known as the *Wolffian ducts* to form the male tubing, in the form of the *epididymis*, vas deferens and ejaculatory duct, all concerned with the passage of semen. The second hormone secreted at this time by the embryonic and still abdominal testis is 'Mullerian inhibitor' that actively inhibits growth of the female Mullerian ducts. Thus, not only is the male tubing actively promoted by one hormone, testosterone, but the embryonic female tubing is actively suppressed by another hormone, the Mullerian inhibitor. The male chromosome is taking no chances!

3.2 External Genitalia

These in the early embryo consist of two cellular aggregates in the pubic region. If there is no Y-chromosome, then these will automatically form into a vagina and a clitoris respectively. But, if Y-induced testosterone is present, then the would-be vagina will heal-up, as it were, and form the scrotum. Note that the skin of both the scrotum and the external vagina is similarly pigmented, wrinkled and hairy; also, the scrotum has a central line (the 'median raphe'), which is where the original vagina healed over. Also, instead of a clitoris, a penis will form, both containing erectile tissues (Money and Erhardt 1971; Sharp 1997).

4 ANATOMICAL ASPECTS

4.1 Body Dimensions

The average British woman is 1.6 m (5 ft 4 in.) tall, compared to 1.7 (5 ft 9 in.) for men, but whatever the height of a race or tribe, men are about 7% taller. This applies also virtually throughout the animal kingdom, with the main exception of the spotted hyena, in which the bitches are larger—probably an evolutionary adaptation to the fact that the males have a tendency to cannibalize the pups. Girls may temporarily be larger—and stronger—between 10 and 12 years, due to their earlier growth spurt, which occurs just over two years earlier in girls. By around 13, the boys forge ahead on average as their growth spurt carries them up to about 10% beyond the girls in many of the physical dimensions.

4.2 Upper Body

Men end up with broader shoulders, longer arms and narrower hips, both in terms of absolute measures, and relative to body height. The shoulder and arm difference usually leads to men being relatively stronger than women in the upper body compared to the lower. The longer arms in men give better biomechanical leverage, which is shown to particular effect in throwing events and racket games, where the terminal velocity of the hand, or of the head of the racket, is the critical factor in determining the speed of missiles leaving either. Longer arms also give men a leverage advantage in rowing and canoeing events. Hence it is entirely reasonable that men perform most of the lifts in dance and ice-dance.

Women tend to have more of a *valgus angle* to their arms than men, whereby their arm is not as straight as men's. That is, if the arm is held down by the side with palms facing forwards, their lower arm angles away from the body (Fig 11.1). Or, when the arm is held extended forward from the shoulder, it is clearly seen to angle out at the elbow in many, but not all, female dancers. It is one reason why many women tend to throw objects, such as balls, stones or snowballs, 'round arm'. The feature is due to a greater male development of the lateral humeral epicondylar cartilage at the elbow. This cartilage has receptor sites specifically programmed to respond to testosterone at puberty, and acts to straighten out the male arm. Normally, this is not important in dance, but a woman with a pronounced valgus (or 'carrying angle') who wished to become a good javelin thrower, might find herself predisposed to elbow injuries. Of the three main athletic throwing events, shot, javelin and discus, and taking into account the different weights of implements which the two sexes throw, women are farthest behind in the javelin, and closest to men in the discus. The latter is what one might expect, given

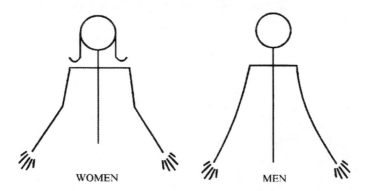

Fig. 11.1 The valgus angle (or 'carrying angle') between the upper arm and the forearm, which may vary from being very pronounced in some women to minimal in others, and which is present to only a very small extent in men

that women's greater spinal flexibility allows more rotation, which is especially important in the discus event.

4.3   Lower Body

The broader hips of women, both in absolute measurement in many cases, and indeed as a proportion of body height, result from a broader pelvis (due to its cells in turn bearing receptor sites responsive to *oestrogen*). This leads in general to a woman's femur tending to make a greater angle medially (the *Q-angle*—see Fig. 11.2) as it inclines towards her knee, which is the main reason why many untrained women throw their heels out when they run. In athletic clubs, such a running style is easily modified, if necessary.

However, a more important implication of this greater medial angulation of the femur relates to the angle of force of the powerful quadriceps

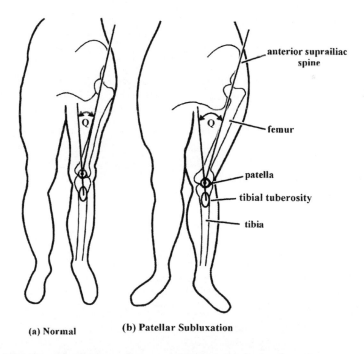

(a) Normal   (b) Patellar Subluxation

Fig. 11.2   The Q-angle between femur and tibia, which may be more pronounced in women due to their broader hips, and more pronounced in broader-hipped women. This may lead to a 'bowstring' effect whereby the kneecap may be pulled sideways out of alignment—patellar subluxation—and to knee pain

muscles as they insert onto the patella or kneecap. The bulk of this muscle group is located laterally, that is on the outer side of the thigh. Thus when it contracts it exerts a strong 'bowstring' effect on the patella tending to pull it sideways (known as subluxation), out of the intercondylar groove on the femur in which it normally tracks (Figs 11.2 and 11.3). This misalignment may lead to excessive wear on the cartilage underside of the patella (the retro-patellar cartilage), resulting in the aching condition of *chondromalacia patellae*. Often known as 'runner's knee', it may occur in dancers, although it is more common in broader-hipped women (Fig. 11.3).

This may also tend to happen in women with a tendency to 'knock-knees', who have too large a Q-angle, which is measured as follows: if you draw a line from the anterior suprailiac spine (the front of your hip bone) to the centre of your patella, and another one from the centre of your patella to your tibial tuberosity (the bony bump just below your knee), the angle these two lines make with each other is the Q-angle (Fig. 11.2). In men it should be less than $10°$, and in women less than $15°$. If it is greater than these, this increases the mechanical advantage of the outside quads, as mentioned above, and it lessens the ability of the one inner quadriceps which acts to counter this bowstring force—the vastus medialis. Thus, overlarge Q-angles lead to bad patellar alignment and tracking in the groove, and increase the possibility of patellar subluxation and of chondromalacia patellae. So, ideally a woman dancer—and runner—should have reasonably narrow hips, and fairly straight legs.

The vastus medialis just mentioned is the one member of the quadriceps muscle group which inserts onto the patella from the opposite direction—medially rather than laterally. And it acts to stabilize the patella in its groove, and to counter the bowstring effect to some extent. If you put your hand on the inner side of your knee, and slowly straighten your leg into full extension, then you will feel the vastus medialis tensing

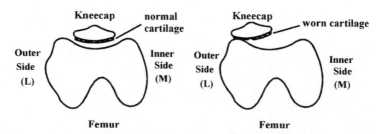

Fig. 11.3 Showing subluxation of the patella, whereby the kneecap is pulled off-line from the groove on the femur in which it normally tracks, with consequent wearing of its underlying cartilage

up as it comes into action just before full extension. Thus, exercises to strengthen the medialis must always involve straightening the leg fully, and slowly, so that there is no swing effect initiated by the other quadriceps muscles. Straightening the leg while seated, and holding it hard *isometrically* (i.e. tensed but not moving) will also strengthen the medialis. This should be done five times on each side, and held for 10–15 seconds, two or three times daily. Otherwise a visit to the 'quads station' of a multigym, with an appropriate demonstration from the instructor, will provide effective training.

4.4 The Foot

Almost, although not completely, confined to female classical ballet dancers is point work. And for this the shape of the foot has important implications. Ideally, viewed from the side, the toes en pointe lie on a line dropped from the mid-patella to the ankle of a well-arched foot (Fig. 11.4). Here, the metatarsal bones of the foot are a straight continuation of the tibia.

If the ankle and/or arch of the foot are not flexible enough, the centre of gravity may fall behind her toes, giving a tendency to fall backwards, unless she bends her knees, which is simply aesthetically impermissible. If the ankle and foot are unusually flexible, with the centre of gravity tending to fall in front of the toes (Fig. 11.4), there is a risk of ligament or

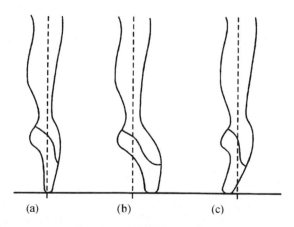

(a)   (b)   (c)

Fig. 11.4 The foot en pointe. (a) The ideal ankle and foot, with the centre of gravity falling along the lines of the weight-bearing toes. (b) An over-stiff ankle and foot, with the centre of gravity falling behind the toes. (c) An over-flexible ankle and foot, with the centre of gravity falling in front of the toes

tendon strain in the hyperextended foot. However, this can be prevented by attention to correct style, with less extension.

The toe bones (or *phalanges*) are also important in point work, ideally with the big toe and its two neighbours being of near equal length, for even weight distribution. Female classical dancers must strengthen the flexor and extensor muscles of the feet, to prevent hyperflexion or hyperextension of the toes while en pointe. Feet which are weak may, in the female classical ballet dancer, predispose to *stress fractures* at the base of the second metatarsal bone, that is the ankle end of the foot bone leading to the second toe, although there is controversy as to exactly why the stress fracture is located there.

4.5 Body Fat

Young women have a considerably greater percentage of their body as fat, compared to men (Table 11.1). As Paul Pacy has indicated above, expressing body fat as a percentage is not especially reliable. Nevertheless, it can be a useful rough guide. The leanest individuals can be found among elite distance runners and gymnasts. Their percentage body fats are in the range from 5 to 8% for men, with very few equivalent women below 16%, and ranging up to 21% (compared to a normal student population of between 12–18% for men, and 22–30% for women).

Until the age of around 10, there is little difference in body fat between boys and girls, but when both sexes go through puberty, the boys tend to lower their body fat percentage, and the girls tend to gain fat. The gain in the women is a natural hormonally induced part of the growth process. The difference in body fat between the 'average' young man and woman

Table 11.1 An approximate comparison of body fat percentages between men and women in their twenties

Men	Women	Fat (%)
Slim		7–11
Average		12–17
Plump	Slim	18–25
Fat	Average	26–30
	Plump	31–36
	Fat	Over 36

is of the order of 70 000 kilocalories (or 300 000 kilojoules), which is just about the energy cost of producing a full-term human infant.

As indicated previously, body fat is primarily an energy store. And men and women tend to store their fat differently. In men, the main fat store is in the abdomen, so a fat man will have a varying degree of 'beer belly', even though he may have quite slim legs. For women, the fat depots are thighs, hips, bust and back of the arm. It makes sense for women not to store fat in their abdomen, which becomes full enough during pregnancy.

This gender difference in average body fat certainly aids survival in extremes of cold and starvation, indeed Scott of the Antarctic may well have reached the South Pole had he and his team been women. It often leads to better performance by women in long-distance sea, lake and loch swims, in many of which women hold the all-comers' records. In part this is because the greater amount of fat acts as an insulation under the skin, and in part it floats women higher in the water, as fat is lighter than water. (Drop a piece of lean meat and a piece of fat—such as butter—in water; and see which sinks, and which floats.) Floating higher makes for easier swimming. However, the greater fat is a handicap in weight-bearing activities involving running or jumping. And often in dance men are not overly appreciative of their women partners carrying excess body fat—which they then may have to lift. This is one of the several pressures towards a degree of female leanness in dance, which may be very harmful if taken to extremes, as described in earlier sections.

The gender difference in body shape, much of it accounted for by body fat distribution, leads to many women having a lower centre of gravity. This may be part of the reason for their better balance, as seen on the balance beam in gymnastics, a discipline for women but not for men, and possibly shown in sailing, where women crew members are often noted as being better balanced in their movements around the boat.

A certain degree of fat is essential to the body; partly this is in terms of acting as a packing material around vital organs, the ovaries for example. Also, fat is important in hormone-processing. It is thought that one reason why women who are very thin stop menstruating may be that they do not have enough fat to fully activate their oestrogen precursors.

5 PHYSIOLOGICAL ASPECTS

5.1 The Cardiorespiratory System

Women have proportionately less blood (65 ml/kg bodyweight compared to 75 ml) than men, and lower haemoglobin concentration (13.9 g/

100 ml compared to 15.8 g). Working maximally, women need 7 litres of blood to carry a litre of oxygen, compared to men's 6 litres, yet proportionately their hearts are about 8% smaller, although maximum heart rates are the same. The net effect is on the *maximal oxygen uptake* (or $\dot{V}O_2$ max), which at elite levels is around 85 ml O_2/kg bodyweight/min for men, and 75 ml for women. As indicated before, it is this $\dot{V}O_2$ max which is responsible for 'aerobic fitness' or overall stamina—the ability to continue strenuous practice or rehearsals for one or two hours—or more. However, in most cases, dance is not a maximal aerobic activity (such as marathon running or 10 000 metre track running), so the sex difference matters relatively little.

5.2   Muscle

Between 10 and 11, many girls are stronger than their boy peers, but boys end up stronger on average. This is partly because the cross-sectional area of their muscles is greater, through *androgen* hormone effects, among other factors—and partly due to the longer levers of their limb bones. There is little difference in muscle quality between the sexes, both tend to generate about 30 *Newtons (N)* of force per square cm of untrained muscle tissue. 30 N is a force of about 3 kg.

   In terms of muscle endurance, women appear to have better low-grade local muscle endurance, for example on repetitions of 50% of their maximum muscle force (see Table 11.2). This may be of benefit in sports such as swimming and cycling, which consist of very large numbers of relatively low-grade contractions. And both are sports where women approach much closer to men's performance than weight-bearing sports such as running—where the forces at each stride are much greater. Although not related to dance, it is of interest to note briefly that women have much better fine manipulative skills, for example as on keyboards, or in electronic assembly.

5.3   Heat Regulation

Exercise such as dance generates considerable heat. About two thirds of food energy appears unavoidably as heat in muscular work, and this must be lost almost as fast as it is generated, or collapse from heat stroke would occur. We live closer to heat death than to cold death. Normal core body temperature is around 37 °C, but much above 43 °C may be quickly fatal. To lose heat in exercise, men tend to sweat more per square metre of skin surface than women do (e.g. 800 ml/hour/m^2 compared to

Table 11.2 Elbow flexion strength, and the number of repeated lifts achieved at loads corresponding to 50–90% of each individual's single maximum load (average values: 409 N for the men, and 190 for the women). Note that as the load becomes progressively lighter, the women's endurance increases over that of the men, that is the women have better lower grade endurance than the men

Percentage of the maximum load (%)	Average number of lifts before fatigue	
	Men	Women
90	3.5	3.7
80	8.0	9.1
70	12.0	17.0
60	20.0	33.3
50	34.8	66.5

Source: Data courtesy of Professor Ron Maughan, University of Aberdeen

600 ml/hour/m^2). However, women tend to lose more heat by radiation. This benefits women in very humid conditions, where sweat cannot evaporate very readily into air already saturated with water vapour. Under such conditions, and not being so reliant on sweating, women tend to radiate more of their heat away, through a warm skin, red with dilated blood vessels radiating the heat like tiny electric fire-bars. Men benefit in dry heat, as their sweat can be evaporated. Sweat which drops off is simply wasted, as far as cooling is concerned, because it is when the sweat changes from liquid into water vapour (i.e. steam), that heat energy is taken from the skin, or, more accurately, from the warm blood circulating through the skin.

Thus women thermoregulate better in wet heat, and men better in dry heat. Men will tend to be more severely affected in a hot humid studio, and women in a hot dry studio. However, their greater sweat production implies that men tend to suffer more quickly than women from *dehydration*. Men may also die quicker than women from dehydration, for example in desert accidents, or if shipwrecked in mid-ocean. In both sexes, sweat patterns change through exercise and training, covering more extensive areas of skin, and occurring sooner. It comes as a surprise to some, that fit people sweat sooner, as experienced by many dancers or athletes at parties or receptions. In both sexes the levels of salts (or *electrolytes*) in sweat drop markedly, the higher their fitness levels, as shown in Table 11.3. In other words, the fitter you are, the better you conserve your body salts.

Table 11.3 Levels of electrolytes (salts) in blood, and sweat of untrained, trained and highly trained athletes or dancers. Note that the fitter the subject, the more dilute sweat they secrete, that is the better they conserve their blood electrolytes (the unit is 'milli-equivalents per litre')

	Electrolytes (m.eq/litre)			
	Sodium (Na)	Chloride (Cl)	Potassium (K)	Magnesium (Mg)
Blood	140	100	4	1.5
Sweat (untrained)	60	50	5	3.0
Sweat (trained)	40	30	4	1.5
Sweat (highly trained)	30	25	2.5	1.0

5.4 Flexibility

Women have greater flexibility than men, as may be seen when asking a group of untrained men and women to plantar flex their foot, that is 'point their toe'. This enhanced flexibility is, of course, much featured in gymnastics and many forms of dance (and in modern circuses, for example the Chinese National Circus, and the Cirque du Soleil). In part the flexibility of women is due to slight differences in their joints. In part it may be due to the presence of the hormone *relaxin*, which appears to act on the ground substance of *collagen*, the vital structural element in ligament and tendon, imparting a greater degree of elasticity. Relaxin comes into its own during childbirth, when it has a major function in acting on the *symphasis pubis* joint. This is where the two pubic bones meet each other at the bony floor of the pelvis—between the legs. Normally there is very little space between the two pubic bones, nor do they normally move, but under the influence of relaxin, the connecting collagen may allow a considerable widening between the pubic bones, thus enlarging the birth canal.

5.5 The Special Senses

Men have better visual acuity on average, that is they can differentiate two points as being distinct about 10% farther away than women. This implies that, on average, men will read the destination of an oncoming bus slightly earlier than women. However, women appear to be better at colour differentiation (which may be important in matching colour in painting stage sets), especially in the blue–green range. Therefore if a set involves matching shades of turquoise, it would perhaps be better to have a woman on the job! (unless the audience is expected to be entirely male). Women may hear quieter sounds than men, and also appear better at differentiating fine changes in musical tones, so they may complain earlier than men of instruments being off-key. Finally, and this would only come into play after the performance is over, women appear to have a better sense of taste, for example in wine tasting.

6   CONCLUSIONS

Men in general are bigger than women, although there is considerable overlap. This alone gives them a strength and leverage advantage. Most anatomical differences between the two genders are due to different roles in the reproduction process. Women carry proportionately more fat, which gives them a modest weight handicap, but they are more flexible and have better balance. Women thermoregulate better in wet heat, and men better in dry heat. However, their greater sweat production implies that men tend to suffer more quickly than women from dehydration. Finally, men have better visual acuity than women, whereas the latter appear to be better at colour differentiation, can hear quieter sounds, and have a better sense of taste than men.

7   FURTHER READING

Most texts of exercise physiology have chapters on gender issues, but a very good comprehensive account is:

Christine Wells (1995) *Women, sport and performance: a physiological perspective.* Champaign, IL: Human Kinetics

REFERENCES

Money J, Erhardt A (1971) *Man, woman, boy, girl.* Baltimore, MD: Johns Hopkins
Sharp NCC (1995) Body fat and weight management. In: Bean A, Wellington P (eds), *Sports nutrition for women.* London: A & C Black: ch. 6

Sharp NCC (1997) The new sexual dimorphism. *British Journal of Sports Medicine,* **31**: 82–3

Wilmore JH, Costill DL (1994) Gender issues and the female athlete. In: *Physiology of sport and exercise.* Champaign IL: Human Kinetics: ch. 19

Chapter 12

Children and Dance

Colin Boreham

1 SUMMARY

For the young dancer, adolescence is a critical period, ushering in a multitude of physiological and anatomical changes that have profound implications for dance performance and health in general. Males become leaner, more muscular and powerful, resulting in enhanced performances on most tests of physical fitness (the important exception being flexibility) Females tend to develop broader hips and relatively narrower shoulders with an increased proportion of body fat, and consequently demonstrate little or no improvement in physical performance. The timing of the various processes of maturation at puberty varies from one individual to the next. Thus, early-maturing males and later-maturing females tend to enjoy temporary advantages in performance over their peers who are average or late maturing. Such advantages however, are not permanent, and teachers should be sensitive to the needs of those who mature somewhat later.

In general, young dancers (as athletes in an artistic setting) will benefit from supplementary training, for example strength or power exercises, away from the dance studio. Such training need not be extensive (as few as two short sessions of weight training each week has been shown to enhance strength in adolescent males) and will aid performance and reduce the risk of musculoskeletal injury, both acute and chronic. Due to certain thermoregulatory characteristics of children, young dancers should wear loose, light clothing and should be encouraged to drink little and often throughout practice and training sessions, particularly if performed in a warm environment. Dance experts and teachers should adhere to well-tested principles of physical training when planning schedules, and should strive to maintain interest and enthusiasm through the key elements of variety and enjoyment.

2   INTRODUCTION

Dance is a form of physical activity enjoyed by almost all children at one stage or other. Some may develop into talented performers, and be subject to the same pressures and physical strains imposed upon top athletes.

While dance in general is an excellent form of physical activity for children, and will confer general health benefits upon its practitioners (such as enhanced leanness, physical fitness, bone density and motor skill levels), there are also a number of potential pitfalls to be avoided. Given the aesthetic nature of elite dance with its stereotype of the ideal shape, it is perhaps not surprising that reports of eating disorders such as *anorexia nervosa* and *bulimia nervosa* indicate a prevalence in female dancers of up to 25%, compared with only 1 or 2% for the general female population. Great care must be taken, particularly over the adolescent period from 12 to 16 years, to prevent such eating disorders becoming manifest, as they are not only dangerous in themselves (between 5 and 18% of cases may result in death) but are also implicated in menstrual dysfunction and loss of bone mass (more about the latter appears in Chapter 10 above).

An appreciation of some of the specific issues associated with children and dance is important for at least three reasons. Firstly, almost every child is exposed to dance, whether formally in the school setting, or informally in the family circle or local community. Secondly, there is a growing appreciation of the importance of overall physical activity to the current and future health of the child, and dance is in many ways the ideal vehicle for the promotion and maintenance of such activity. Thirdly, for the elite performer, *childhood* is the seedbed for later excellence, and as such, is a critical period in the development of dance talent. As childhood is also a time of rapid physical, intellectual and social change, it is important to review some of the processes of *growth* and *maturation*, and how these may impinge upon performance in the young dancer. Particular attention will be paid to the period of adolescence (approximately between the ages of 10 and 18 years) when the pace of change is at its most rapid, and the consequences of growth and maturation for dance at their most acute.

3 GROWTH, MATURATION AND PHYSICAL PERFORMANCE

Growth following birth may be divided into four periods: infancy (birth to one year), early childhood (pre-school), middle childhood (to around the age of 10) and adolescence (10 to 18 years). Although children may be engaged in dance from a very young age, this involvement will seldom be at a high level until the pre-adolescent and adolescent period of childhood. The remainder of this chapter will therefore concentrate upon the *adolescent growth period*, paying particular attention to gender differences arising from the processes of accelerated growth and differential maturation at this time.

In general, physical differences between boys and girls that may influence dance performance are minimal before adolescence. Girls, however, begin their adolescent growth spurt, on average, two years before boys (12 versus 14 years, respectively). This can give a temporary physical advantage to girls, who for a year or two may be slightly taller and heavier than their male counterparts. Thus, in ballet, it may be easier for a 12-year-old girl to perform a lift on her male partner than vice versa. However, within one or two years, this situation becomes reversed, with interest, as the male growth spurt takes over, and the average boy surpasses his female counterpart in most physical dimensions (height, weight, muscle mass) and fitness measures (strength, speed, endurance, power).

The relatively minor differences in size and shape between the sexes that are evident before adolescence also become magnified during this period. Following the growth spurt, girls generally display a broader pelvis, with a proportionately longer trunk:legs ratio. *Body composition* also changes, with the average girl accumulating about 5% of her body weight as fat (increasing from about 20 to 25% of total body weight), while the average boy loses 2 or 3% of his body fat (falling from about 18 to 16%) over adolescence. In children, levels of activity and fitness are closely associated with the amount of fat deposited around the body (Boreham, Twisk, Savage *et al.* 1997), so it is not surprising to learn that young dancers are much leaner than the 'average' figures quoted above. For adult female and male ballet dancers, body fat percentages of 18–20% and 12–15% respectively have been reported (Hergenroeder, Fioretto and Klish 1991). Such relative leanness accounts at least partly for the particular growth patterns of female ballet dancers (Fig. 12.1) who tend as a group to be of average height but well below average weight. If taken to extremes, this emphasis on leanness may contribute to medical complications in young girl dancers, as previously discussed in this book.

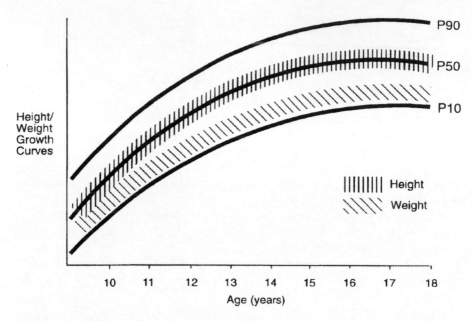

Fig 12.1   Approximations of growth curves for heights and weights of female ballet dancers. Note that while height is close to the average (*P*50 = 50th percentile), weight is well below average throughout adolescence
Source: Adapted from Malina (1994)

In addition to becoming leaner over the adolescent period, boys also experience a dramatic rise in their muscle mass, shoulder width (by maturity, the male shoulder:hip ratio is 1.45, compared with 1.35 for females) and leg length. Such differences between the sexes—the boys being generally leaner, more muscular, broader shouldered and narrower hipped, with relatively longer legs and straighter limbs—have obvious implications for dance, and it is no surprise that patterns of dance and gender roles within dance have evolved accordingly. Some examples of how boys and girls evolve over the period of adolescence are given in Fig. 12.2.

At this point, it may also be appropriate to say something about the concept of 'adolescent awkwardness'—that temporary disruption of co-ordination and balance that seems to occur during the growth spurt. There is some evidence (Beunen and Malina 1988) that such an increase in clumsiness may appear, especially in boys, lasting for about six months. This may affect up to one third of boys, and is probably caused by the disproportionate growth of trunk over legs (resulting in a 'top-heavy' frame). Whatever their origins, these symptoms soon disappear.

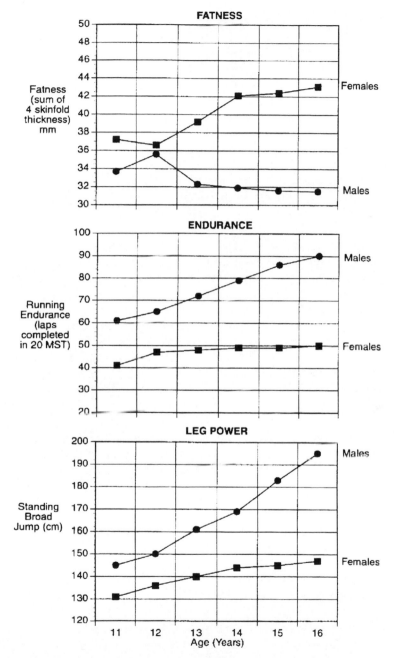

Fig 12.2 The development of certain aspects of physical fitness over adolescence
Source: Data are from the Northern Ireland Fitness Survey (1990)

4   INDIVIDUAL DIFFERENCES IN MATURATION

A casual glance at any group of young teenagers—say at 13 years of age—reveals a startling feature which is not apparent at any other stage in the lifecycle. While some boys may be relatively muscular, with deep voices and a beard (the so called 'early maturers'), others will be slight in build, speaking in treble voices and displaying no facial hair at all (the 'late maturers'). A similar situation holds with girls of course, with the commencement of *puberty* in the early maturers occurring as much as 5 years before that of the late maturers in extreme cases (Armstrong and Welsman 1997). Given the far-reaching physical changes (outlined in Chapter 10) that accompany puberty, whether a given child is an early, late or average maturer can have major consequences for their perform-ance in dance over the adolescent period.

The early maturing male dancer—with his increased strength, power, leanness and height—may well find himself at a physical advantage over his peers who mature at an average or late age. Obviously, care must be taken to nurture and encourage these late developers, who, given appro-priate guidance and patience, may well catch up, and even surpass (if their inherent skills are superior) their early maturing peers by their late teens. For females, the situation is reversed, with the leaner, lighter and more linear late maturers (who, incidentally, also usually tend to perform better on *motor tasks*) being at a distinct advantage (Malina and Bouchard 1991). It is therefore not surprising that elite ballet dancers' menarche (i.e. their first period) tends to be 1–2 years later than average (Fogelholm, Lichtenbelt, Ottenheijm and Westerterp 1996). Such a delayed menarche may be partly inherited, given that the mothers of such girls also display a tendency towards late menarche (Brooks-Gunn and Warren 1988). However, delayed menarche is also a feature of sports characterized by high training loads and an emphasis on weight control, such as gymnas-tics, ice-skating and diving (Claessens, Malina, Lefevre *et al.* 1992). The potentially damaging—but not inevitable—effects of high training loads and insufficient food intake in the young female dancer are covered by Roger Wolman in Chapter 10.

5   HEALTH BENEFITS OF DANCE IN CHILDREN

In general, regular physical activity, such as that experienced by the young dancer attending three or four sessions each week will fulfil the recommendations recently adopted for healthy physical activity in chil-dren (Sallis and Patrick 1994). As a result, such activity will probably lower the risk of developing 'lifestyle' diseases such as coronary heart disease later in life, particularly if continued into adulthood (Boreham, Twisk, Savage *et al.* 1997; Raitakari, Taimela, Porkka *et al.* 1997).

Regular dance participation will also help to develop overall physical fitness. Padfield, Eisenman and Leutkemeier (1993) tested the physical fitness of 40 adolescent females divided into recreational (less than 5 hours of dance per week) and performing dancers (greater than 5 hours per week). In comparison with their sedentary peers, both groups displayed superior flexibility, muscularity and *aerobic* and *anaerobic* capacities, indicating that just a few hours of dance each week may improve overall fitness for everyday activities and other sports and pastimes. Providing further experimental evidence for such benefits, Flores (1995) reported that 12 weeks of thrice-weekly aerobic dance sessions in 10–13-year-old children, significantly improved their relative leanness and resting heart rates. Even the foetus is not immune to the benefits of dance—40 minutes of low-impact aerobic dance in pregnant women proved more effective in raising foetal heart rate than walking at the same relative intensity (McMurray, Katz, Poe and Hackney 1995).

In addition to these benefits, the single greatest contribution that dance activities can make to the health of the child is likely to lie in the area of bone health. The most common disease of bone is *osteoporosis*, a condition in which the strength of bone is diminished, due largely to a progressive loss of mineral content (mainly calcium). Osteoporosis usually affects middle-aged and elderly females and may be responsible for up to 150 000 fractures of the hip, wrist and vertebrae (spine) each year in British women alone. Bone mass in later life (and hence, the risk of fracture) is primarily determined by two factors: (1) the peak bone mass achieved in early adulthood (which represents a 'bone bank'); and (2) the rate of loss of this bone mass experienced throughout adult life. Both processes may be influenced by exercise—in particular, achieving an optimal peak bone mass in early adulthood may be significantly influenced by the amount of physical activity during adolescence. Most notably, the years from about 9 to 15 (when one third of the bones' total mineral content is accumulated) are critical. The type of exercise is also important, with studies indicating that activities that incorporate sudden changes of direction and high impact forces—as in jumping—are most effective for strengthening bones in females. Thus, dance in all its forms would appear to be the ideal vehicle to promote bone health in young females, and to delay, or prevent altogether, osteoporosis in later life. This potential for prevention is illustrated schematically in Fig. 12.3.

Such mechanisms have some support from experimental research studies. Khan, Bennell, Crichton *et al.* (1997), for example, showed that classical ballet classes undertaken around 10–14 years of age were

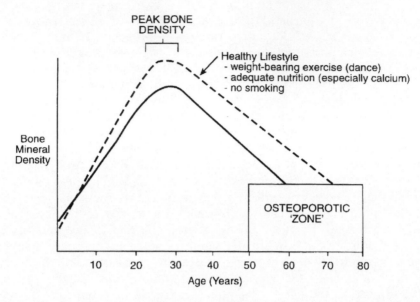

Fig 12.3 A model showing the likely influence of a healthy lifestyle (weight-bearing exercise such as dance, adequate nutrition and calcium intake) during childhood and adolescence on the achievement of an optimal peak bone density. Note that a higher peak bone density in early adulthood may delay the onset of osteoporosis in later life

associated with increased hip *bone density* in retired dancers, irrespective of the subjects' levels of activity in adulthood. Other studies (for example Heinonen, Kannus, Sievanen *et al.* 1996) have confirmed that as little as 18 months of regular (3 times weekly), high-impact exercise in middle-aged women can significantly improve bone mineral density when compared with results from a control group which did no exercise. It seems therefore that a lifelong dance programme in females, beginning in early adolescence and carrying on into middle age, may be one of the more feasible and enjoyable ways of optimizing and maintaining bone health. However—and this is an important qualification to the above positive health message—such benefits as improved bone mineral density may not apply for the minority of dancers in whom training loads and dietary control are taken to extremes, particularly if associated with menstrual irregularities. The features and dangers of this so-called 'female athlete triad' (consisting of disrupted eating, menstrual dysfunction and bone mineral disorders), were again addressed more fully in Chapter 10.

6 TRAINING FOR DANCE IN CHILDREN

6.1 General Principles

Training for dance may start at a young age. In general, regular training will be a positive influence in a young person's development, enhancing skills, various aspects of fitness including flexibility, strength and leanness, and introducing order and self-discipline and a sense of purpose within a social environment. Although a detailed review of dance-training practices in children is outside the scope of this chapter, some general principles guiding practice should be borne in mind:

- Individuals in positions of influence over young dancers should be aware of, and sensitive to, the complex changes that dominate the adolescent's life. Progress should always be viewed in relation to the individual's stage of biological development.
- Progress should be gradual, with the early emphasis on the acquisition of basic skills and physical fitness. Large volumes of work in classes, rehearsals and performance should not be imposed before late adolescence.
- For all dancers, but particularly for elite young dancers, basic skills training should be augmented by specific fitness training, to improve strength, power and endurance. Such training will aid performance and help to reduce injuries.
- Normal growth and development should not be interfered with in any way. Particularly for adolescent female dancers, healthy nutritional practices should be encouraged, and an undue emphasis on an 'ideal' body weight and shape avoided.
- Dance training for the young must be varied and it must be fun. In this respect it is a challenge to the teacher of dance to combine basic skills and fitness training with a sense of enjoyment.

6.2 Injury and Children—Dance and Training Implications

Although there is a scarcity of information on the types and rates of injury for many forms of dance, studies on ballet indicate surprisingly few injuries in young participants. Less than five injuries per 1000 hours of participation have been recorded (Backx 1996), which is far less than some of the more popular forms of childhood activity such as soccer, tennis, swimming and field hockey. Why this should be so is open to speculation, but the emphasis on lengthy and thorough warming-up, involving stretching and *calisthenics*, in ballet might be one factor preventing injury. Indeed, there is some evidence (Kokkonen, Eldredge and Nelson 1997) that regular stretching training (40 minutes, three times weekly) may improve general athleticism, as well as reducing the risk of injury (Fig. 12.4).

Other factors which have been thought important in *primary prevention* of sport—and dance—injury in children (Backx, 1996) include the provision of a safe environment (e.g. appropriate dancing surfaces) and specific fitness training for the activity concerned. By introducing specific strengthening activities (such as simple weight training), power exercises (such as jump training, or *plyometrics*) and endurance training (some stationary cycling, or jogging) young ballet dancers should, in theory, reduce their susceptibility to injury. A fitter young dancer will not fatigue as rapidly (the risk of injury increases with fatigue), and will be able to perform well within their 'limits of tolerance', unlike the unfit dancer who may be required to perform at (or beyond) their physical capabilities. However, supplementary fitness training for young dancers should probably not be started before secondary school age (11+).

Strength training should initially be confined to simple body weight exercises (sit-ups, press-ups and so on) and single-station strength

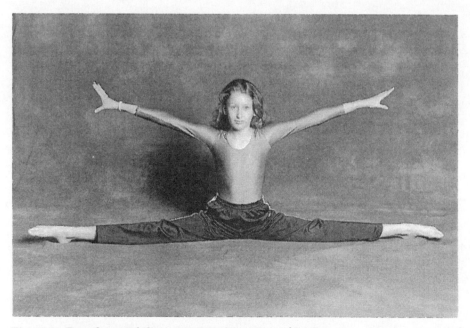

Fig 12.4 Regular mobility training in young dancers may improve general fitness and reduce susceptibility to injury

machines of the type now found in the majority of fitness suites and health clubs. Such training should take place two or three times each week, should last no more than 30 minutes or so, and should ideally be performed immediately following a dance session (thus alleviating the need for warm-up). Simple strength-training exercises should be performed with loads that allow 10–15 repetitions for each set of exercises, with the exception of 'body weight' exercises, such as sit-ups, which should be performed with higher repetitions (say 20–30). Three 'sets' of each exercise are optimal, with lighter loads on the first warm-up set of exercises. A balanced strengthening programme should attempt to exercise all major muscle groups, with the emphasis in young dancers on the legs and trunk. Exercises such as: bench press, press behind neck, leg extensions/leg press, hamstring curls, sit-ups and back hyperextensions, would provide such a programme. Strength training has been shown to be very effective in young children and adolescents (Pfeiffer and Francis 1986; Ozmun, Mikesky and Surbury 1994), but should not be undertaken without the benefit of advice and supervision from qualified experts.

In many ways, the young dancer should be viewed and treated as a young athlete. The developments of skills and physical fitness go hand in glove, and both require considerable experience and knowledge in their integration for optimal performance. Above all, the health and happiness of the young dancer should be the prime concern of those in positions of authority, be they coaches, trainers, choreographers or parents.

7 TEMPERATURE REGULATION AND FLUID BALANCE

During activities such as dance, the working muscles produce large amounts of metabolic heat. The resulting excess heat must be dispersed to the environment to avoid serious problems. This *thermoregulation* is accomplished by the following mechanisms: convection, radiation and evaporation (via sweating). In a warm environment, sweating is the main mechanism for heat loss, and there is some evidence that the sweating rate of children is lower (by about 30–40%) than that of adults. Also the child's larger ratio of body surface area to body mass, means that the child will tend to absorb heat from the environment in hot conditions and lose heat in cold conditions more rapidly than the adult. Such differences in thermoregulation between adults and children should encourage caution in this regard towards the young dancer. Some sensible guidelines include:

- Ensure full hydration before exercise by encouraging children to drink water or a sport drink at least 20 minutes beforehand.

- Provide for, and encourage regular drinking of small amounts during the dance sessions. Don't wait until thirst manifests itself.
- Drinks should be chilled, preferably flavoured (especially for children) and not too concentrated.
- Vigorously discourage weight loss through sweating. Clothing for exercise should be light and loose, with an adequate exposure of skin.
- Ensure the young dancer is educated in, and adheres to, the above principles.

8 CONCLUSIONS

It is clear that for children, dance is a worthwhile activity with many potential benefits to health, enjoyment and skill development. However, teachers, coaches and parents (as well as the young dancers themselves) should be aware of the complex and far-reaching physical changes that occur over the period of adolescence—changes that can influence performance to a much greater extent than any regime of dance training. Consequently, progress in certain individuals during adolescence may be simply a product of early maturation, while others lag behind only to catch up or surpass their peers at a later time. Great care must be taken to ensure that undue pressures are not exerted on young female dancers to conform to an 'ideal' weight or shape at a time when rapid changes in these parameters are naturally occurring. Adequate food intake must be encouraged, and if necessary, training loads moderated to ensure that normal menstruation commences and is maintained into adulthood. Finally, young dancers should be encouraged to undertake moderate amounts of supplementary training, away from the studio, to help minimize risk of injury and maximize performance.

9 FURTHER READING

Armstrong N, Welsman J (1997) *Young people and physical activity*. Oxford University Press

Backx FJG (1996) Epidemiology of paediatric sports-related injuries. In: Bar-Or, O (ed.), *The child and adolescent athlete*. Oxford, UK: Blackwell Science: pp. 163–72

Khan KM, Bennell KL, Crichton KJ *et al.* (1997) Childhood ballet classes, not adult ballet training predicts adult hipbone density in former dancers. (Abstract) *Medicine and Science in Sports and Exercise*, **29** Suppl.: S59

Malina RM, Bouchard C (1991) Growth, maturation and physical activity. Champaign, IL: Human Kinetics

Raitakari OT, Taimela S, Porkka KVK *et al.* (1997) Association between physical activity and risk factors for coronary heart disease. *Medicine and Science in Sports and Exercise*, **29**(8): 1055–61

Sallis JF, Patrick K (1994) Physical activity guidelines for adolescents. *Pediatric Exercise Science*, **6**: 302–14

Sharp C (1991) The exercise physiology of children. In Grisogono V, Sharp C, Griffin J. *Children and sport: fitness injuries and diet.* London, UK; John Murray.

REFERENCES

Armstrong N, Welsman J (1997) *Young people and physical activity.* Oxford University Press

Backx FJG (1996) Epidemiology of paediatric sports-related injuries. In: Bar-Or, O (ed.) *The child and adolescent athlete.* Oxford, UK: Blackwell Science: pp. 163–72

Beunen G, Malina RM (1988) Growth and physical performance relative to the timing of the adolescent growth spurt. In: *Exercise and sports sciences reviews.* American College of Sports Medicine Series, New York: Macmillan: Vol. 16, ch. 15

Boreham CAG, Twisk J, Savage MJ *et al.* (1997) Physical activity, sports participation, and risk factors in adolescents. *Medicine and Science in Sports and Exercise*, **29**(6): 788–93

Brooks-Gunn J, Warren JP (1988) Mother–daughter differences in menarcheal age in adolescent girls attending national dance company schools and non-dancers. *Annals of Human Biology*, **15**: 35–43

Claessens AL, Malina RM, Lefevre J *et al.* (1992) Growth and menarcheal status of elite female gymnasts. *Medicine and Science in Sports and Exercise*, **24**: 755–63

Flores R (1995) Dance for health—improving fitness in African-American and Hispanic adolescents. *Public Health Report*, **110**: 189–93

Fogelholm M, Lichtenbelt WVM, Ottenheijm R, Westerterp K (1996) Amenorrhoea in ballet dancers in the Netherlands. *Medicine and Science in Sports and Exercise*, **28**: 545–51

Heinonen A, Kannus P, Sievanen J *et al.* (1996) Randomised controlled trial of effect of high impact exercise on selected risk factors for osteoporotic fractures. *Lancet*, **348**: 1343–7

Hergenroeder AC, Fioretto ML, Klish WJ (1991) Body composition in ballet dancers measured by total body electrical conductivity. *Medicine and Science in Sports and Exercise*, **23**: 528–33

Khan KM, Bennell KL, Crichton KJ *et al.* (1997) Childhood ballet classes, not adult ballet training predicts adult hipbone density in former dancers. (Abstract) *Medicine and Science in Sports and Exercise*, **29** Suppl.: S59

Kokkonen J, Eldredge C, Nelson AG (1997) Chronic Static Stretching improves specific sports skills. (Abstract) *Medicine and Science in Sports and Exercise*, **29** Suppl.: S63

Malina RM (1994) Physical growth and biological maturation of young athletes. In: *Exercise and sports sciences reviews*, American College of Sports Medicine Series. New York: Williams & Wilkins: Vol. 22, ch. 13

Malina RM, Bouchard C (1991) *Growth, maturation and physical activity.* Champaign, IL: Human Kinetics

McMurray RG, Katz VL, Poe MP, Hackney AC (1995) Maternal and fetal responses to low impact aerobic dance. *American Journal of Perinatology*, **12**(4): 282–5

Northern Ireland Fitness Survey (1990) *The fitness, physical activity, attitudes and lifestyles of Northern Ireland post primary schoolchildren.* Division of Physical and Health Education, The Queen's University of Belfast

Ozmun JC, Mikesky AE, Surbury PR (1994) Neuromuscular adaptations following prepubescent strength training. *Medicine and Science in Sports and Exercise*, **26**: 510–14

Padfield JA, Eisenman PA, Luetkemeier MJ, Fitt SS (1993) Physiological profiles of performing and recreational early adolescent female dancers. *Paediatric Exercise Science*, **5**: 51–9

Pfeiffer RD, Francis RS (1986) Effects of strength training on muscle development in prepubescent, pubescent and post-pubescent males. *Physician and Sportsmedicine*, **14**(9): 134–43

Raitakari OT, Taimela S, Porkka KVK *et al.* (1997) Association between physical activity and risk factors for coronary heart disease. *Medicine and Science in Sports and Exercise*, **29**(8): 1055–61

Sallis JF, Patrick K (1994) Physical activity guidelines for adolescents. *Paediatric Exercise Science*, **6**: 302–14

Chapter 13

Life After a Professional Dance Career

Susie Dinan

1 SUMMARY

Current dance education and training programmes still fail to prepare dancers for the world of dance, transition and retirement. This leaves the transition between dance and the 'life after' to a combination of the dancer's own resources and luck. Today, we need a more responsible and holistic approach to dance training to include specialist support services focusing on the artistic, personal, psychological and physical development of the dancer *as well as* transferable skills and lifelong learning.

The international dance community is the key to this change. This chapter outlines how that community, through its embryonic transition movement, is beginning to address the inequalities dancers suffer in artistic, professional and financial status and dispel the myths and misconceptions held by society and dancers alike about dance and its performers. It must alert dancers to the implications of sudden physical inactivity and the vulnerabilities the dancing years may leave. Above all, it must make them aware that—like all of us—they cannot escape the ageing process but that, through sensitive and appropriate physical training systems, they can achieve optimal health and success both in their performing years and in the life they want to lead 'afterwards'.

2   INTRODUCTION

The average age for the active dancer has dropped, puzzlingly and dramatically, over the last decade from mid to late thirties to mid to late twenties. Injuries account for only 11% of this early retirement phenomenon as the decision to retire is often based on a wide range of factors which will vary depending on the genre and country in which a dancer works. 'Change of interest' was the most frequent reason given for retirement (22%) followed by 'difficulty finding work because of age' (18%) and further down the scale, 'financial problems' (14%) (Leach 1997). Nevertheless, despite this seemingly bleak situation, one thing is abundantly clear: there *is* Life after Dance!

This chapter is a celebration of dancers in transition; of the growing evidence that dancers can make extraordinary transitions to 'ordinary' careers and to fulfilling healthy later lives if they, and those responsible for their training, prepare early enough for this part of a dancer's life. It is a celebration of the fact that today's dancers are part of a fundamental, unprecedented movement in the history of dance—a movement that no longer perceives life after dance merely as the 'twilight years' but, rather, as the beginning of a new life of fulfilment and opportunity. Above all, this chapter celebrates the growing acknowledgement that the more holistic and integrated the approach to dance education and training, the fitter and healthier will be the dancer, the transition, the new life, and dance as a whole.

As a subject, 'dance transition' relates to a wide range of aspects integral to dance life, such as early education, methods of training, causes and prevention of injuries, dance physiology and psychology, nutrition and healthcare as well as the status of dancers within society and the artistic community. It provides valuable insights into the intrinsic and extrinsic factors that affect dancers' development and their continuing health status and quality of life. It serves to highlight both the strengths and the weaknesses in the dance tradition and, most importantly, the need to view the development of the whole person and the artist as the core aim of dance training. It is this concern for the whole person of the dancer—with its parallel developments of the body and the mind—that will move dancers towards a better understanding and control of their own health and positive well-being during and after their performing years. Their achievement of optimal, lifelong health and fitness depends upon it.

Neither the immediate future of the art form, much less the long-term future of the dance, will be best served by solely shaping the bodies of competent technicians. Neglect of intellectual curiosity and of the development of practical and social skills encourages the dancer's tendency to become isolated and obsessive within the confines of the dance world. The art of dance, its artists and society need the surefooting of well-developed minds. In this chapter, selected physiological, sociological, and psychological aspects in relation to the ageing dancer will be discussed, while suggestions will be made on how dancers will be better equipped for the years following retirement.

3   INTERNATIONAL RECOGNITION OF THE NEEDS OF DANCERS IN TRANSITION

The need for change in the management of retiring dancers was first signalled in the late 1960s and early 1970s by the foresight of individuals in both commerce and dance. There was concern that the experience of retirement was often so profound that it temporarily and, in many cases permanently, impaired the dancer's sense of identity and ability to make the transition to another valued career. While it was acknowledged that the transient, highly committed nature of the dancer's life would involve pain in the passing, the degree of disorientation and depression expressed both during the dancing years (Brinson and Dick 1996) and in transition (Leach 1997) seemed in due proportion to the lack of preparation for these events. Moreover, there was concern at the wastefulness of failing to redeploy such valuable resources as, after a lifetime of dedication and distinction, many dancers remained unemployed after retirement.

Britain and the Netherlands were the first to formalize a system of support, and were quickly followed by Canada and the US. Their initial resettlement strategies took the form of financial assistance to facilitate retraining and extensive, informal, individual mentoring. Counselling services were added but it soon became evident that, although these measures had done a great deal, a large part of the solution lay in the dance education and training process itself, as well as in the way that society tends to view dance and the dancer. Although considerable growth and innovation took place in the resettlement programmes between 1973 and 1988, the proportionally small numbers, as well as the insularity and the traditions that still characterize the dance community, meant that international collaboration was necessary to effect fundamental change.

In 1993, the International Organization for the Transition of Professional Dancers (IOTPD) was established at the University of Lausanne under the patronage of UNESCO. It currently comprises 17 countries committed to raising awareness of, and support for, the specialist needs of dancers in transition throughout the world. The IOTPD organizational objectives were established in the first international symposium in May 1995. They are:

> - Accident and illness insurance for all dancers from the start of their training to completion of their transition—with a special guarantee of financial support where incapacity leads to loss of career
> - Career counselling service
> - Financial solutions to the problems of transition
> - Equal social protection for employed and self-employed for all dancers
> - Pension rights related to length of service/career not age
> - Supplementary accident insurance schemes for dancers
> - Adequate medical care
> - Adequate academic education, alongside dance training, to better prepare dancers for their eventual transition

This emphasis on transition seeks to effect the necessary changes to ensure that dancers receive a training that nurtures them as people as well as artists and equips them with a range of life skills, knowledge and specialist resources. It aims to provide dancers with the confidence that their training, dedication and discipline are highly prized, transferable skills that provide a solid foundation for a future outside the world of dance.

4   THE DANCER'S DILEMMA

4.1   Changing Work Patterns and Early Retirement

Today, there is no such thing as a standard dance career. There are as many career patterns as there are genres and styles and, with very few exceptions, the dancer's career is intense and increasingly short-lived. Where previously there was greater security in the classical idiom than in music theatre and variety, *all* dancers' career paths are now more and more characterized by short-term or even single production contracts won by audition.

Many established companies have difficulty providing full-year contracts, let alone contracts which offer security over a full career span. Less than half offered 46 weeks in one financial year. The most common pattern is 37 weeks. Rare exceptions are the major, generally classical, state companies in Scandinavia, France and Italy where full security and a fixed pension age of 40–45 are enjoyed by the dancers. Dancers in these countries who do not work for state companies often have little or no contractual security or pension.

In addition to shorter work seasons and, consequently, longer unemployment periods, there are fewer opportunities. Dancers now travel widely to compete for contracts; this international mobility not only increases competition, but further jeopardizes the dancer's security. Insufficient working periods can also mean that the dancer fails to meet minimum requirements for access to health insurance, unemployment compensation and pension coverage in the countries where he or she is working.

4.2 Ageing, Burnout and Early Retirement

'Ageism and aestheticism in our society prevent people seeing the real beauty in older peoples' movement' (Tajet-Foxell 1997). These words pose a powerful challenge to the dance community, especially when dancers are unnecessarily and unjustly propelled out of the profession at a wastefully young age.

In the independent sector in particular, UK dancers feel that audiences and promoters fail to value the older dancers' experience (Brinson and Dick 1996). Preference is given to the 'fresh and new' so that at a time when, theoretically, dancers should be at the peak of their physical and emotional capacity, they are already incurring physical damage and feelings of rejection and lack of reward for years of hard work.

As discussed in Chapter 10, intense physical activity during adolescent growth spurts may compromise physical development and predispose the dancer to bone and joint problems in later life. As a further consequence of the demanding time schedules, intellectual and emotional maturity can be severely underdeveloped by the start of a full-time career that itself leaves little time or energy for healthy maturation. Women are also more likely to leave the dance profession because of age and burnout and are less likely to leave because they positively want to change careers. Lack of opportunity in this female-dominated profession is often cited as an early retirement incentive.

These points raise crucial issues that challenge the core assumptions of modern training for both male and female dancers. In addition to the implications of burnout which were discussed in earlier chapters, the main questions that must now be addressed are:

- Whether this burnout is due in part to excessive physical regimes and in part to the relentless pursuit of youth and perfection
- Whether dancers, particularly ballet dancers, begin serious training too young

> • Whether the current pattern of entry into companies at 16, 17 and 18 places the development of the dancer above that of the person

(Leach 1997)

4.3 The Issue of Professional Status

To become a professional dancer takes years of training. This dedication, however, has yet to be recognized. The dancer continues to be viewed by society and, sadly, by the artistic community itself, as a lesser member of the arts world. This has a debilitating effect on his or her perceived status as a professional and, equally importantly, on his or her psychological and physical well-being.

Much of this actual and perceived professional inequality is historical and is based on myth and lack of understanding. Colomè, for example, is convinced that it stems from 'an unfounded, persistent notion that dancers' morals are as loose as their limbs' (in Leach 1997). Whatever the case, dancers are viewed by some as romantic figures and by others as people who play rather than work. Dance is not seen as a legitimate occupation and, though this is true of all arts careers, it seems to be particularly so for the dancer. The parents of many a serious dance student, for example, often ask, 'What are you going to do for a career?'

Yet, a tangible mixture of delight and fascination always seems to greet the discovery of a dancer at a social gathering. As most of us seem instinctively to recognize in dance the expression of the spirit and the soul brought to physical reality, dance is seen to be more than a profession—it is a vocation. As such, it requires years of study, dedication and a high degree of specialization. In this respect, it is very similar to medicine.

Unlike medicine, however, it elicits little respect as a salaried profession. Its contribution to society cannot be conventionally measured, analysed, understood and, ultimately, *applied* for 'the good of mankind'. As a profession, dance cannot, in the eyes of society, be slotted into any accepted definition of the term and the dancer, therefore, remains of value only in aesthetic terms.

On the level of economics, an artist who is seen to be concerned, therefore, with material return or even security is not only a lesser artist but is of less value aesthetically. This powerful but misguided concept of the devoted artist putting his or her art before financial gain not only actively prevents the dancer from achieving the status of an appropriately respected professional but can erode his or her self-esteem, confidence and ability to recognize his or her own value.

In addition, historically, dancers are considered to be dispensable. This

view is prevalent in music theatre, the most profitable area of live enter-
tainment where dancers are very moderately paid when working and,
when injured or no longer sufficiently youthful looking, are simply
discarded. Indeed, dancers are particularly vulnerable in their thirties. At
a time when other professionals are normally 'getting into their stride'
even the injury-free dancer is compelled to retire from active performance work. It is virtually impossible for most people to understand, let
alone accept, that the 25-year-old dancer is actually comparable in terms
of training, experience, standards and expectations of performance to the
average 40-something 'other' professional. Finally, the dance community
itself possesses an insularity, intensity, single-mindedness and curious
determination to avoid interaction with the wider community.

4.4 The Cost of Professional Status

It is just as difficult to translate the complex facts of a dancer's life into
levels of salary, social security and pension benefits in order to place
them on an equal footing with other highly skilled, experienced, elite
professionals. Even compared with other performing artists, the majority
of dancers receive an entirely inadequate income from their professional
activities. They simply do not have the finances to compensate for and to
deal with the lack of security, high cost of travel and accommodation and
higher insurance premiums to sustain them in the face of accidents,
illness, unemployment and legal fees.

Dancers face greater chances of suffering permanent disability than
most other elite competitors. They may be too old for general student
loans, too fit for disability pensions or allowances or have too limited an
education and practical skills for short retraining programmes. This
economic dilemma is exacerbated by the higher non-working subsistence
costs demanded in the financial outlay for daily classes and various
therapeutic treatments necessary for them to remain employable.

With fewer performing years, longer working hours per week, higher
professional maintenance costs and levels of physical risk, dance wages
are among the lowest in the performing arts and reflect the relatively low
status dancers possess—all of which has dire implications for their quality of life and later years.

4.5 Redressing the Balance

The dance world itself must share responsibility with society for this
lamentable situation. Clearly, the balance must be redressed for the

dancer to achieve parity of status, artistically, economically and socially with other performing artists and members of society. Myth must be replaced by reality.

The dancer's current professional status must therefore be reviewed according to agreed criteria and subsequently examined in relation to the present dance world in order to help define the dancer for society. Happily, the IODPT has recently proposed a set of criteria which begins this process:

- Specialized/technical training
- Level of income
- Time invested in career

This major shift in focus is a challenge that is best achieved through representation by the international dance and 'friends of dance' community. Dancers themselves need to play their role in these changes by taking responsibility for continued learning and preparation for transition in their own lives.

5 THE DANCER'S DESTINY

5.1 Strengths

Evidence shows that dancers consistently achieve very high academic averages and are highly successful in a wide variety of new careers. Their

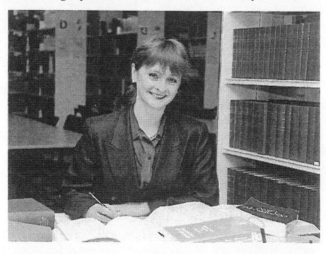

Fig. 13.1 Rosie O'Donnell, retired dancer, now a solicitor. (Photo by Elaine Mayson)

training and experience as performing artists develops a rare blend of positive work-related skills and qualities that are transferable to many new fields and that are of high value in the workplace.

Analysis of these strengths can give confidence and focus. Therapists, psychologists and career counsellors report a remarkable concurrence in their assessment of the dancer's profile, which includes aspects such as:

- Discipline
- A will to succeed
- A desire for excellence
- Resilience
- Resourcefulness and loyalty

All of these are valuable commodities in any workplace. Suzie Jary, staff member for Career Transition for Dancers, has further qualified these by identifying the following core attributes which she believes are common to dancers:

- The ability to work independently or as a member of a team
- The ability to take directions
- The ability to concentrate and focus mentally
- Dedication and persistence
- High motivation to achieve excellence by improving and perfecting skills
- Flexibility and adaptability to change
- Ability to think quickly on their feet and under pressure
- Energy, physical stamina and an engaging presence

These findings have also elicited a high degree of resonance with current and former dancers who, armed with them, can begin to change their self-perceptions in order to see themselves as highly employable, versatile and responsible people.

5.2 Weaknesses

> Resettlement was seen as a negative, the end not the beginning of the next life. Until recently, dancers themselves were very reluctant to think or talk about this almost taboo subject
>
> (Hamilton in Leach 1997)

The goal-oriented nature of dance training means that many aspects of personal development are submerged or undeveloped. Just as important as possessing and optimizing positive skills and traits is the ability to identify and acquire missing skills.

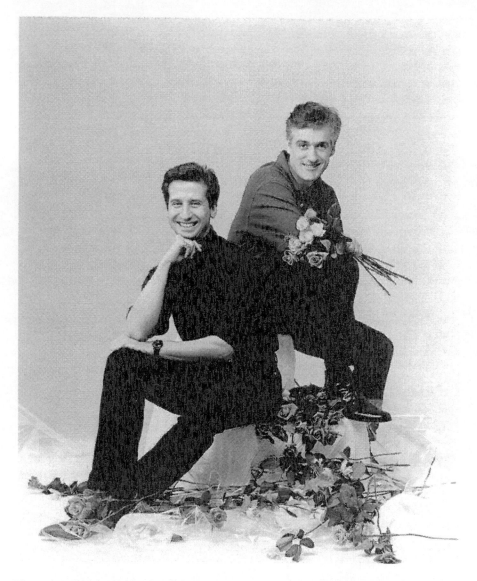

Fig. 13.2 Mark Welford and Stephen Wicks retired from dancing and now have their own business as florists. (Photo by Bill Cooper)

Verbal communication, for example, is often poor initially. Learning to dance requires kinesthetic intelligence and develops exceptional movement and memory skills incorporating many rhythms, modalities and patterns. These can only be mastered by spending many silent hours experiencing the movements, observing one's own movement in the mirror and sensing how to master a pattern or translate a teacher's correction into improved technique or expression.

Such skills transfer well to the single-minded completion of task-oriented projects but act as barriers to the dancer developing his or her interpersonal skills. More time must be apportioned to encourage confident verbal communication and can only enhance—throughout life—the dancer's effectiveness as a role model, teacher, choreographer, artist, and professional.

The ability to receive and apply criticism and instruction positively and productively while taking individual responsibility is also very attractive to any employer. Greben (in Leach 1997) however, notes that, despite such ability, dancers do not feel autonomously competent but depend too much upon the leadership and opinion of others. They tend also to define themselves too much by the approval of others so that self-esteem is often felt only when they are dancing well or when told they are dancing well.

Dancers don't know how to integrate into society, and simple things such as knowing how to pay taxes or what their rights are remain unknown facts of life. This can be exacerbated by low income. Consequently many dancers do not have a car, own no property and have no experience with banks, lawyers or accountants.

Since as much as 80% of a young dancer's time is spent in physical training, early academic opportunities and the acquisition of these life skills are easily and misguidedly sacrificed. Only when dancers begin to understand that these life skill gaps are not the failure of the individual dancer but a very real resistance within the dance education system itself, will education take its rightful place in the dancer's development. This resistance has caused life skills education to be viewed as something to be fitted in or even worked around within the dance curriculum as a whole.

5.3 The Inner Self

> I didn't know who I was any more because I was no longer a dancer.
> (attributed to Monica Mason Company UK Royal Ballet, in Brinson and Dick 1996)

Most dancers do not plan for the future beyond their final curtain call. According to research undertaken by psychologist Catherine Glenfield, 57.4% of dancers have no idea what they wish to do when they retire. This lack of preparation means that, after years of training and performing, the end of what is often an intense but brief career can be something of a shock. Often, dancers who are injured will not face the finality until far beyond the point at which retirement is obvious to those around them. Many find the transition physically and psychologically 'harrowing'.

The core dilemma for the dancer is the level at which dance is part of the personality structure or identity and, therefore, unlike most jobs, it cannot simply be discarded. There is a bereavement process that dancers go through as they lose not only their work and a career but also their way of life, their community and, perhaps most crucial of all, their identity. This is a situation similar to that of many former professional sportspersons, especially cricketers.

Specialists point out that dancers need much more than career counselling to cope and adapt to retirement from performance. Loss of identity can overwhelm, leading to feelings of powerlessness and an inability either to identify appropriate new directions, meet the demands of new roles or modify new roles to suit their talents. It can also can lead to hasty, irrational, ill-advised or inappropriate decisions (Yates, personal communication).

Loss of identity is a key problem for both male and female dancers. The longer and narrower the experience, the more difficult the transition. Successful dancers face the loss of prestige, respect, satisfaction and artistic identity. Unsuccessful or injured dancers face the emptiness and disappointment of having failed to achieve their goal. For both, hard won physical mastery and regimen is lost and, with it, confidence, the outlets for physical energy, dramatic expression and musicality disappear. Other losses may include friends, familiarity of studio, sharing the adventure of the creative process and high degrees of discipline.

Feelings of panic, fear, terror and anxiety are common and powerful. The trick is to balance and combine these with the positive feelings of elation, excitement and anticipation as the process of transition unfolds. This can only be achieved by training and practice.

Within the dance culture, psychological training is often neglected. Greben reports that 'dancers have often been directed to ignore, suppress or deny their own spontaneous feelings and desires. An important part of self-esteem derives from being able to identify and respect feelings within oneself' (Leach 1997). Consequently, society and even the dance world itself labour under two particular misapprehensions—that dancers are neither intelligent nor stable.

This self-doubt that dancers often feel—given the single-minded, goal-oriented training and frequent lack of wider-reaching interests—is partly self-ignorance. It seems there is something in the feedback between dancers, teachers, peers and the general public that is creating a mythology that doesn't stand up to analysis. Nevertheless, the intelligence curve of the typical dancer in Canada actually peaks at a point equivalent to the top 15% of the normal population.

The notion that dancers are prone to anxiety is also belied by reality. Evans (in Leach 1997) has shown that, despite the extraordinary physical and emotional demands on the professional dancer and the fierce competition for scarce jobs, dancers' scores on the Cattell 16 Personality Questionnaire demonstrate appreciably greater mental equilibrium than other performing artists and slightly above average for general populations. He concluded that dancers may internally feel insecure and low in self-esteem and externally believe some of the mythology that they are poor communicators and are unqualified for anything but dance.

5.4 Bridging the Belief–Reality Gap: Lessons from Sport Psychology

In sport, psychological training has been shown to have a significant role in enhancing performance and preventing injury. Canadian research, for example, highlights the positive relationship between developing psychological skills such as anxiety, control, concentration, motivation, interpersonal skills and winning Olympic medals (Tajet-Foxell 1997).

To work with athletes at national or international level, coaches must understand factors affecting performance such as anxiety, tension, fear, and inappropriate thoughts. They must also know the most effective techniques for preparing the athlete mentally for performance. Even at less competitive levels, coaches are required to understand and use praise, constructive criticism, task setting, evaluation and feedback, visualization, and mental rehearsal techniques.

Despite growing interest in applying physical sports training techniques, however, psychological cover in the dance world is still remedial rather than preventive. Two thirds of dancers surveyed used counselling services to manage injury and of 25% who have suffered stage fright, none have sought help (Brinson and Dick 1996). Another significant feature common to dance is the 'tension experienced with other people'. For many, these feelings endured, albeit less intensely, in retirement.

The need for a supportive environment is, therefore, critical. Two thirds of ballet dancers felt that their teachers' criticism had affected them negatively (Brinson and Dick 1996). The same survey reported that negative criticism seemed to be firmly established in many teachers' minds as the surest way of bringing out the best performance. Yet it is clear that excessive external discipline fails to encourage personal responsibility and works against the development of self-esteem.

Such a negative approach has serious implications for the personal development of the dancer. Lessons should be learned from educational psychology and sports psychology by emphasizing the importance in a teaching environment of establishing empathy, warmth, and unconditional positive regard. Tajet-Foxell (1997) has also advocated an all-inclusive model of dance training in which injury management and nutrition are incorporated with physical, technical *and* psychological training. This model should, therefore, support dancers medically, physically and psychologically to the same standards as other sports professionals.

Although differences do exist between one dance form and another and between dance and other forms of athletic activity, it is the similarities between the disciplines of sport and dance that count. By acknowledging and defining the overlap we can begin to adopt appropriate findings (Tajet-Foxell 1997).

6   CURRENT INITIATIVES IN DANCE EDUCATION

> I went through school with no education on fitness, but slowly the dance world is dragging itself into the twentieth century; it has been turned on to sports medicine, performance preparation, injury prevention and so on.
> (Deborah Bull, Royal Ballet Company, UK, Zest 1998)

Throughout the dance world today, there are striking examples of endeavour to revitalize dance training in a physical sense. Earlier chapters, for example, have advocated cross-training, rest and relaxation and education programmes that acknowledge the dancer as an athlete *and* an artist. These include a number of disciplines to equip him or her to meet the wide-ranging technical and stylistic demands of today's choreography, and simultaneously train all-round fitness for optimal functional capacity and health status. Although often inconsistently practised and as yet unknown in music theatre and ballroom dancing, these physical training initiatives are thoroughly researched, applied and taught by sport and exercise science and sports medicine or by dancers who have studied or even trained in the teaching of these techniques.

With regard to the artistic development of the dancer, it is the *balance* of several complimentary techniques that matters. The inclusion of specific rehabilitation techniques such as *Pilates* and interior work such as *Alexander*, *Feldenkrais* and *Tai Chi* as well as sports psychology, stress management and relaxation techniques should certainly also be advocated along with the above recommendations.

Interestingly, several contemporary dance-training programmes have long incorporated Tai Chi and integrated arts approaches. In most cases, this has been due more to the instinct and wisdom of individual directors than accepted educational practice. Such programmes must be expanded, improved and applied throughout the dance world. As will be seen later in the chapter, Tai Chi is particularly useful as it can be practised throughout life.

More importantly, however, in the current context, there are now exciting initiatives that address the problems of transition early in the dancer's career. At company level, New York City Ballet (USA) and Northern Ballet (UK) have negotiated the right for dancers to take time off to attend college during their performing schedules. At professional level, the National Ballet School of Canada has introduced smaller academic classes and tutorials to encourage verbal participation skills. Its innovative 'Rap' groups (where each class meets once a month with a trained counsellor) have had 'a profound, unquantifiable effect on students' well-being' (Leach 1997).

Several worldwide school surveys have also shown a significant drop in the incidence of eating disorders following the employment of psychologists specializing in this field. Other educators have recommended the introduction of a second language. Mastery of such relevant academic skills not only assists the dancer, professionally, personally and socially but also creates enduring attributes and gives confidence for future learning tasks.

7 SUPPORT AND SUCCESS FOR DANCERS IN TRANSITION

Transition confusion often arises due to a combination of lack of preparation and underestimation of the enormous scale and instability of the life transition. Dancers today need to know that they are intelligent, inherently stable people with a range of highly transferable skills and that whatever they set their minds to, provided it is appropriate for their talents, they are highly likely to succeed. This kind of positive reinforcement can turn what Yates (Personal Communication 1998) calls the 'can't, won't, shan't, mustn't' attitude of many dancers in transition to positive effect.

Although transition implies artistic, emotional, physical and spiritual losses, it is *the process* that creates the anxiety, not the dancer. As dancers are goal oriented from an early age and as the 'research phase' of moving from familiarity into the unknown feels like an absence of structure for them, they are inclined to rush into decision-making simply to create a sense of security. Many dancers undermine their abilities by choosing careers that do not necessarily reflect their capacity. Again, this is a learned skill that is not prioritized in the relentless pursuit for learned perfection.

The dancer in transition needs a positive, practical and supportive outlook. The need for specialized psychological guidance, practical support, reassurance and, above all, calm is paramount. A skilled, resourceful professional with time to listen, with whom to sound things out, brainstorm, set goals and plan provides an invaluable, educational, and positive process. As the resettlement period is all about change, acknowledgement, development, enhancement and moving on, the earlier this process begins the better the outcome for the dancer.

Feedback from present and former dancers confirms the growing reputation of Transition Centres in facilitating successful transitions as well as greater openness about transition in the dance community. Yates emphasises (in Leach 1997) that a Transition Centre must be:

- A safe place (confidentiality)
- Independent
- Skilled
- Empathetic
- Experienced

Confidentiality is essential as it protects the dancer from the fear of being sidelined or misinterpreted should it become known that a second career was being considered. Independence ensures objectivity in awarding assistance based on the criteria of length of service, specialized training and level of income, thereby protecting the dancer from having to go 'cap in hand' in the event of imperfect relationships with company management. Independence also ensures emotional protection when voicing something, often for the first time, so uncomfortable as the idea of leaving dance.

Many dancers tend to choose artistic and sensitive occupations in particular hands-on work with a creative bent. In the UK, between 1992 and 1995, second career choices have shifted from dance (30%) and the caring professions (20%) towards academic pursuits (20%) and entrepreneurial employment (30%). Canada's Dancer Transition Resource Centre also reports a greater preference for university study than in the past, where 30% of 'resettled' dancers retrain in dance-related fields such as choreography, teaching or notation. The remainder have chosen such diverse careers as:

- graphic design
- theatre design
- interior decorating
- floristry

- photography and picture framing
- physiotherapy, osteopathy
- movement or exercise therapy
- reflexology
- acupuncture
- and, recently, medicine, architecture and law

8 AGEING AND THE DANCER

The physiological impact of the changes of the ageing process may seem very far away for the young dancer. An understanding of this process can, however, make the dancer more aware of how the exercise and lifestyle choices of today will strongly influence the dancer's health tomorrow. Indeed, if dancers were to think of their life as an elite, ongoing performance and were to invest in it the energy and skills they invest in the dance, they would ensure their own lifelong optimal health and well-being.

8.1 The Decline in Physical Performance

> Just like the Olympic athlete, the elderly person must perform frequently and consistently at the very limit of their physical ability.
>
> (Young, 1997)

Young's distinctive analogy which likens the older person to the Olympic athlete may be sufficiently intriguing and familiarly challenging to engage the dancer's interest in scientifically preparing for his or her later years. He points out that the decline in physical abilities associated with old age means that many elderly people are forced to perform at the limit of their physical ability just to meet the physical demands of everyday life. For many people over 80 everyday tasks demand maximal musclar forces or levels of oxygen use. The need to perform frequently and consistently at the limit of their physical ability means that the Olympic athlete and older people may have a lot in common.

Training at any age is about improving physical performance. In old age, it is particularly focused on functional performance since the ability to perform everyday activities is central to well-being. Exercise studies on very elderly, older and younger people have clear evidence of improvements in selected performance and health-related issues (Harridge and Young 1998; Shephard 1997) including:

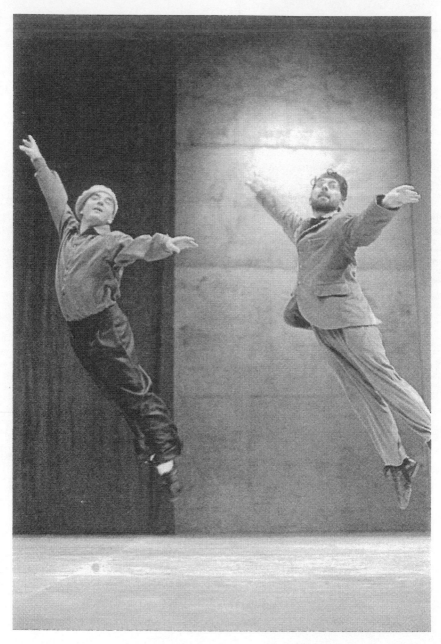

Fig. 13.3 Brian Bertscher and Fergus Early in Green Candle Dance Company's 1996 production 'Tales from the Citadel', in which all the company were dancers between the ages of 45 and 85. (Photo by Hugo Glendinning)

- Bone strength
- Muscle strength and power
- Joint range and pain control
- Aerobic capacity
- Balance co-ordination
- Reaction time
- Pain control
- Improved immune function

In every individual, each biological system ages at a different rate and it begins much earlier than we think. Ageing is not a process with a

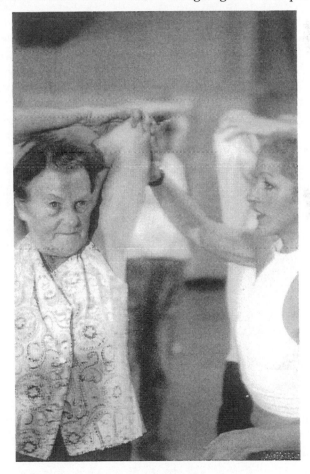

Fig. 13.4   Susie Dinan, clinical exercise practitioner who is a retired dancer, with one of her older clients

sudden onset at 40, 50 or 60. It is rather a process of slow onset which begins in the womb and continues throughout life (Dinan and Sharp 1997). However, as we age, it is important to do everything possible to ensure that the body's physiological functions remain above critical threshold levels (Fig. 13.5). Bone mass, for example, declines towards a fracture threshold, muscle mass towards a series of functional thresholds necessary for everyday independent mobility (Fig. 13.6). The adoption, therefore, of a lifestyle that incorporates the necessary physical activities is potentially a very important element of personal health promotion (Kennie, Dinan and Young 1998). It will assist older persons to maintain safety margins between maximal function and critical thresholds of function which, generous in youth, are constantly being eroded (Young 1997).

Although dancers are undeniably ahead in some aspects of fitness, these are transient as fitness cannot be stored. To a dancer, the risks may seem distant enough to be ignored and, although the body will respond at any age to exercise and training (Young and Dinan 1994), the earlier this training begins, the better the investment returns. Time spent in learning about and committing to the benefits of fitness throughout life will not only enlighten the performing years but will counter many dance-related deficiencies and will ensure optimum health, function and quality of life with age.

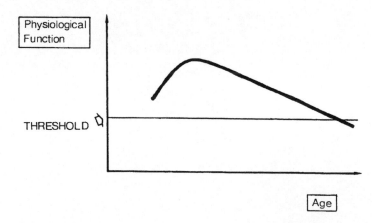

Fig. 13.5 Diagrammatic pattern of change of physiological functions with increasing age
Source: Reproduced from A. Young (1997), Ageing and phyiological functions. *Philosophical Transactions of the Royal Society of London*, B: 1836–40, with permission from The Royal Society

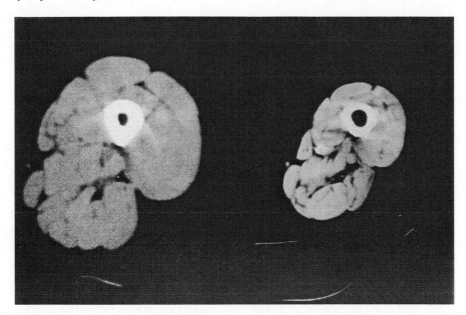

Fig. 13.6 Cross-sectional images at mid-thigh from a healthy woman in her twenties (a) and a healthy woman in her eighties (b), to the same magnification
Source: Reproduced from A. Young (1997), Ageing and physiological functions. *Philosophical Transactions of the Royal Society of London*, B: 1836–40, with permission from The Royal Society

The physical transition itself requires particular attention. Dancers in retirement must be alert not only to the implications of cessation of daily physical activity and the dance lifestyle legacy of less than ideal nutritional and health status but also to the fact that they cannot escape the normal ageing process.

8.2 The Loss of Movement

The loss of a physical way of life goes well beyond the loss of a familiar regimen. The physical activity patterns of dancers in retirement tend towards a scaled-down regimen of dance classes, Pilates or a combination of these two. Even in self-selected retirement, the swift loss of physical mastery means that, for many, a dance class becomes an increasingly psychologically and physically uncomfortable experience and it is finally abandoned. The reported negative psychological effects associated with retirement are similar to those connected to injury periods, and are often underestimated and unanticipated:

- Depression
- Decreased self-esteem and confidence
- Inability to cope with stress
- General anxiety
- Fatigue
- Lethargy
- Disturbed sleep
- Joint aches and pains
- Feeling old

The key for the dancer is to understand that it is the loss of physical activity just as much as the loss of creative movement that is the catalyst for these negative changes. Muscles cannot 'know' if they are doing a series of triplets or running on a treadmill—they respond in the same way. The challenge for the dancer, therefore, is to replace the performance goal with a fitness for life goal.

This should involve an exercise programme that is comprehensive, balanced and sufficiently fresh to enable the dancer (perhaps for the first time) to view physical activity as a pleasurable leisure time pursuit. Certainly such a programme would be the more effective in achieving optimal levels of fitness for the rest of a dancer's life. There are many options to help achieve this and, indeed, dance may not be one of them.

8.3   Bone and Joint Function

Chapter 10 clearly maintained that it is critical for all women—in particular, those known to be at high risk (including elite performers such as dancers and endurance athletes)—to do everything possible to prevent the onset of *osteoporosis* and to stay above the bone-fracture threshold. This becomes exponentially more important with age. Osteoporosis is currently the major cause of bone fractures in post-menopausal women and older people and it is associated with a high personal and medical cost (Rutherford 1997).

At every age, the maximal load a bone can withstand without fracture is positively related to its bone mineral density. Women reach *critical fracture thresholds* much younger than men. In the wrist, for example, the threshold is thought to be reached at about age 60–65 in women but possibly not until after 90 years in men. Similarly, white women are thought to reach 'at risk' thresholds for vertebral crush fractures in their sixties (Young 1997). In other words, men seem to have a 'bone age' some

15 years younger than the women of their age group. Interestingly, as mentioned in Chapter 10, many dancers go on to develop osteoporosis in their fifties, about 15 years earlier than normal.

Nicola Keay's (1995) work with retired dancers reinforces this strong message about the dangers of poor menstrual status with age. She demonstrated that those who had had the fewest periods, or whose weight had dropped furthest below the ideal weight for their height, had the lowest spinal bone density. Despite the resumption of normal periods in retirement, many of the subjects had not recovered sufficiently to match the bone density norms for their age.

To stay above the fracture threshold throughout their lives, female dancers must, therefore, ensure that in addition to regulating their menstrual cycle, they also commit to a physical training programme that is effective in 'loading' the bones.

Although more study needs to be done to identify optimal intensity, frequency and form of exercise, the most effective method of stressing bone is thought to be through a varied programme of dynamic and weight-resisted activities that target the whole skeleton, and in particular the vulnerable fracture sites of the spine, wrists and hips (Rutherford 1997). The importance of targeting with the over fifties (especially the female dancer) cannot be overemphasized.

Significant increases in bone density in 50–76-year-old subjects were demonstrated with a single year of a moderate intensity weight-training programme on the femoral neck (hip) and lumbar spine (Nelson, Fiatarone, Morganti *et al.* 1994). Squeezing tennis balls and other resistance exercises were shown to be effective for the wrist. General fitness sessions containing a combination of low and medium impact work, step training and resisted conditioning exercises with a high proportion of back extension work appear to be able to improve spinal bone density in old age.

The exercise protocol clearly needs to be designed specifically for the age and health (bone and general) of the individual and supervised by the appropriate medical or exercise professional. In addition, as advocated in Chapter 10, bone scanning is essential as a further precaution after the age of 50 for all female dancers and endurance athletes as well as other groups at risk from osteoporosis.

Osteoarthritis is another development of ageing and almost certainly an occupational hazard in dancers. Recent studies have done much to establish the benefits of exercise in preserving optimum joint function and have also helped to allay concerns as to whether there is a negative impact of exercise (Ettinger, Burns, Messier *et al.* 1997). Both the aerobic and the resistance training programmes showed a reduction in disability scores and pain and an increase in functional tasks such as walking, lifting and carrying.

8.4   Muscle Function

From middle age onwards there is a steady loss of muscle strength, even in completely healthy individuals. In the muscles of the leg, for example, this loss of strength equates to approximately 1–2% per annum in those over 60 years of age. Between 70 and 80 years, the muscle groups of the lower limb are able to generate only 60% of the force generated by 20–30 year olds (Fig. 13.7).

This loss of muscle strength results primarily from a loss of muscle mass (*sarcopenia* or *muscular cachexia*), due, principally, to a reduction in the number of muscle fibres which, in turn, is related to the progressive loss of *motor nerves*. In addition to a reduction in the number of muscle fibres, there may also be a reduction in the size of the remaining fibres. This is especially noticeable in the presence of illness following immobilization and also in advanced old age. Moreover, older muscle may also be weak for its size. The degree of loss of muscle is masked, however, in many older people, because there is an increase in the amount of fat stored around the muscle. Size and body weight, therefore, can be deceptive.

To overcome a fixed resistance, such as body weight, elderly people must use a greater proportion of their maximum strength. To do this, the muscle contracts more slowly. This phenomenon partly explains why,

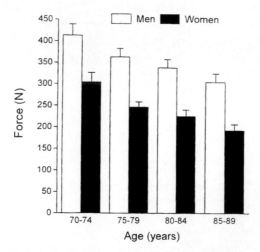

Fig. 13.7   Progressive decline in maximum voluntary static strength in healthy men and women aged 70–89 years
Source: Redrawn from Skelton, Greig, Davies *et al.* (1994). Reproduced by permission of Oxford University Press

with increasing age, *muscle explosive power* declines at an even greater rate (3–4% p.a.) than strength (1–2% p.a). Elderly women are particularly vulnerable because they have lower power/weight ratios than elderly men of the same age. Large numbers of healthy, elderly women, for example, have strength and power below or near to functionally important thresholds and have lost, or are in danger of losing, the ability to perform everyday tasks such as stepping up and down and getting in and out of chairs.

Although it is not possible to influence the number of fibres or to compensate completely for their loss, ageing muscle is highly trainable. Older individuals who continue to train for strength show isometric and general strength, speed of movement and cross-sectional muscle similar to that of young control subjects (Fig. 13.8).

The physiological benefits of physical training could be equivalent to 15–20 years' rejuvenation. In general, resistance training should no longer be resisted by the dancer—in particular, the female—or the older person. Given the wide range of training equipment from multigym to weights to balls and bands (or even baked bean tins!), retired dancers have every opportunity to optimize muscle and bone health as they age. Increasing the size of an older person's muscle not only benefits contractile function but also serves to provide an ultimate source of fuel for fighting illness, as well as producing heat (Harridge and Young 1998).

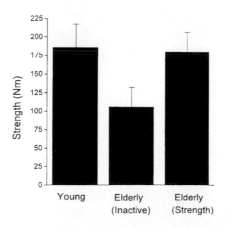

Fig. 13.8 Averages of knee extensor strength in healthy non-trained young (28 years), non-trained elderly men (68 years) and elderly men (68 years) who had strength training over the past 12–17 years. No differences were found between the young non-trained group and the older trained group
Source: Data from Klitgaard, Mantoni, Schiaffino (1990)

8.5   Aerobic Power

Another aspect of physical performance that declines with age is maximal *aerobic power* (sometimes referred to as *maximal oxygen uptake or* $\dot{V}O_2$ *max* and extensively discussed in Part II). The ability to perform continuous dynamic exercise (e.g. running, brisk walking) without fatigue or discomfort (never the dancer's forte!) depends heavily on the individual's maximal oxygen uptake. The decline in aerobic power (approximately 10–15% per decade after the age of 35 in both men and women) may be due, in part, to the diminishing total muscle mass and to a reduction in cardiac output, the latter due primarily to the decline in maximal heart rate. These age-related changes limit the ability to perform everyday activities and can be seen even in veteran endurance athletes who have trained during their entire adult lives (Harridge and Young 1998).

The resulting decline means that many elderly people (particularly women) need only a small further deterioration in aerobic power to render some everyday activities (e.g. walking, getting dressed) either impossible or unpleasant to perform. This is especially true when coupled with the effects of disease. As with muscle strength, however, it seems that up to at least 70 years of age, a 10–20% improvement in aerobic power can be expected from endurance training. This is equivalent, perhaps, to 10–20 years' rejuvenation. New information demonstrates that, even beyond the age of 80 years, endurance training achieves a meaningful gain that can make everyday aerobic activities easier to perform (Malbut-Shennan, Dinan, Verhaar *et al.* 1995; Young 1997). For the dancer as well as the older person, it is time to discover the benefits of aerobic exercise.

8.6   Notions about Exercise

Unfortunately, although dancers seem fairly open to 'softer' forms of exercise, many tend to fight shy of more vigorous exercise (aerobics, step workouts, power walking, jogging, etc.) and equipment-based forms of cardiovascular training (bike, rowers, steppers). Furthermore, misconceptions such as 'dancers never run or do aerobics', 'running builds up the wrong muscles' tend to endure in retirement.

There are even more myths surrounding resistance training. For the female dancer, for example, resisted upper body moves are rare and specific weight training almost unheard of. Although male dancers increasingly include strength work, female dancers are very resistant, often through an unfounded fear that they are building the 'wrong' muscles or 'unsightly' muscles.

Free weights, body bars and therapy bands and balls tend to get a more positive response, although, again, with female dancers the amount of resistance used is usually too light to be effective. This reluctance may be partly due to the non-aesthetic, overtly fitness 'feel' of the exercises but it is more likely to be due to ignorance about the myriad benefits of these particular forms of training for the dancer at every stage of life. Bone strength, joint integrity, muscular balance and strength as well as aerobic power are always at a premium as they are not fully achieved through dance training and they become particularly important with age.

Another benefit of such resistance exercises is *fall prevention*, as falling is responsible for the majority of osteoporotic fractures in old age. Learning correct lifting and carrying techniques may be helpful in reducing risks of fracture resulting from biomechanically unsound positions. Such training strategies are core to all specialist exercise work for older people and, although dancers have high levels of skill in many of these, lifting and other body management techniques are advisable for them as they age (Wolfson, Whipple, Derby *et al.* 1996). Learning the dangers of the much-loved straight-legged trunk flexion when lifting from the floor, for example, can teach the dancer to avoid using this and other similar movements in everyday life. Finally, sleeping patterns show significant improvement in 50–76 year olds following weekly aerobic exercise training programmes (King, Oman, Brassington *et al.* 1997).

8.7 Dance is not about Health

We know that elderly athletes have the potential to remain functionally independent longer than their sedentary counterparts and, today, the number of elderly athletes is steadily increasing. Veteran elite dancers who still perform are, however, extraordinarily rare.

As discussed earlier, this stems more from a combination of the aesthetic ideal and the current dance training and education culture than the ageing process itself. Like their athletic counterparts, ageing dancers lower their physical output on retirement. Unlike many of their counterparts, however, they tend to do significantly less activity or, sometimes, even nothing at all. Indeed, as with their performance training, there seems to be a reluctance to integrate other forms of movement into their exercise patterns.

Even at the height of their powers, dancers' bone and joint integrity, muscular balance and aerobic power are the Achilles heels of the dance-only fitness system. This absence of 'complete fitness', the legacy of injuries, the lower levels of activity after retirement in addition to the normal ageing process may mean that dancers run the risk of being far less healthy than their counterparts in sport or even the more sedentary members of the general public. Indeed, it would be foolish to assume that dance has ever been about health.

To ensure optimum health and functional independence well into their seventies and eighties, dancers must, therefore, acknowledge health as a prime motivator. They must also acknowledge that physical activity is central to health. It is vital that dancers, together with the international dance community, take responsibility for developing and implementing appropriate physical activity programmes that focus on fitness for life, rather than dance only, as the goal for their performing, transition and retirement years.

9 CONCLUSIONS

The key to transition is to address it before it becomes an issue. Current initiatives prove that dance transition is a passage to new beginnings. Through education, the dancer can become confident of his or her own ability and authority as a valued and respected member of society who possesses a fit and healthy body as well as a range of highly developed, eminently employable, transferable and enduring skills.

Today, there is an urgent need to challenge the belief systems of the dance world and of society. The perpetuation of notions of youth—the adoration of the 'sylph'—and the denial of the ageing process—the fear of the 'fossil'—are myths out of step with today's world. These entrap, de-skill and disrespect dancers and they deny them optimal health and fulfilment as dancers and human beings. Despite these shortcomings, dancers are better conditioned for change than most professionals. Dance education owes it to them to become more open-minded, holistic and honest in its approach. It must develop a curriculum of a broader physical training programme with a broader base of academic learning which prioritises the acquisition of technical, psychological and life-management skills. This must also involve the study and experience of other art forms as well as exposure to other professional areas that may offer inspiration during transition. Most importantly, it must do this within the context of the dancer as a human being who is as subject to the ageing process as the rest of us.

10 FURTHER READING

Dinan S, Sharp C (1997) *Fitness for life*. London: Piatkus Books
Shephard RJ (1997) *Ageing, physical activity and health*. Champaign, IL: Human Kinetics
Thomasen E, Rist RA (1996) *Anatomy and kinesiology for ballet teachers*. London: Dance Books

ACKNOWLEDGEMENTS

I particularly want to thank Pernille Ahlstrom, Archie Young, Stephen Harridge, Linda Yates, Celeste Dandeker, Christopher Bannerman, Peter Wilson and my many dance colleagues and friends who have helped in my own transition and in the preparation of my chapter.

REFERENCES

Brinson P, Dick F (eds) (1996) *Fit to dance?* The Report of the national inquiry into dancers' health and injury. London, UK,Calouste Gulbenkian Foundation
Dinan S, Sharp NCC (1997) *Fitness for life*. London: Piatkus Books
Ettinger WH, Burns R, Messier SP *et al.* (1997) Randomised trial comparing aerobic exercise and resistance exercise with a health education program in older adults with knee osteoarthritis. *Journal of the American Medical Association*, **277**: 25–31
Harridge SDR, Young A (1998) Skeletal muscle. In: Pathy MSJ (ed.), *Principles and practice of geriatric medicine*, (3rd edition). Chichester, UK: Wiley: in press
Keay N (1997) The healthy dancer. *Dance Theatre Journal*, London, reprinted 1997
Kennie D, Dinan S, Young A (1998) Health promotion and physical activity. In: Brockelhurst J, Tallis R, Fillit H (eds), *Textbook of geriatric medicine and gerontology* (5th edition). London: Churchill Livingstone: in press
King AC, Oman RF, Brassington GS *et al.* (1997) Moderate-intensity exercise and self-rated quality of sleep in older adults. *Journal of the American Medical Association*, **277**: 32–7
Klitgaard H, Mantoni M, Schiaffino S *et al.* (1990) Function, morphology and protein expression of ageing skeletal muscle. A cross-sectional study of elderly men with different training backgrounds. *Acta Physiologica Scandinavia*, **140**: 41–54
Leach B (ed.) (1997) *The dancers' destiny*. Based on the 1st international symposium of the International Organization for the Transition of Professional Dancers. Lausanne: International Organization for the Transition of Professional Dancers
Malbut-Shennan KE, Dinan SM, Verhaar H *et al.* (1993) Maximal oxygen uptake in 80-year-old men. *Clinical Science*, **89** (suppl. 33): 31
Nelson ME, Fiatarone MA, Morganti CM *et al.* (1994) Effects of high intensity strength training on multiple risk factors for osteoporosis fractures. *Journal of the American Medical Association*, **272**: 1909–14

Rutherford OM (1997) Bone density, physical activity. *Proceedings of the Nutrition Society*, **56**

Shephard RJ (1997) *Ageing, physical activity and health*. Champaign IL: Human Kinetics

Skelton DA, Greig CA, Davies JN *et al.* (1994) Strength, power and related functional ability of healthy people aged 65–89 years. *Age and Ageing*, **23**: 371–7

Tajet-Foxell B (1997) Learning from sports psychology. In: *Sidelines*, The Royal Ballet School, London: **10**: 2

Wolfson L, Whipple R, Derby C *et al.* (1996) Balance and strength training in older adults: intervention gains and Tai Chi maintenance. *Journal of American Geriatric Society*, **44**: 498–506

Young A (1997) Ageing and physiological functions. *Philosophical Transactions of the Royal Society of London*, **B**: 1836–40

Young A, Dinan S (1994) Fitness for older people. *British Medical Journal*, **309**: 331–4

Glossary

Actin: Along with myosin, actin is the main protein of the sarcomere involved in contraction. There are two sets of actin molecules in each sarcomere, each set attached to a z-line. Actin is pulled past myosin by the myosin cross-bridges, rather like the oars in a rowing eight, and the two z-lines are pulled together, so shortening the sarcomere. At full muscle extension, when the sarcomeres are at their longest, the minimal overlap means only a few cross-bridges make contact, so the force developed is very low.

Acupressure: Acupuncture is well known as the insertion of needles leading to a blockade of nerve impulses at the point of entry to the spinal cord. Acupressure is a very similar principle, except that pressing or squeezing with the fingers is used instead of needles. The best known example is pressing your upper lip to prevent a sneeze. Or rubbing your shin when you have banged it against a piece of scenery.

Adenosine triphosphate (ATP): High-energy compound used as energy supply for muscle and other biological functions.

Adolescent growth period: A period of accelerated growth associated with puberty.

Adrenaline: The first discovered hormone, adrenaline stimulates the heart action and raises blood pressure and prepares the body for action. At the same time it inhibits digestion and excretion, and reduces blood flow except in the muscle and heart.

Aerobic: Literally 'with air', but taken to mean 'with oxygen', and is applied to exercise where the energy is liberated from the fuel source by oxygen, which itself is conveyed to the muscle via the cardiorespiratory system of heart, lungs, blood and blood vessels.

Alexander Technique: A method for improving posture designed by F. Matthias Alexander. It is used widely to ease chronic back pain, painful periods and postural and breathing problems. It is particularly popular amongst actors and singers.

Allergens: Proteins that can cause an allergic reaction.

Amenorrhoea: Complete absence of menstruation.

Amino acids: Are one of 20 compounds which form the building blocks of protein. They are subdivided into essential (i.e. the body is unable to make these amino acids) and non-essential or dispensable (i.e. body can make these amino acids). There are 8 essential amino acids in adults and 10 in infants.

Amphetamines: A group of psycho-stimulant drugs ('uppers') which also may suppress appetite.

Anaemia: A debilitating condition in which the level of haemoglobin, the oxygen carrier in the red blood cells, is below what are considered to be the normal limits. 'Sports anaemia' (or 'pseudo-anaemia') is where the level of haemoglobin is indeed just at or below the low end of normal. However, this is entirely due to the fact that, following months of aerobic training, the volume of the blood plasma increases more than the cells. So the total amount of haemoglobin in the circulation is the same or higher, but its concentration is lower. This is a normal physiological response to aerobic training.

Anaerobic: Literally 'without air', but taken to mean 'without oxygen', and is applied to exercise or energy pathways in muscle which do not require oxygen. Phosphocreatine releases its energy to ATP without oxygen. The cycle of glycolysis processes glucose to pyruvic acid also without oxygen; and if there is more pyruvic acid than the mitochondria can oxidize, it accumulates and is transformed to lactic acid.

Anaerobic endurance: The ability to sustain anaerobic power output for periods between 10 and 40 seconds.

Anaerobic glycolysis: All glucose goes through a preparatory process called glycolysis before entering Krebs cycle, and about 8% of the glucose energy is released. Oxygen is not needed for glycolysis, hence it is called 'anaerobic'. Pyruvic acid is its normal end product, which enters Krebs cycle. An overaccumulation of pyruvic acid leads to its being transformed to lactic acid.

Anaerobic power: The rate of work produced by the two anaerobic sources of energy, phosphocreatine and glycolysis.

Anaerobic threshold: This is a name that many physiologists don't like, but it is a very convenient term. They prefer the acronym OBLA, for 'Onset of Blood Lactate Accumulation'. Either way, it refers to the highest level of sustained aerobic exercise which can be performed without a fatiguing rise in lactic acid.

Androgen: A collective name for 'male' hormones (such as testosterone), but androgens are also necessary in women, in whom they are secreted by the cortex of the adrenal gland. 'Oestrogen' is the collective female equivalent.

Anorexia: Derived from the Greek word *orexi* meaning yearning, with the prefix 'an' signifying lack of. Used to signify lack of appetite.

Anorexia nervosa: An eating disorder causing a loss of appetite, more common in young women, which can lead to a variety of medical complications.

Anterior suprailiac spine: The ilium (along with the ischium and pubis) is one of the three bones that make up the pelvis. It forms the hip bone. Its anterior spine is the front part of the top of the hip bone.

Antibody: A large protein produced by cells of the immune system in response to antigens.

Antigen: A protein that is foreign to the body.

Antigen presenting cell: A cell of the immune system that presents antigens to T-cells for recognition.

Antioxidants: Are substances (e.g. vitamins C and E) that can protect the body from certain harmful effects of oxidation.

Arthritis: Inflammation in a joint causing pain and loss of movement.

Athletic amenorrhoea: Amenorrhoea that occurs in athletes and dancers related to intense traning and dietary restrictions.

Atopic: Having a disease condition involving susceptibility to developing allergies.

Autonomic nervous system: An ancient part of the evolved nervous system. It is divided into two parts, the sympathetic, which actively assists physical activity during performance; and its opposite partner, the parasympathetic, which keeps us alive in terms of general housekeeping of the body.

Axonal fibres: These are otherwise known as nerve fibres.

β-agonist drugs: Agents which bind to β receptors and mimic the actions of noradrenaline.

B cells: Cells of the immune system that produce antibodies.

Biopsy: This is a small sample of tissue removed under anaesthetic for analysis. It may be muscle—or it may be suspected tumour tissue, from anywhere.

Body composition: The relative proportions of fat and lean tissues within the body.

Body-fat stores: Thighs, bust, back of arms and hips are the main sites for body-fat storage in women, and the upper back and abdomen in men.

Body mass index: Represents the weight (kilograms) of an individual divided by the height (metres) squared, i.e. kg/m^2.

Bone density: A measure of the calcium concentration in the bone.

Bronchoconstriction: Narrowing of airways.

Bronchodilation: Widening of the airways.

Buffer: This is a chemical that acts to mop up hydrogen ions, so lessening the damaging effects of acids. Fitter dancers will have higher levels of blood and muscle buffers.

Bulimia nervosa: Is a neurosis of—mainly—young women. The patient eats well, having normal or even excessive appetite, but food is removed through voluntary vomiting.

Caffeine: A French word used to describe the bitter white crystalline xanthine found in coffee, tea, etc. It dilates blood vessels, speeds up the heart and promotes urine formation as well as causing improved concentration.

Calisthenics: General exercises relying on body weight for resistance.

Carbohydrates: These are foods containing sugar or starch. Much of the sugar is ultimately glucose, and starch is simply a string of glucose molecules (as is glycogen).

Carbohydrate loading: There two popular methods used mainly by sportsmen and women to increase their muscle glycogen content. The original (or classical) method requires prior glycogen depletion through exercise; the modified method does not require such depletion.

Cardiac output: The amount of blood which the heart is pumping at any given time, usually expressed in litres per minute. It is about 5 litres per minute at rest, and may go above 20 on hard exercise. The cardiac output is determined by the heart rate multiplied by the stroke volume, which is the amount of blood pumped from the left ventricle at each beat; e.g. 100 beats per minute and a stroke volume of 120 ml would give a cardiac output of $100 \times 120 = 12\,000$ ml $= 12$ litres per minute.

Cardiovascular (or cardiorespiratory) system: Is the system responsible for the extraction of oxygen from the atmosphere and its transportation inside the body. It contains vital organs such as lungs, heart, blood vessels and blood.

Carnitine: Is a compound which is required to transport long chain fatty acids into the mitochondria where the fats are oxidized to produce energy. Canitine is obtained from foods (animal sources richer than plant sources) as well as from synthesis in the body.

Childhood: Period between first birthday and the onset of puberty.

Cholesterol: A substance of a fatty nature found in all animal fat and oils. Vital for manufacture of steroid hormones. Harmful in excess.

Chrondromalacia patellae: Damage to the cartilage layer at the back of the knee-cap. A cause of knee pain.

Chromosome: The form which DNA adopts just before the cell divides. DNA contains all the information for the cell's function, and in humans there are normally 23 pairs of chromosomes in each cell. Two of them, the X and the Y chromosome, carry the information relating to sex determination and function.

Collagen: The collagen molecule is a long protein fibre which forms the material from which tendons and ligaments and all fibrous tissue in the body is made.

Complex carbohydrates: The term describes foods high in starch such as bread and vegetables. Complex carbohydrates consist of more than two 'sugar' components.

Concentric: Contraction that involves shortening of the muscle (e.g. dumb-bell curls for biceps).

Cortisol: An adrenal cortical steroid essential for life.

Creatine: Found mainly in skeletal muscle where it exists either as creatine (found in acutely fatigued muscle) or creatine phosphate (found in rested muscle). Creatine phosphate serves as a means for the immediate regeneration of ATP, which is responsible for muscular contraction.

Critical fracture threshold: The point at which bone cell and mineral loss reaches a minimum of density and strength thereby compromising bone function and increasing the risk of fracture.

Daily reference value (DRV): Is the recommended daily intake for various food components. On a food label, the DRV is based on a 2000-kcal diet.

Dehydration: A loss of body water (in dancers, usually from sweating—but also from diarrhoea or vomiting). During strenuous exercise it is accompanied by weakness and inco-ordination—and a possibly rising temperature (possibly leading to hyperthermia).

DEXA Scan: A computerized X-ray scanner that accurately measures bone density.

Diastole: The period in the heart's cycle when it is relaxing and filling. It lasts about twice as long as **systole**.

Dietary fibre: Plant food that cannot be broken down by the human digestive system.

Dietary reference values (DRVs): A general term used to cover the terms 'estimated average requirement', 'lower reference nutrient intake', 'reference nutrient intake' and 'safe intake'.

Disaccharides: The second simplest form of carbohydrate containing two 'sugar' components.

Dorsi-flexion: Is a term usually applied to the foot, when you bend it upwards ('dorsally') towards your shin. The opposite, when you point your toe, is called 'plantar-flexion'.

Dynamometer: Mechanical or computerized apparatus used for strength assessments.

Eccentric: Contraction that involves lengthening of the muscle (e.g. landing after a vertical jump).

Elastic connective tissue: Flexible and relatively light tissue present mainly in the muscle. Large amount of this connective tissue positively affects, *inter alia*, levels of muscle flexibility and, therefore, joint mobility.

Elastin: A protein which helps to determine the 'elasticity' of muscle and connective tissues.

Electrolytes: Are substances that, in solution, conduct an electric current. They usually dissociate into particles carrying either positive or a negative electric charge. Vital for generating the electrical impulses of brain, nerves and muscle. The main electrolytes present in sweat (and thus the ones normally needing most replacement) are sodium, chloride, potassium and magnesium.

Electromyography: All muscles are triggered into action by nerve signals. These are themselves electrical, and they in turn trigger an electrical signal along the muscle cell itself. These signals may be detected by electrodes, and amplified, to give an idea of the sequence and intensity of muscle action.

Electron transport: A series of chemical reactions which convert the hydrogen ions, spun off by glycolysis and Krebs cycle, into water, producing yet more energy.

Enzymes: Proteins produced by living cells. They are the workforce of all body cells as they are involved in a number of biological functions (e.g. energy production).

Eosinophils: White blood cells that are involved in allergic inflammatory reactions.

Epiphysis: The separate bony growth plate at the ends of the long bones responsible for the growth seen in childhood and adolescence. It fuses with the rest of the long bone towards the end of the adolescence.

Epithelium: The internal lining of the airways, consisting of **epithelial cells**.

Ergometer: Equipment used in the laboratory to make subjects work in a controlled way. A treadmill is an ergometer, as is an exercise cycle, together with rowing machines and canoe simulators. An ergometer is a work machine.

Essential fatty acid: A fatty acid needed by the body for health but which it cannot make, so it must be supplied from food.

Estimated average requirement: For energy or a nutrient this is the amount which, on average, any stated group of individuals will require. Usually half of the individuals will need more, while the other half will need less than estimated average requirement.

Exercise-induced asthma: Asthma symptoms following a bout of exercise.

Extrinsic: Caused by an outside agent.

Fallopian tubes: The tubes that connect the ovaries to the uterus, and through which the ova pass. In the embryo, they form from the **Mullerian ducts**.

Fascial sheaths: Membrane-like structures that cover muscle fibres, separating them from the rest of muscle.

Fat: An abundant substance in nature used mainly as energy source and store; stored in the body when energy intake is greater than energy output.

Fatty acid: The most basic unit of fat. It is obtained from the breakdown of fats, and is the form in which body cells (including muscle) use fat to produce energy.

Feldenkrais: A mind–body technique designed by Moshe Feldenkrais that focuses on physical and mental exercises to achieve functional integration.

Fibrous connective tissue: Strong tissue full of tough collagen fibres that keeps other tissues or organs in place. Following muscle trauma, the body uses fibrous connective tissue to repair it. Frequent soft tissue (muscle) injuries may negatively affect local flexibility levels due to large amounts of this connective tissue present, as 'scar tissue' which tends to shorten as part of the healing process, but can be lengthened.

Free fatty acids: Found mainly in the blood, fatty acids are obtained from the breakdown of fats, and are the form in which muscle uses fat.

Free radicals: These are atoms or molecules which contain an unpaired electron. Normally electrons are balanced in pairs, and are not very reactive. But unpaired electrons are highly reactive. Within a cell they may react with structures and damage them; e.g. they can make tendons more brittle, or inactivate enzymes, or damage DNA or injure the cell membrane. However, cells are equipped with antioxidants, such as vitamin E, and DNA repair mechanisms—and it may be that 'electron transport' was originally evolved to deal with free radicals.

Forced expiratory volume in the first second (FEV_1): The volume that can be exhaled during the first second of a maximal expiration.

Fracture: A break of the bone.

Gene: A particular length of DNA (see **chromosome**). A gene contains a complete set of instructions for making a protein, such as collagen, or an enzyme, or a hormone, or a receptor on a cell surface. If the item to be instructed for is not a protein, the particular gene or genes code for proteins that then make the item. For example, the sex hormones (testosterone, oestrogen) are not proteins, but a class of chemicals called steroids.

Genetics: The science of heredity, i.e. the characteristics, physical or mental, with which we are endowed by the information carried in the chromosomes.

Glucose, and Blood glucose: Glucose is by far the most important simple sugar into which carbohydrate is broken down in the small intestine. It is vital that the level of glucose in the blood is kept within narrow limits:

too high or too low, and you lapse into a coma. In between meals, the liver supplies the glucose for the blood. The reason muscle slowly stores glucose (as glycogen) during rest is to prevent it taking all the blood glucose within a few minutes of work, as it could. Glucose is the only brain fuel.

Glucose polymers: Carbohydrates containing chains of 4–20 glucose molecules produced from boiling starch (e.g. cornstarch) under controlled commercial conditions. Useful as energy source during exercise.

Glycaemic index (GI) of a food: Is the rate of glucose release into the blood from the gut, after the consumption of a food, compared to that of a corresponding quantity of pure sugar (glucose).

Glycerol: A clear syrupy liquid. Combines with fatty acids to produce triglycerides, the storage form of fat.

Glycogen: A polysaccharide that is the storage form of carbohydrates (glucose). Primarily found in muscles and in the liver as *muscle* and *liver glycogen* respectively.

Glycolysis: The term has a Greek origin (glycolysis = splitting of sugar) and literally means 'breakdown of sugar'.

Glutamine: Is an amino acid produced in muscle; it is an important fuel for some cells of the immune system and may have specific immunostimulatory effects.

Golgi tendon organ: Called after its discoverer, this is a sensor located in tendons. It relays information to the spinal cord and brain regarding the tension being developed in the tendon, and hence applied by the muscle.

Goniometry: Meaning the 'measure of an angle' the term derived from the combination of the Greek words angle (= gonia) and to measure (= metró). A goniometer consists of a 180° protractor to measure joints.

Growth: Increase in the size of the body or its constituents.

Haemoglobin: A large iron-containing protein molecule, many of which are carried in the red blood cell. Their function is mainly to transport oxygen, and 1 g of haemoglobin can transport 1.34 ml of oxygen. A normal range for men is between 14 and 16 g per 100 ml blood, and for women around 12 to 14. Haemoglobin has a smaller sister-molecule, myoglobin, in muscle cells, to help transport and store the oxygen.

Hormone: A chemical secreted by a gland directly into the blood, and affecting target tissues all over the body. Examples of hormones are testosterone, oestrogen, insulin, growth hormone, thyroid hormone and relaxin.

Hydrogen ion: Often written as [H^+], and also called a 'proton' this is the very active particle which comes from acids. They interfere with many cellular functions, and are the cause of fatigue from the high-intensity work that results in lactic acid production. 'Strong' acids give off a lot of

[H$^+$], 'weak' acids give off only a few. In the body, lactic acid may be regarded as relatively strong.

Hydrolysis: A Greek word meaning 'in the presence of water'.

Hypermobility: Excessive mobility of joints, often regarded as potentially hazardous to their healthy functioning.

Hyperreactive airways: Used to describe airways that respond in an exaggerated fashion to a minor irritant.

Hyperthermia: Is said to occur when the body temperature rises to the point where normal body function is compromised, as in lack of co-ordination or even collapse.

Hypertrophy: Enlargement of muscle, usually as a result of intensive physical training.

Hypoglycaemia: Blood sugar levels lower than normal.

Hypothalamus: A region of the brain below the third ventricle, i.e. in the floor of the front part of the brain between the cerebral hemispheres. It may act as a link between the conscious forebrain and hormone release, via the pituitary gland, i.e. a link between mind and body.

Immune system: Is the body's defence against disease. Immunity can be *innate* (from inherited qualities) and it can be *acquired* actively or passively, naturally or artificially.

Immunoglobulin E: A specific type of antibody involved in allergy.

Inflammatory mediators: Active molecules that have a range of actions, which produce the symptoms of inflammation, heat, swelling, redness and pain.

Insulin: Facilitates the storage of excess sugar as liver and muscle glycogen, thus maintaining optimal blood sugar levels. Also facilitates transfer of glucose into all cells including muscle.

Interstitial fluid: The fluid in between all body cells.

Intrinsic asthma: Asthma symptoms caused by an unknown internal mechanism.

Isokinetic machines (or isokinetic dynamometers): Technologically advanced equipment for assessing muscle function. Individuals are tested under controlled conditions, such as speed of movement, type of action (e.g. concentric, eccentric), range of movement, etc. The term 'isokinetic' is a combination of two Greek words meaning the 'same speed'.

Isometric: The term comes from two Greek words *iso* (= same) and *metro* (= length) and it refers to a type of muscle contraction where tension (i.e. strength) is developed but there is no movement, as in a male dancer holding his partner above his head.

Kinesiology: The term derives from the Greek word *kinisis* (= movement), and describes the body of knowledge concerned with the structure and function of the musculo-skeletal system of the human body.

Krebs' cycle: The biochemical process for energy production with the presence of oxygen; water and carbon dioxide are released during this process.

Lactic acid: Glucose is first metabolized to pyruvic acid, which is taken up by Krebs cycle. If too much pyruvic acid is produced, it is reversibly formed into lactic acid, which is a major cause of high-intensity fatigue and muscle pain.

Lactovegeterians: Vegetarians who also consume dairy products.

Lipolysis: Meaning 'breakdown' of fat, the term is the combination of the Greek words *lipos* (= fat) and *lysis* (= breakdown).

Lower reference nutrient intake: For protein, vitamin or mineral represents the amount of the nutrient that is sufficient for only the few people in a group who have low needs.

Mast cells: Cells of the immune system that release and synthesize inflammatory mediators when activated.

Maturation: Progress towards the mature biological state.

Maximal oxygen uptake: Often abbreviated to '$\dot{V}O_2max$', this refers to the highest rate at which a dancer or athlete can utilize oxygen, so it is a measure of the functional limit of the oxygen delivery system—heart, lungs and blood—and of the oxygen uptake system in muscle. Used as a measure of aerobic fitness.

Maximal strength: The highest value obtained at a given set of conditions (i.e. type of muscle contraction, speed of the contraction, position of the body, etc).

Medulla: The central zone of a gland or other organ. The term also refers to the lowest part of the brain.

Menarche: The onset of the first menstrual period, usually between 11 and 14 years.

Menopause: The time when menstruation ceases, usually between 45 and 55 years.

Metabolic heat: Heat generated as a by-product of muscular contraction.

Metabolically active: Usually refers to body-composition elements that require increased amounts of energy during exercise (i.e. muscle mass plus associated tissue components).

Metabolically inactive: Usually refers to body-composition elements that require no extra energy during exercise (i.e. fat, bone).

Metatarsal: This refers to the five long parallel bones that connect your five toes to your ankle. They form the arch of your foot.

Minerals: The term is referred to 21 known metallic elements occurring in nature.

Mitochondria: Are rice-grain shaped organelles in all body cells (except red blood cells), especially muscle cells. Their function is to generate energy, via Krebs cycle, which uses carbohydrate (in the form of pyruvic acid), fats (in the form of free fatty acids), and proteins (in the form of some amino acids).

Monosaccharides: The simplest form of carbohydrate; contain a single 'sugar' component.

Motor nerve: The nerve fibre which supplies the motor unit. The latter is a group of muscle fibres activated by the same motor nerve

Motor tasks: Activities involving movement.

Mullerian duct: A paired set of cellular tubes in all embryos, which will form the internal genitalia if the embryo develops as a female.

Muscle fuels: A collective term used to describe phosphocreatine, carbohydrates, lipids (or fats) and, to lesser extent, proteins in muscle.

Muscle power: A combination of force generation and speed of movement. Factors in addition to muscle size (e.g. muscle length and type of muscle) also influence power production.

Muscle spindles: These are receptors lying in among the muscle fibres, sensitive to stretch. They themselves are controlled by nerves which alter their degree of sensitivity. They are much involved in the control of muscle movement and trigger the 'knee-jerk' reflex, for example.

Myocardium: This is the muscle of the heart. It approximates to 'slow' muscle, generates its own rhythm, virtually never becomes anaerobic, and responds to training by becoming larger and stronger. It forms the four chambers of the heart, which is in effect two hearts: a right heart pumping blood from the body to the lungs for oxygen, and a left heart pumping oxygenated blood from the lungs to the body.

Myoglobin: This is a muscle chemical similar to haemoglobin in the red cells, although about a quarter of its size. It is partly what gives red meat its colour. When oxygen finally comes off haemoglobin within the muscle capillary, it diffuses across the capillary wall, across the interstitial fluid which lies between all cells, through the muscle cell membrane—and is then avidly picked up by myoglobin, which assists its transport deep into the muscle cell.

Newton: This is a unit of force. You exert about 10 Newtons of force when you lift a weight of 1 kg

Non-essential amino acids: Amino acids that—under normal conditions—can be formed inside the body. Therefore, there is no need to obtain them from diet.

Noradrenaline: Known in the US as *norepinephrine*, is a hormone that functions in conjunction with *adrenaline* (the first hormone to be discovered—1894). For example, while adrenaline acts during emergencies and prepares the body for action, noradrenaline does the routine jobs such as maintaining an even blood pressure, by adjusting the diameter of the small arteries, and hence their resistance to blood flow.

Occupational asthma: Asthma symptoms usually caused by an irritant in the work place.

Oestrogen: A group of female hormones produced mainly by the ovary and responsible for menstruation and important for maintaining the skeleton.

Oligomenorrhoea: Irregular, infrequent menstrual periods.

Osmolality: Is a measure of the number of dissolved particles in a fluid. Intakes of drinks with high osmolality cause water to move from the body into the gut resulting in delayed absorption. In contrast, ingestion of drinks with low osmolality causes water to move from the gut to the blood resulting in fast fluid (drink) absorption.

Osteoarthritis: See **Arthritis**

Osteoporosis (or brittle bone disease): Is primarily a disease of the elderly, but is also found in young and very active females including dancers. The disease indicates loss of bone density due to excessive loss of calcium and phosphorous, leading to brittle bones with an increased risk of fracturing.

Ovary: Female reproductive organ.

Ovovegetarians: Vegetarians who eat plant foods, dairy products and eggs.

Oxygen debt: Is a popular term for the extra oxygen that you use after a fairly short bout of very heavy exercise. Exercise scientists use the term 'post-exercise-oxygen-consumption'—as not all of it is 'debt'. Some of the extra oxygen is needed as your metabolic rate has risen because of the exercise: the 'after-burner effect'.

Pacemaker (or sino-atrial node): Cells in the right atrium which both initiate the heart beat, and determines its rate. The pacemaker is influenced by sympathetic nerves, which speed it up, and parasympathetic nerves which slow it down. We gradually lose pacemaker cells as we get older, and our maximal heart rate drops, about one beat per year after   20.

Parasympathetic nervous system: A branch of the autonomic nervous system involved in the control of basic bodily functions at rest.

Peak bone mass: The point at which the bone reaches its maximum density and strength, usually in the twenties.

Peak expiratory flow rate (PEFR): The maximum flow rate that is achieved during a maximal expiration.

Periodization: Planned variations of load, frequency and duration of physical training, aiming to increase levels of fitness. These variations may occur in one-week intervals to intervals lasting for several months or years.

Phalanges: These are the sets of bones which make up the fingers or toes.

Phosphocreatine (PC): Energy-rich compound that backs up ATP in providing energy for fast and powerful muscular contractions.

Photosynthesis: The term originates from the Greek words *fos* (= light) and *synthesis*, and indicates the process whereby green plants manufacture their own food, mainly from carbon dioxide, with the help of sunlight.

Pilates: A rehabilitation technique designed by Joseph Pilates specifically for dancers. The technique focuses on key postural muscles to establish core stability, in this way providing a support system for movement. In recent years, Pilates technique has been increasingly used with the general public and in clinical settings.

Pituitary: Gland in the brain that controls the function of many other glands and is under the influence of the hypothalamus.

Plyometrics: Hopping and bounding exercises done to improve muscle power.

Pneumotachograph: A device that measures the flow rate of air exhaled and inhaled during breathing.

Polysaccharides: Carbohydrates that contain more than two 'sugar' components.

Primary amenorrhoea: Occurs when the menarche is delayed beyond the age of 16 years.

Primary prevention: Prevention of a condition or disease before it manifests itself.

Progesterone: Female hormone produced by the ovary and partly responsible for menstruation

Progestogens: Substances that have an action like progesterone.

Proprioceptors: Nerve receptors which help in the control of movement. Two important types of proprioceptor are: (1) **muscle spindles**, which are sensitive to a change in length as well as to the rate of change in length of the muscle fibre; and (2) **Golgi tendon organs**, which detect changes in tension, i.e. in the force the muscle is applying through the tendons.

Prostaglandins: A family of compounds that are potent inflammatory mediators.

Puberty: Period of rapid changes associated with maturation of the sexual organs to the adult state.

Pyruvic acid: The end-point of anaerobic glycolysis. If too much of it accumulates, it is formed into lactic acid.

Q-angle: If one 'straightens one's leg' fully (i.e. into full extension), the leg is very rarely completely straight. There is usually an angle between the thigh and the lower leg. This angle is termed the Q-angle, and it is usually greater in women than men.

Receptor: A specific chemical pattern on the surface of a cell, which is 'recognized' by a hormone, which then exerts its effect. Without the receptor, the hormone cannot act.

Thermoregulation: The control of body temperature.

Thyroxine: The principal hormone of the thyroid gland. Its main function is to maintain or raise energy expenditure. A deficiency results in tiredness, lack of concentration and in a tendency to gain weight.

Torque (or twisting force): Measured in Newtons per metre (N m), torque is another way of expressing muscular strength. Approximately 10 N.m is 1 kg.

Training set: Used mainly in strength training programmes, the term is synonymous to 'round'. A training set indicates the number of different exercises that are executed in a single round.

Triglycerides: The storage form of fats formed by the union of glycerol and fatty acids.

Unsaturated fats: Fats that can accept hydrogen atoms in their chemical structure; soft at room temperatures. Mainly vegetable fats are more acceptable in health terms.

Valgus angle: In many women, the upper and lower arm often do not form a straight line when the arm is held 'straight' or fully extended. The valgus angle is the angle between the upper and lower arm. It is also known as the 'carrying angle'.

Vasoconstriction: Narrowing of the blood vessels.

Vegans: Strict vegetarians who eat only foods from plant sources. However, such individuals must take B12 supplements, as this vitamin is not found in plants.

Venule: Minute vein, receiving blood from capillary vessels.

Vital capacity (VC): The maximum usable volume of the lungs.

Wolffian ducts: A paired set of tubes in all embryos, but which only develop in the male. They form the male ducts (known as epididymis, vas deferens and ejaculatory duct) which transmit the sperm and secretions, which collectively make up semen, from the testis and other glands to the penis.

INDEX

AAT

Using Accounting Software

Level 2

Foundation Certificate in Accounting

Combined Text and Question Bank

For assessments from September 2017

Second edition 2017

ISBN 9781 5097 1236 6

British Library Cataloguing-in-Publication Data
A catalogue record for this book is available from the British Library

Published by

BPP Learning Media Ltd
BPP House, Aldine Place
142-144 Uxbridge Road
London W12 8AA

www.bpp.com/learningmedia

Printed in the United Kingdom

> Your learning materials, published by BPP Learning Media Ltd, are printed on paper obtained from traceable sustainable sources.

We would like to thank Sage for giving us permission to use screenshots from their software within our materials.

We are grateful to the AAT for permission to reproduce the sample assessment(s). The answers to the sample assessment(s) have been published by the AAT. All other answers have been prepared by BPP Learning Media Ltd.

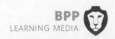

Contents

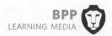

Introduction to the course

This unit provides students with the knowledge and skills needed to carry out typical bookkeeping transactions and tasks using accounting software. In the modern business environment, processing data and information into accounting software is a necessary task in most finance roles. This unit teaches students the practical steps for processing accounting information electronically and will allow students to reinforce their understanding of the sequence in which bookkeeping tasks are carried out.

On completion of this unit, students will have the practical ability to enter accounting transactions into accounting software and to perform bank reconciliations accurately. Students will be able to enter information into accounting software and understand the main features of accounting software. They will learn how to set up general ledger accounts for new and existing businesses and process the typical bookkeeping entries expected of students at this level, including the processing of sales and purchase documentation, recording bank and cash entries and carrying out bank reconciliations accurately. Students will also learn how to produce reports using the software, and understand the purpose of these reports.

Students must have access to a suitable specialised accounting software package, as part of their study for this unit and for the assessment. Spreadsheet software will not allow full unit content coverage, so cannot be used for study or assessment of this unit.

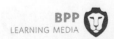

Test specification for Using Accounting Software unit assessment.

Assessment type	Marking type	Duration of exam
Computer based assessment	Human marked	2 hours

Learning outcomes	Weighting
1. Set up accounting software	25%
2. Process sales and purchases transactions	35%
3. Process bank and cash transactions	20%
4. Perform period end routine tasks	15%
5. Produce reports	5%
Total	**100%**

AAT qualifications

The material in this book may support the following AAT qualifications:

AAT Foundation Certificate in Accounting Level 2, AAT Foundation Certificate in Accounting at SCQF Level 5 and Certificate: Accounting Technician (Level 3 AATSA).

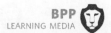

Sage software

Why does this Combined Text and Question Bank refer to Sage 50 and Sage One?

To explain and demonstrate the skills required in this unit, it is necessary to provide practical examples and exercises. This requires the use of computerised accounting software.

Chapters 1 and 2 of this Combined Text and Question Bank have been written using examples taken from **Sage 50**.

Chapters 3 and 4 of this Combined Text and Question Bank follow the same content as Chapters 1 and 2 but have been written using examples taken from **Sage One**.

When working through the chapters, you should only refer to either Chapters 1 and 2, or Chapters 3 and 4.

After the chapters, you should then work through the whole of the remainder of the Combined Text and Question Bank as this can be worked through using either software package.

Do students have to use Sage to complete this unit?

No. Students **do not** have to use Sage in their AAT *Using Accounting Software* assessment.

The AAT recognises that a variety of accounting software packages is available and can be used. The only stipulation the AAT makes is that the package used must be capable of performing the procedures outlined in the learning outcomes and assessment criteria.

Do students need access to Sage software to use this Combined Text and Question Bank?

Students that don't have Sage software may still pick up some useful information from this book, for example the practice assessments.

However, those students with access to Sage will find it easier to work through the practical exercises than users of other accounting software packages.

Refer to the next page for details of how Sage software may be bought, for educational purposes, at very reasonable prices.

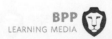

What version do I need?

The illustrations in Chapters 1 and 2 of this Combined Text and Question Bank are taken from Sage 50 Accounts Essentials. The illustrations in Chapters 3 and 4 of this Combined Text and Question Bank are taken from Sage One.

Sage One is an online or 'cloud' based program and is quite different to traditional desktop Sage products such as Sage 50 and Sage Instant. If you are using Sage 50 or Sage Instant you should refer to the Sage 50 section of this book.

For Sage 50, many features and functions remain the same from version to version. For this reason, it is expected that this Combined Text and Question Bank will remain valid for a number of future versions of Sage.

For Sage One, updates are more regular and therefore some screens and menus in this book may appear slightly different to the version you are using, but you should be able to work your way through the tasks. A full list of updates to Sage One can be found by visiting the Sage One website:

http://uk.sageone.com

How do I buy Sage software?

Colleges

If this book is used by students in a college environment, the college will need Sage to be available on student computers. This publication is based on both Sage 50 Accounts Essentials, which will be installed from disk, and Sage One, which is available over the internet, and students can use either product to study for this course. If a college is using Sage 50 Accounts Essentials, they may use a different version of Sage or a different Sage product such as Sage Accounts Instant. Sage 50 and Sage Instant packages are very similar in their operation If a college is using Sage One the software is constantly up to date.

Colleges wanting to purchase Sage One should contact sageonepartners@sage.com for other Sage products colleges should contact Sage in the UK. Contact details can be found at www.sage.co.uk.

Individual students

Individual students are able to buy:

Sage One by visiting the following site:

http://info.uk.sageone.com/aat-computerised-accounting

Sage 50 Accounts Essentials from BPP Learning Media. This must be for educational purposes. For details you should contact BPP Learning Media customer services on 0845 075 1100 or email learningmedia@bpp.com

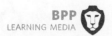

Are Sage data files provided with this book?

No. Sage data files aren't provided because the material is written in such a way that they aren't required.

New instances of Sage allow users to access a blank ledger suitable for experimenting. Instructions are provided in this Combined Text and Question Bank that enable a new blank ledger to be created.

Skills bank

What do I need to know to do well in the assessment?

Using Accounting Software is a practical syllabus that is assessed by a single scenario involving accounting transactions in a specific period for a business organisation. The scenario comprises a series of tasks that will be completed using accounting software. Your success will depend on the accuracy of your reports.

The tasks can be summarised as being in three phases:

- Set-up (of accounts and balances)
- Input (of transactions such as invoices and payments)
- Output (of various reports including an Audit Trail)

In order to start, however, there are other practicalities that you will need to know but are not directly assessed within the Learning Outcomes:

- How to launch the software
- How to create a company
- How to correct errors

As a comparison, when you use word processing software you will be presented with a blank screen and before writing your text you would be well advised to plan your layout!

In the *Using Accounting Software* unit the templates are already designed for you within the software package. Therefore your first task is to familiarise yourself with the templates. Then you will know where to enter data.

One more factor that will help you is understanding double entry bookkeeping. While you can operate the software without this knowledge, knowing <u>why</u> you are performing the tasks will help you to master them more efficiently.

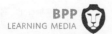

Logical approaches to tasks

You will be assessed on:

1   Accuracy of data such as dates, net and VAT amounts
2   Selection of appropriate codes (nominal, bank, customer, supplier)
3   Accurate completion of processes (such as bank reconciliation)
4   Selection of appropriate reports (trial balance, etc)
5   Screenshot evidence of some tasks

Entering data

Accuracy is the key here so it important that any data entered is accurate and complete. It is always worthwhile checking that your data is the same as any data given to you on the assessment as it can be easy to transpose figures, for example entering 213 instead of 123.

Appropriate codes

Understanding double entry principles should help you to select appropriate account codes. Accounting software often contains many account codes so that it is useful to know all the most commonly used codes (sales, purchases, bank, etc). Furthermore, if you know the logic of the coding system (eg, 4 digits, first digit relating to the account category) this will help you to look in the right sequence for the code.

Completing processes

When performing an involved process such as a bank reconciliation, ensure that you know how to check that it is accurate and that it has been completed.

Appropriate reports

Most accounting software contains many pre-designed reports that can be selected. Many can look similar but contain brief or detailed versions of the same type of report.

Ensure that you understand what the task requires, and very importantly, when you preview or print it, look at it to see if you understand it, and if it meets the task needs.

Screenshots

Some tasks require you to take a screenshot of the accounting software at certain points. When pasting into software such as Microsoft Word ensure that it is as you intend and that it is readable.

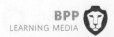

BPP Learning Media's AAT Materials

Supplements

From time to time we may need to publish supplementary materials to one of our titles. This can be for a variety of reasons. From a small change in the AAT unit guidance to new legislation coming into effect between editions.

You should check our supplements page regularly for anything that may affect your learning materials. All supplements are available free of charge on our supplements page on our website at:

www.bpp.com/learning-media/about/students

Improving material and removing errors

There is a constant need to update and enhance our study materials in line with both regulatory changes and new insights into the assessments.

From our team of authors BPP appoints a subject expert to update and improve these materials for each new edition.

Their updated draft is subsequently technically checked by another author and from time to time non-technically checked by a proof reader.

We are very keen to remove as many numerical errors and narrative typos as we can but given the volume of detailed information being changed in a short space of time we know that a few errors will sometimes get through our net.

We apologise in advance for any inconvenience that an error might cause. We continue to look for new ways to improve these study materials and would welcome your suggestions. If you have any comments about this book, please email nisarahmed@bpp.com or write to Nisar Ahmed, AAT Head of Programme, BPP Learning Media Ltd, BPP House, Aldine Place, London W12 8AA.

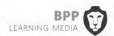

Sage 50 – Part 1

1

Chapter coverage

You will be required to prove your competence in the use of computerised accounting software by completing an assessment. Assessments are likely to include a series of exercises, for example, entering customer and supplier details, posting transactions such as journals, invoices and credit notes, and generating and saving reports.

This chapter explains how you might complete the hands-on computerised accounts parts of an assessment. It is by no means a comprehensive guide to computerised accounting.

The illustrations in this chapter and the next chapter are from Sage 50 Accounts Essentials, which is just one of many packages that you might use. We use a Sage package because these are popular among small/medium-sized businesses in the UK; and with colleges, for training purposes.

There are a large number of illustrations in this chapter, so don't be put off if it seems long – it should be relatively quick and easy to work through.

The topics covered in this chapter are:

- Accounting software
- Assessments
- Company data and the general (nominal) ledger
- Customer and supplier data
- Journals
- Entering invoices
- Help!

1 Accounting software

Accounting software ranges from simple 'off the shelf' cash book style software to heavy-duty Enterprise Resource Management systems used in large organisations. Very large organisations often have a system that has been built specifically for them, made up of components from a variety of software suppliers, or written for them on a one-off basis.

Obviously, we cannot even begin to cover the vast range of available software, but we can illustrate the features of a typical package, and the most popular one in the UK among small to medium-sized businesses is Sage.

Sage produces a variety of accounting software and this book deals with Sage 50 Accounts Essentials, from which the illustrations in this chapter are taken. In the remainder of this chapter, we will just use the word 'Sage' to refer to Sage 50 Accounts Essentials.

1.1 Hands-on

The illustrations in Chapters 1 and 2 are taken from Sage. The tasks you are required to carry out are set in the period of January 2016.

Sage upgrades its software regularly. However, many features and functions remain the same from version to version. Some training centres may use different Sage packages or different versions of Sage. The different Sage packages for small and medium-sized businesses are based on common principles and are very similar in their operation when it comes to performing the tasks included in this Text. Some screens and menus may appear slightly different, depending on the age or version of the product you are using, but you should be able to work your way through the tasks.

If possible, we strongly recommend that you sit at a computer equipped with a version of Sage as you read through this chapter. Most of the activities assume that you are doing this and can complete the tasks we describe as you go along.

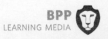

1.2 Finding your way about: terminology

We'll assume that you know what we mean when we say 'menu' and 'button', but there may be some other terms that you are not sure of, so here is a quick guide. In this chapter, we will use bold text when referring to something that you will see on screen, such as a button or a menu or a label beside or above a box. We also use arrows to indicate a sequence of actions. For example, we might say choose **'Settings > Change Program Date'**. This means click on the **Settings** menu and then click on **Change Program Date**.

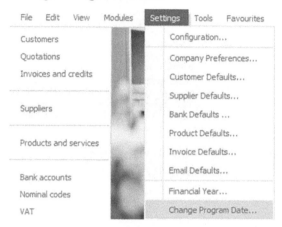

While you can use the buttons on the toolbars as your main starting point, it is useful to familiarise yourself with the Settings and Modules buttons, as the content of these rarely changes, although the layout and position of the buttons can vary between different versions. Here is the main toolbar that you can see at the left of the screen when you open up Sage, with the **Customers** button highlighted.

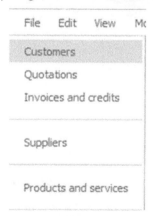

When the **Customers** button is highlighted, the following toolbar appears at the top of the screen.

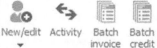

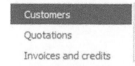

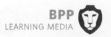

Most of what you do involves you making entries in **fields** – for example the **A/C** field and the **Date** field in the next illustration.

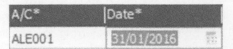

A/C*	Date*
ALE001	31/01/2016

We also refer to 'drop-down lists' which are lists of items to select from within a field. A drop-down list is indicated by a downward arrow button next to the field. The screenshot below shows a drop-down list for the field **Type**, in the account codes area of Sage.

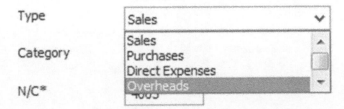

Type   Sales

Category   Sales
            Purchases
            Direct Expenses
N/C*   Overheads

Sometimes you need to select a 'tab' to view the part of the program we refer to. For instance, in this example the **Activity** tab is selected.

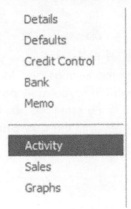

Details

Defaults

Credit Control

Bank

Memo

Activity

Sales

Graphs

Finally, make sure that you know where the **Tab** key is on your keyboard. It looks similar to this.

Also that you are aware of the function keys (**F1**, **F2** and so on, usually along the top).

Note. On some keyboards the function keys only operate by holding the **Fn** key at the same time. In this Text we refer to actions using the function keys and assume that these will operate directly by pressing them. However if they do not work, you may have to hold the **Fn** key at the same time.

The **Esc** key is also very useful for closing windows quickly.

1.3 Defaults

Computerised packages make extensive use of '**defaults**', which are the most common entries. When you start entering data you will often find that Sage has done some of the work already, using the default options that would normally be chosen. This saves a great deal of time, but you should always glance at the default entries in case they are not the ones you want. This will become clearer as you start using the package.

1.4 Screenshots

During the assessment, for certain tasks, you will be asked to 'save a screenshot' of a screen to provide evidence that you have completed the task correctly. This means you need to capture and save an image of a particular screen shown on the computer.

To take a screen capture of an entire screen, on your keyboard press **Print Screen** or **PrtScn**. To capture the active window only, press **Alt +Print Screen** or **ALT + PrtScn** (on some keyboards the key may be labelled PrtSc).

The image can then be pasted into a document using an application (using **CTRL + V**) such as **Word** from where the document can be saved as a file (**CTRL + S**).

1.5 Exporting to PDF file

You will also be required to generate various reports from the accounting software. To provide evidence that you have generated the reports, you should export these to PDF (Portable Document Format) files if your accounting software program allows this. If not, you should take screenshots of the full report on screen and paste these to a document. You should save your files to your computer. Reports are covered in Chapter 2.

To export a report to a PDF file, click on the **Export** button at the top of the screen that the report is shown in.

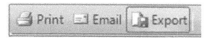

This brings up a box that asks you for the location on the computer where you want to save the PDF file to, and the name of the file. Specify the location and name of the file and click on Save. In the assessment you will be told the location of where to save the file and the type of name to use.

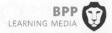

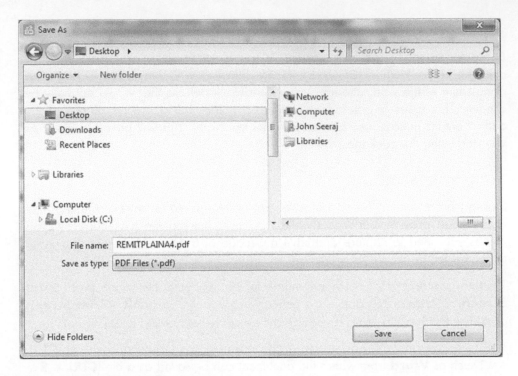

1.6 Uploading files

You will be required to 'upload' the documents or PDF files you have saved. This means that in the assessment, there will be an option on screen to upload files saved in your computer. Selecting this option brings up a box similar to that shown below, which asks you choose the file you wish to upload from your computer.

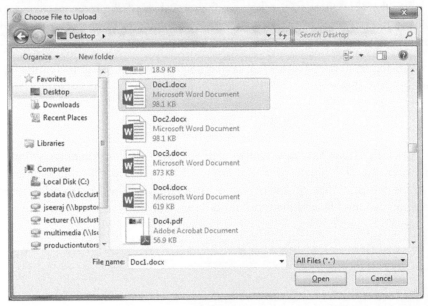

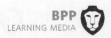

1.7 Accounting entries

This module assumes you have a basic understanding of double entry accounting, the fundamental principle of which is that **each and every transaction has two effects**.

So for every transaction that a business makes, there must be:

- **Debit entries** in particular ledger accounts
- An equal and opposite value of **credit entries** in other ledger accounts

Ledger accounts are accounts in which each transaction is recorded – there will be a ledger account for different types of transaction such as sales and purchases, and for every type of asset and liability.

The **general ledger** (also referred to as **nominal ledger**) is the accounting record which forms the complete set of ledger accounts for the business.

To know when to use debits and credits, use the following general rules:

- An **increase** in an **expense** (eg a purchase of stationery) or an **increase in an asset** (eg a purchase of computer equipment) is a **debit**.

- An **increase** in **revenue** (eg a sale) or an **increase in a liability** (eg buying goods on credit) is a **credit**.

- A **decrease** in an **asset** (eg making a payment from the bank) is a **credit**.

- A **decrease** in a **liability** (eg paying a creditor) is a **debit**.

In this book, we often refer to 'posting' a transaction. This simply means recording the transaction in the ledger accounts.

2 Assessments

Your AAT assessment will involve a number of practical tasks that test your competence in the assessment criteria.

2.1 Before you start...

Before you start, you should find out from your assessor what the arrangements are for:

- Opening the accounting software and logging in, if necessary
- Changing any overall company details or settings, if required
- Creating new accounts, as necessary
- Posting transactions and completing other assessment tasks
- Exporting and saving your work

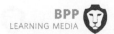

Example

The following example is based on a past sample simulation issued by the AAT (simulations were used before assessments).

SITUATION

SFE Merchandising is a new business that has been set up by Charlize Veron, one of Southfield Electrical's former marketing staff. Charlize is an expert on store layout and management of inventories (stocks) and she intends to sell her skills and knowledge, on a consultancy basis, to medium-sized and large retailers to help them to optimise their sales.

Charlize has started her new venture as a sole trader and has taken on some of the risk herself. However, SFE Merchandising is part-financed by Southfield Electrical, and may well be acquired by them if this new venture is a success. Initial enquiries have been so promising that Charlize has already voluntarily registered for VAT and intends to run the standard VAT accounting scheme. (Assume the standard VAT rate is 20%.)

The business commenced trading on 1 January 2016.

Tasks to be completed

It is now 31 January 2016 and you are to complete the tasks in Chapters 1 and 2.

There will be 13 tasks in the real assessment involving setting up data, entering journals, posting sales and purchase transactions, generating reports and so on.

You will be provided with a series of documents such as invoices and cheques. We'll show you how to deal with all of this in the remainder of this Text.

You should now have Sage open on your computer and follow through the activities.

Task 1

Preliminary

This exercise starts with a new installation of Sage or a 'clean' company which contains no transactions.

Your college will tell you how to install Sage afresh or from where to restore the clean company.

If you are studying at home and are installing Sage for the first time on a particular computer, follow the on-screen installation instructions for a standard installation – then **go to the New Set Up instructions below**.

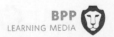

If you are studying at home and **have an existing Sage ledger**, you may **create a new installation and a blank ledger** by following the steps below.

- Click on the **File** button along the top menu and select **Maintenance.**

- Click on the **Rebuild** option and untick all the options on the left hand side. In some cases, you may need to keep the nominal ledger accounts ticked to maintain the **chart of accounts**. This will vary from version to version.

- Once the rebuild is complete, you will be asked to enter the month and year of the company being worked on. This is given in the scenario. If no year is given use the current year.

- Now go to the settings options and overtype the name of the existing company with that of the new company and change the program date if required to do so.

Two important points to note:

- **You will not be required to set up a new company in your real assessment. We cover this here to enable us to create the same starting point in Sage for all students.**

- **If installing the program for the first time, you will need to know its Serial Number and Activation Key, often found on the CD or packaging**

New Set Up

The first time you open the package you are presented with a company set-up wizard. A wizard is a type of software assistant that presents a user with a sequence of boxes that guide the user through a series of steps.

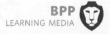

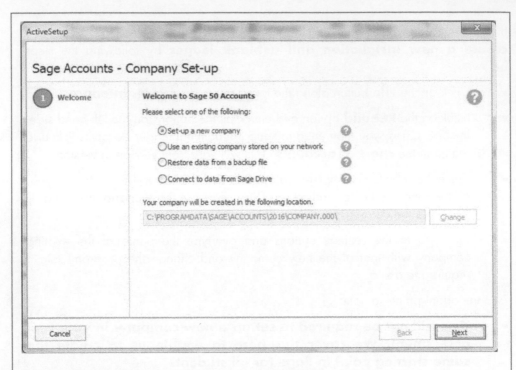

Select **Set-up a new company** and press **Next**.

If your Sage installation does not start at the set-up wizard, you can enter the company information by accessing **Settings > Company Preferences** from the menu at the top of the screen.

Note. Sage generally refers to a business as a 'company' in its menus (eg Company Preferences). However, this is just the terminology used by Sage, and Sage can be used for sole traders and partnerships, as well as limited companies. Where menus and references in this book refer to 'company', take this as meaning 'business' unless otherwise stated. Therefore, such references can encompass sole trader businesses as well as companies.

2.2 Back up and Restore files

It is sensible to create a copy of your work at regular intervals, and at the end of sessions. You will then be able to restore the work later.

Go to **File>Back up** and then choose an easy to find location to store the back up file. The Browse button will help you find a location.

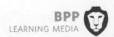

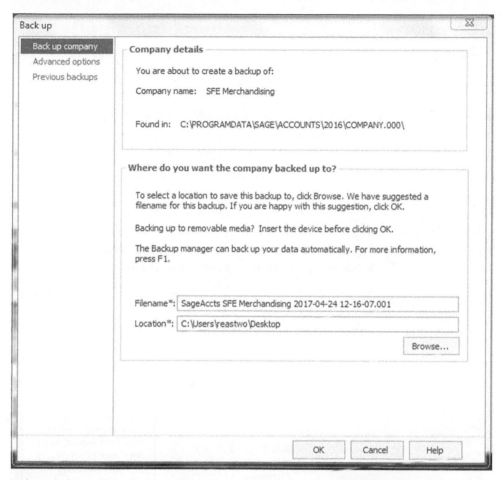

When re-launching Sage software, it will list the last used data files. As below, select SFE Merchandising, being the company you wish to restore.

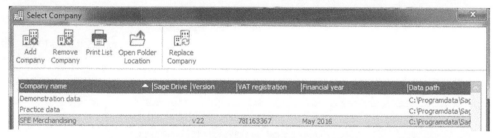

If you are already in Sage and wish to load another back up, go to **File>Restore** and use Browse, or Previous Backups, to find the relevant location and file.

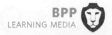

3 Company data and the general (nominal) ledger

3.1 Company data

The name and address of the business should then be entered. This information will appear on any documents you produce with the package, such as reports and invoices, so make sure it is accurate and spelled correctly.

Enter all the information given in the screen below. Use the **Tab** key on your keyboard to move between different lines. Alternatively, click on each line, but this will slow you down, so get into the habit of using the **Tab** key to move from field to field (almost all packages work this way). When you have finished, press **Next** (each time you complete a new screen you will need to press **Next** to continue – you can also use the **Back** button if you need to revisit a screen).

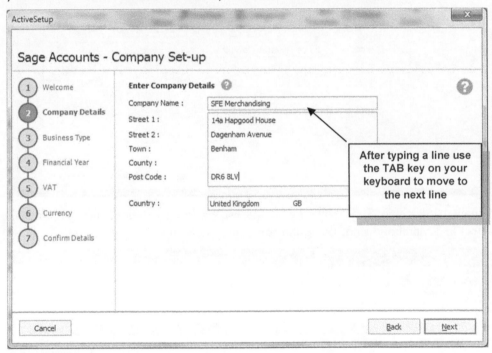

3.2 Accounts in the general (nominal) ledger

As explained earlier, the general ledger is the ledger that contains all the business's ledger accounts. This is also known as the NOMINAL LEDGER and 'nominal ledger' is the term used by Sage.

When a new business is first set up, there is a choice between a number of different 'charts of accounts'. A chart of accounts is a template that sets out the nominal ledger accounts and how they are organised into different categories.

The charts provided are tailored towards the type of business. In Sage 50 Accounts Essentials, you are given a choice between a Sole Trader, Partnership and Limited Company. SFE Merchandising is a sole trader, so you should select this option – **Sole Trader**.

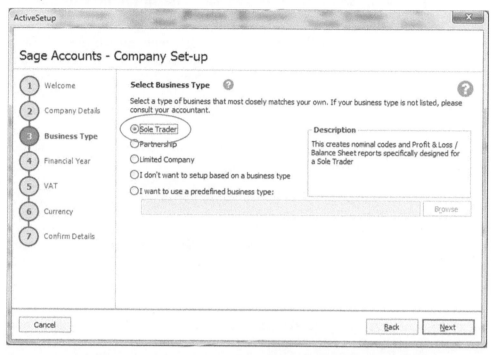

If you are using other versions of Sage, you may be faced with a number of chart of accounts for different types of company, similar to that shown below.

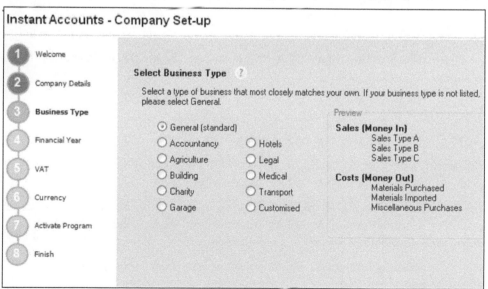

These have accounts tailored for the particular business type.

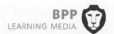

For example, the 'Hotels, Restaurants and Guest Houses' chart includes sales accounts for 'Restaurant Meals' and 'Alcoholic Beverage Sales'.

Many organisations use the 'General' chart, and modify it to suit their needs. If you are faced with the screen above, choose the **General (Standard)** chart of accounts.

Note that you are not confined to using the accounts that you are given by the program when you first set up the company. Certain accounts must always remain because the program will not be able to operate without them – so you will not be able to delete the main bank account, the receivables (debtors) and payables (creditors) control accounts, VAT accounts, and certain other essential accounts. But you can delete any non-essential accounts (so long as you have not yet posted any transactions to them), and you can rename them and add new accounts as required.

3.3 Financial year

Set the start of the financial year to January 2016. This can be done either by progressing through the wizard or by accessing **Settings > Financial Year** from the menu.

3.4 VAT

The business is **VAT registered** (so select **Yes** in the wizard) and is not registered for cash accounting. Using either the wizard or by choosing **Settings > Company Preferences > VAT** enter 524 3764 51 as the VAT number.

Enter the standard VAT rate % as 20.00.

3.5 Currency

Select **Pound Sterling**, either from the wizard or **Settings > Currency** from the menu.

3.6 Complete set-up

You may get an option to customise the company. Ignore this and click **Close**.

If necessary, activate the program by entering the serial number and activation code supplied with the program or by your college.

The final step is the **Confirm Details** step. Check that the details you have entered are correct and if necessary go back and modify them. Once you are happy the information is correct, click on **Create**.

You are now ready to proceed with entering the company's transactions.

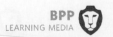

3.7 New accounts and your assessment

You will be presented with a home screen as shown below. There are various options for the purposes of getting started. Ignore these for now. However, if you have the time, there is no harm in looking at these as they contain useful help webinars and demo data.

In your assessment, you may need to add new nominal ledger accounts to complete your tasks. As you work through your assessment, before starting each task, check that the accounts you will need are set up. We recommend you create any new accounts required before starting the task the account is needed in.

If the assessment includes a purchase invoice for stationery, for instance, check that there is already an 'Office stationery' overheads account before you start to post the invoice. The tasks may actually ask you to do this. You can see which chart of accounts has been applied by choosing **Nominal Codes**.

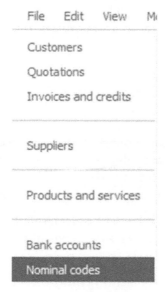

You are then presented with the chart of accounts.

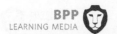

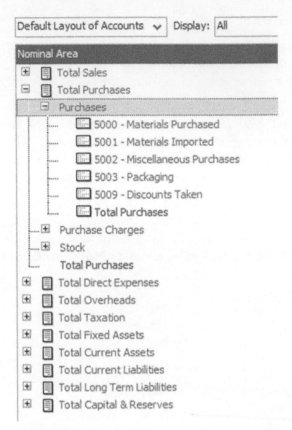

The chart of accounts has been grouped by type of account. These main headings can be expanded by clicking on the '+' sign next to each heading to reveal the accounts contained within the headings. For example '5000 – Materials Purchased' is grouped by 'Purchases', and further grouped by 'Total Purchases'.

If the chart is displayed as a long list of accounts, you can change it to the format shown above by accessing the **Layout** options at the top right of the screen and choosing **Analyser**.

Expand **Total Overheads** and then **Printing and Stationery** and you will see that there is not yet a specific account for 'Publicity material', so we will create one.

Task 2

Create a new account for 'Publicity material'.

Make sure you are in the Nominal Codes function (click on **Nominal Codes** from the left side of the screen). Click on the **Wizard** button

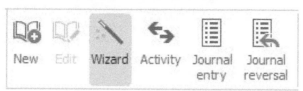

and the program will take you through the Nominal Record Wizard. It is possible to set up new accounts without using the wizard, but we discourage this, because it can very easily lead to problems in the way the program handles your new nominal ledger accounts when it is producing reports and financial statements.

The first step is to decide on the **Name** of your new account (overtype 'New nominal account' with 'Publicity material') and choose what **Type** of account it is.

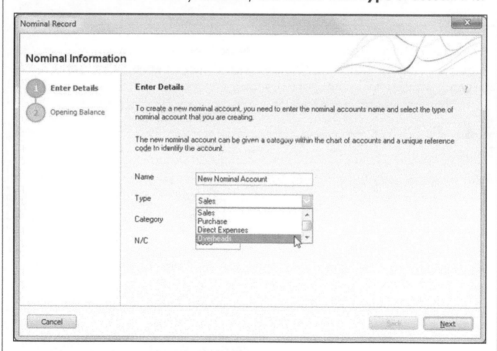

You can further refine the **Category** of account (the options available will depend on the type of account you are setting up – here 'Printing and Stationery') and choose an account code (**N/C**). In fact, the program will suggest a code based on the type and category of account, and we strongly recommend that you accept this.

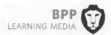

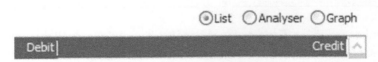

After making your selections and clicking **Next**, you will be asked if you want to **enter an opening balance**. Choose **No** and click **Create**. We cover entering opening balances later in the chapter (directly or via a journal).

Task 3

Vimal was in a hurry to post a transaction. He wasn't sure what nominal account to use, so he created a new account named 'L8R'. Why might this cause problems later on?

It is also possible to change the name of existing nominal accounts. If you are not already in the Nominal Codes module, click on **Nominal Codes**, and then double click on the desired account code. When looking for a particular code, you may find it easier to view the account codes as a list by choosing **List** at the top right of the screen.

⦿List ◯Analyser ◯Graph

Debit | Credit |▲|

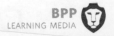

The accounts are then presented as a list as shown below.

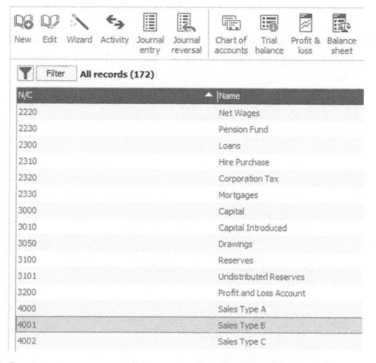

Double clicking on an account brings up the **Nominal Record** screen showing details of the selected account and you can update the name field by typing over the existing name and selecting the **Save** button. (If you cannot see the screen below, make sure the **Details** tab to the left of the screen is selected.) For example, you could change the account '4001 - Sales Type B' to something that is more descriptive of the particular sales to be recorded in that account (eg Overseas Sales).

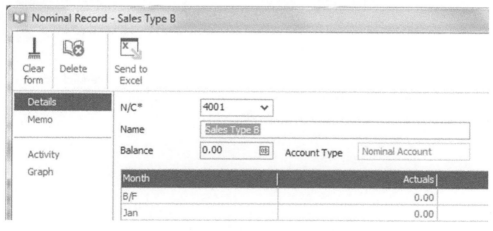

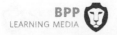

3.8 Entering opening balances in nominal ledger accounts

If you are transferring your business's accounting records from a manual system to a computer system, you will need to post opening balances to your nominal ledger.

Although you can do this using a journal (as we will see later in the chapter), Sage allows you to go directly to the relevant nominal accounts to enter opening balances and makes the accounting entries for you.

To enter opening balances on nominal accounts, find the nominal account you wish to add an opening balance to. For example, you may want to post the opening balance for a property.

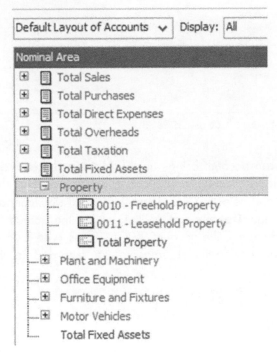

As we saw in the previous section, selecting the account and double clicking on it brings up the **Nominal Record** screen, which includes a 'Balance' field.

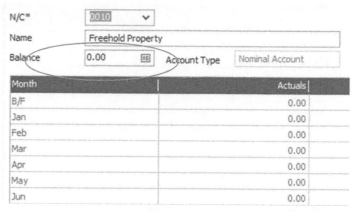

Clicking on the small button to the right of this field marked '**OB**' brings up a screen where you can enter and save an opening balance (although don't save anything now).

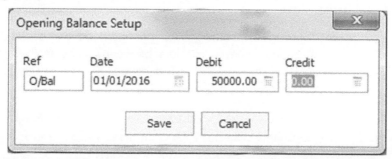

Note that for any entries made using this option, the corresponding entry will be posted to a suspense account. However, since opening balances entered should sum to zero (having the same value of debits and credits), entering all opening balances should result in a zero balance overall on the suspense account.

3.9 Tax codes

3.9.1 Tax codes and VAT rates

When entering transactions, it is important to use the appropriate **tax code** to ensure the VAT is correctly treated. The tax codes in Sage are summarised below. Note that in the assessment, you do not need to know what different rates of VAT are used for. You will be told in the assessment if VAT is applicable, and the rate to use.

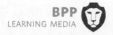

Tax code	Used for
T0	Zero-rated transactions, such as books, magazines and train fares. (Think of the code as 'T Zero' – then you will never confuse it with the code for exempt transactions.)
T1	Standard rate, currently 20%. Some standard-rated items that catch people out are taxi fares (but only if the taxi driver is VAT registered), restaurant meals and stationery. You can only reclaim VAT if you have a valid VAT invoice; if not, use code T9.
T2	Exempt transactions such as bank charges and insurance, postage stamps and professional subscriptions.
T5	Lower/Reduced rate, currently 5% for certain things such as domestic electricity, but this does not normally apply to business expenditure.
T9*	Transactions not involving VAT, for example wages, charitable donations and internal transfers between accounts (for instance from the bank to the petty cash account). Also used if the supplier is not VAT registered or if you do not have a valid VAT invoice.

* The code 'T9' would also be used for all transactions if your business was not VAT registered. However, in this case study the business is VAT registered.

As mentioned above, you will **not** be expected to know the VAT rates for different goods and services. However, you may find the following list of current VAT rates helpful in real life:

www.gov.uk/rates-of-vat-on-different-goods-and-services

3.10 Editing VAT codes and rates

Occasionally, an existing VAT rate is changed. This happened when the rate moved from 17.5% to 20% in 2011. This is easy to manage in Sage and only takes a few moments. The process is set out below and is for your general information. If you decide to try this out and change the VAT rate using the following steps, **make sure you change it back to 20% before you continue** through the Text. Alternatively, click on **Cancel** at the end of Step 4 and do not click Save and your changes will not be saved.

Step 1   Click on Settings, and then select **Configuration**

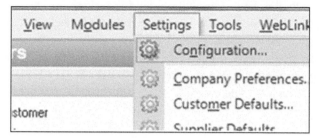

Step 2   Select the **Tax Codes** tab

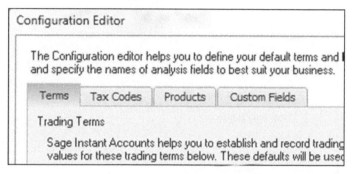

Step 3   In the tax codes tab you will find a list of tax codes. To change an existing code it is best to make the changes on the day it begins to affect your company or the nearest trading day after that, highlight the tax code on the list and then click on **Edit**.

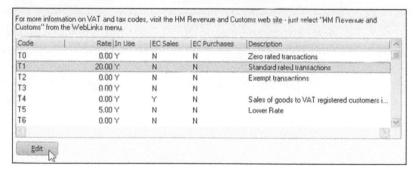

Step 4   The following pop-up screen appears. Simply overtype the existing rate with the new rate (this should be done on the day the rate changes). Once the rate has been updated, clicking OK makes the pop-up screen disappear and the entry will have been amended in the tax code list. Clicking on Save results in the company tax code being updated but you should exit without clicking Save, as we want to keep the VAT rate as 20%.

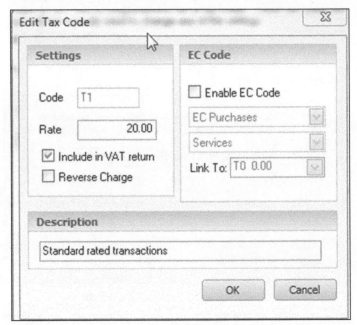

Some companies may prefer to run the older code and newer tax codes concurrently for a short while and in this case, a new code will need to be created. To do this, you would follow the instructions above but instead, at Step 3, a code should be selected that is currently unused (such as T3). The older rate will be entered there, ensuring the **Include in VAT return** box is ticked. Step 4 is unchanged.

If in doubt about which tax code to use when creating new tax codes, check with a manager or your accountant for advice, as all companies are set up differently.

3.11 Trade and non-trade receivables

One thing to note is that the Sage package does not make a distinction between trade and non-trade (or 'other') receivables; anyone to whom you grant credit is simply treated as a customer in Sage. (You can assign different types of customers to different categories and/or to different 'departments', but that is beyond the scope of your present studies.)

Another point to note is that Sage uses old UK GAAP (Generally Accepted Accounting Principles) terminology, rather than IFRS (International Financial Reporting Standards) and new UK GAAP terminology, and therefore uses the term 'debtors' rather than 'receivables'. Therefore, the receivables control account in Sage is named the debtors control account. You will **not** need to post non-trade or 'other' receivables, so you will not need to use Sage's standard 'other debtors' account.

Note. From now on, we will use the same terminology as Sage uses (ie old UK GAAP terminology) for the purposes of navigating through Sage.

4 Customer and supplier data

Before you can post customer and supplier transactions, you will also need to set up accounts in the trade receivables ledger (often referred to as the sales ledger) and the trade payables ledger (often referred to as the purchase ledger).

Note. Customer and supplier accounts are subsidiary accounts of the overall trade debtors ledger account and trade creditors account respectively. Therefore, transactions entered in all customer accounts will be posted to the **one** trade debtors ledger account in the nominal ledger (and the same treatment applies to supplier accounts and the trade creditors ledger).

Once again, we recommend that you set up all the accounts you need before you start posting any transactions.

In an assessment (and in real life) you will find the details you need on the documents you have to hand: the business's own sales invoices and its suppliers' purchase invoices.

4.1 Customer and supplier codes

The first decision you will need to make is what type of codes to use. In Sage, the default behaviour of the program, if you use the wizard to set up the new supplier's record, is to use the first eight characters (excluding spaces and punctuation) of the full name of the customer or supplier, so if you enter 'G.T. Summertown' as the name, the package will suggest that you use the code GTSUMMER.

This is a very clear and easy to use coding system because the code actually contains information about the account to which it refers. If you gave this customer a numeric code such as '1' this might work fine as long as you only had a few customers. However, if you have thousands it is most unlikely that you would know who, say, customer 5682 was, just from the code.

The program will not allow you to set up two customers or two suppliers with the same code, so if you had a customer called 'G.T. Summerfield' as well as one called 'G.T. Summertown' you would get a warning message suggesting that you use the code GTSUMME1. For this reason, many businesses actually introduce numbers into their coding systems. For example, you could use the first five letters

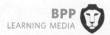

of the name and then the numbers 001, 002 and so on for subsequent customers or suppliers with the same first five letters in their name (GTSUM001, GTSUM002, and so on).

Of course, in your work you would use the coding system prescribed by your organisation. However, in an assessment you will usually be told which code to use. If a task does allow for choice, we recommend an alphanumeric system (a mixture of letters and numbers), as this displays your understanding of the need for understandable but unique codes.

Task 4

Do you think it is possible for a customer and a supplier to have exactly the same code? Explain your answer.

4.2 Entering the account details

We'll now illustrate setting up a supplier account. Please note that the process is identical for customers, apart from the fact that you will be working within the **Customers screens**.

If you click the **Suppliers** button (on the left of screen), this gives you a new set of buttons.

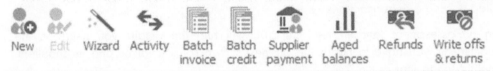

New   Edit   Wizard   Activity   Batch invoice   Batch credit   Supplier payment   Aged balances   Refunds   Write offs & returns

The first way to set up a new account, is to click on **New** and enter as many details as you have available. The details you need will usually be found on the supplier invoice. If the invoice shows an email address, for instance, be sure to type it in, even though you may not have email addresses for other suppliers. Most information is entered in the first three sections listed to the left of the screen **(Details, Defaults** and **Credit Control**). Take care with typing, as always. When you are happy that everything is correct, click on **Save** and a blank record (like the one that follows) will now appear ready for you to enter the next record. Always remember to click **Save** after entering each supplier and when you are finished click on **Close**.

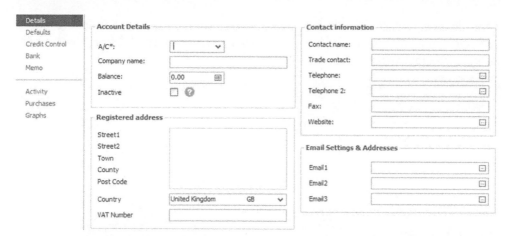

An alternative method for setting up a new account is to click on the **Wizard** button and use the supplier record wizard to enter supplier details. Some people prefer to do this in the first instance, although it can be slower and is not often used in the workplace. Try both methods and decide which is best for you.

Task 5

Set up a supplier account based on the following details taken from the heading of an invoice. Decide on an appropriate coding system yourself.

McAlistair Supplies Ltd
52 Foram Road
Winnesh
DR3 5TP
Tel: 06112 546772 Fax: 06112 546775
Email: sales@mcalisupps.co.uk
VAT No. 692 1473 29

If you use the wizard, don't put anything in for any other data, except for clicking on 'Terms Agreed' in the 'Credit Control' screen.

Remember to **Save** the new account.

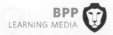

You will see that McAlistair Supplies is now listed as a supplier in the main supplier window. Double clicking on **McAlistair Supplies Ltd** from the list will bring up the following screen:

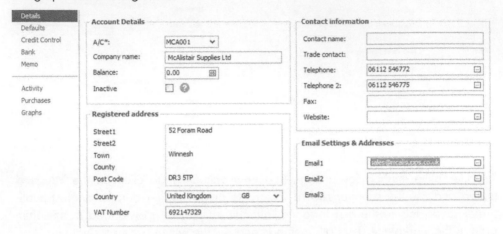

4.3 Entering the opening balance

Earlier in this chapter, we looked at entering an opening balance for a nominal ledger account. The opening balance for the 'Trade creditors' ledger account is made up of the sum of the individual suppliers' opening balances.

You can enter an opening balance for the supplier in this screen by clicking on the **'OB'** icon next to the **Balance** field, once you have set up the supplier. The suppliers you are asked to set up in an assessment task may have opening balances and you can use the screen in the previous section to enter them.

If you see the following message when entering a supplier record:

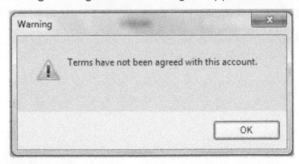

Click on the **Credit Control** section for this record.

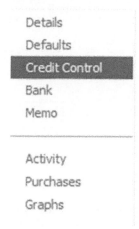

Put a tick in the appropriate checkbox at the foot of the screen, and then save the record. This is simply something Sage requires in order for you to continue entering data for this supplier/customer.

Restrictions

☐ Can charge credit   ☐ Restrict mailing
☑ Terms agreed   ☐ Account On Hold

4.4 Customer and supplier defaults

By default, when you set up a new customer account, customer invoices you enter will be posted by default to the following accounts:

DR   Debtors Control Account (debit gross amount)

CR   Sales Account (credit net amount)

CR   Sales Tax Control Account (credit VAT amount)

For sales, this is probably exactly what you want to happen, unless you are specifically instructed that different types of sales should be posted to different sales accounts in the nominal ledger.

When you set up a new supplier account, the supplier invoices you enter will be posted by default to the following accounts:

DR   Purchase Tax Control Account (debit VAT amount)

DR   Purchases Account (debit net amount)

CR   Creditors Control Account (credit gross amount)

For supplier invoices, however, it would be better to set an appropriate default for the expense for each supplier, depending on the type of purchase. For example, you would want to post a stationery supplier's invoices to the stationery account, but an insurance company's invoices to the insurance account.

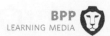

To change the defaults, just open the supplier record and click on the **Defaults** section.

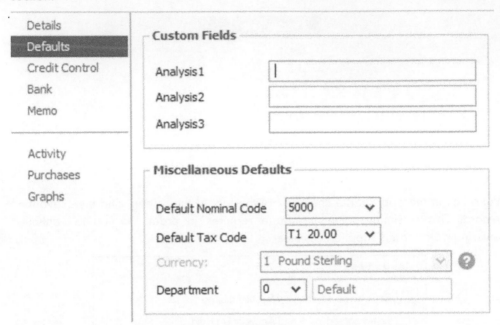

In the box labelled **Default Nominal Code**, you can set the nominal ledger account to which all transactions with this supplier will be posted, unless you specify otherwise when you actually post a transaction. To see a list of all available accounts, click on the arrow 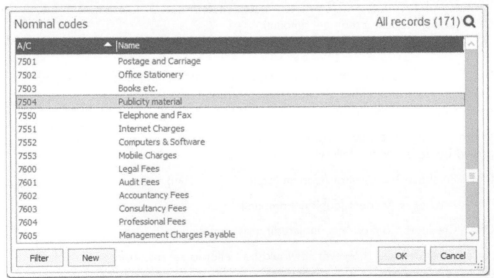 at the right of the box or just press the **F4** key on your keyboard. For example, we may wish to set the default for McAlistair Supplies to 'Publicity Material'.

A/C	Name
7501	Postage and Carriage
7502	Office Stationery
7503	Books etc.
7504	Publicity material
7550	Telephone and Fax
7551	Internet Charges
7552	Computers & Software
7553	Mobile Charges
7600	Legal Fees
7601	Audit Fees
7602	Accountancy Fees
7603	Consultancy Fees
7604	Professional Fees
7605	Management Charges Payable

Nominal codes — All records (171)

Filter   New   OK   Cancel

To do this we would scroll down the list and select the Publicity Material account created earlier (account 7504). If you need a new nominal account to post to, you can set one up from this screen – but we recommend using the Nominal Record wizard, as mentioned earlier.

Payment terms

The default payment terms (ie, how long a supplier gives a customer to pay an invoice) is set to 0 days' credit. If in the assessment you are asked to set up a supplier with payment terms other than 0 days (eg, 30 days), select the **Credit Control** option and enter the number of days in the **Payment Due** field.

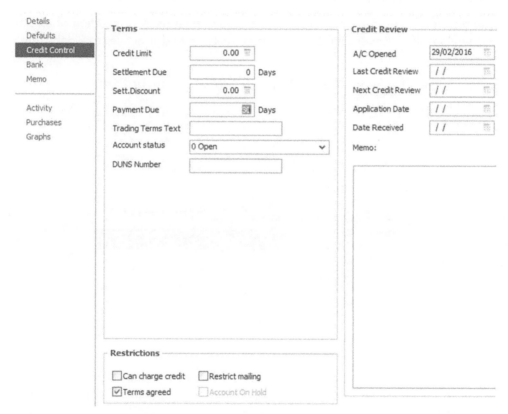

The same process also applies for customers.

Also, a credit limit can also be set for each customer/supplier by entering the amount in the **Credit Limit field**.

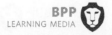

Task 6

Open the McAlistair Supplies Ltd suppliers record and set the default nominal code to 7504, Publicity Material.

Remember to **Save** this change.

5 Journals

If you are setting up a new business, the first entries you are likely to make will be done via a journal, to set up any opening balances (although see also the direct method covered earlier in this chapter for entering opening balances).

Journals are also used for non-routine transactions, such as the correction of errors and writing off irrecoverable debts. Error corrections and irrecoverable debts are covered at the end of Chapter 2.

To post a journal in Sage, choose **Nominal Codes > Journal Entry**.

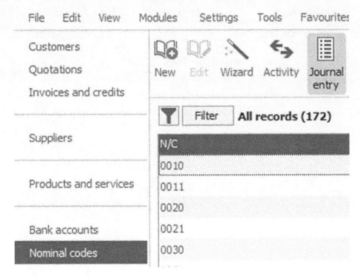

This journal entry screen looks reassuringly similar to a journal slip in a manual system, but all you need to do in a computerised system is to fill in the slip and click on **Save**.

Note. Once saved or 'posted' it is not possible to correct a journal and you will need to input another journal to correct any errors so check carefully before saving.

Let's suppose you want to post the following journal, to set up the opening cash and capital balances.

		£	£
DEBIT	Bank	2,750.00	
DEBIT	Petty Cash	250.00	
CREDIT	Capital		3,000.00

The Nominal Ledger journal input screen is shown below.

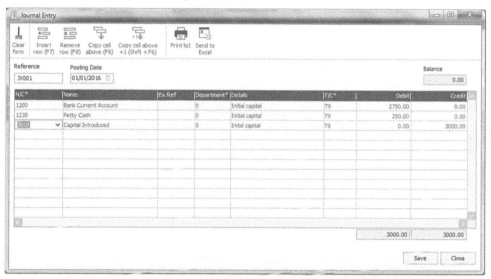

The table below explains what to do as you work through each entry field, in the order in which the Tab key will take you through them.

SCREEN ITEM	HOW IT WORKS
Reference	Type in the journal slip number you are given, if any. Journals should be numbered consecutively, so you may need to check to find out the number of the previous journal. If this is the first ever journal, choose your own coding system and make sure it has room for expansion. For example,'J001' allows for up to 999 journals in total.
Date	By default, this field (box) will show the program date, but you should change it to 01/01/16. Pressing the F4 key, or Clicking the button will make a little calendar appear.
N/C	Enter the nominal ledger code of the account affected, or press F4 or click the button to the right of this field to select from a list.

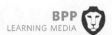

SCREEN ITEM	HOW IT WORKS
Name	This field will be filled in automatically by the program when you select the nominal code.
Ex. Ref	Leave this blank.
Dept	Leave this blank.
Details	Type in the journal narrative. In the second and subsequent lines, you can press the F6 key when you reach this field, and the entry above will be copied without you needing to retype it. This can save lots of time.
T/C	The VAT code, if applicable. For journals, this is likely to be T9 (transaction not involving VAT).
Debit/Credit	Type in the amounts in the correct columns. If it is a round sum, such as £250, there is no need to type in the decimal point and the extra zeros.

It is not possible to post a journal if it does not balance.

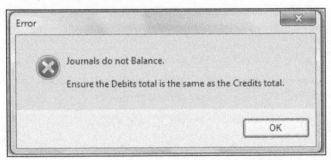

Task 7

Enter the journal shown earlier in this section (DEBIT Bank Current Account 2,750, DEBIT Petty Cash 250, CREDIT Capital Introduced 3,000). Date it 01/01/16 and give a reference of JVI and tax code (T/C) 9. Enter 'Initial capital' in the details field. **Save** then **Close** the journal window.

If you click on Nominal Codes > Balance Sheet > preview > Run

you should see that 3,000 is the total Current Assets and 3,000 is the total Capital & Reserves on the Balance Sheet.

5.1 The importance of dates

By default, Sage sets the date of transactions to the current date according to your computer, but this may not be the date you want to use, especially if you are sitting an assessment.

It is vitally important to enter the correct date when you are using a computerised system, even if you are only doing a practice exercise, because the computer uses the date you enter in a variety of ways – to generate reports such as aged debtors reports, to reconcile VAT, and so on.

If you attempt to enter a date outside the financial year, you will see a warning such as the following.

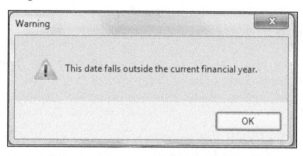

However, if you enter an incorrect date that falls within the financial year, Sage will allow you to do this.

The best way to avoid this kind of error, especially when undertaking an assessment, is to use the facility to set the program date before you enter any transactions. Select the **Settings** menu and then **Change Program Date.**

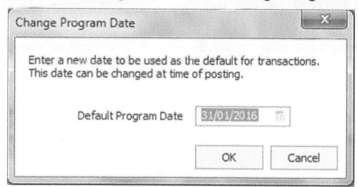

If you are doing an assessment, we recommend that you set the program date to the last day of the month for which you are supposed to be posting transactions. That way, you can never go seriously wrong.

Once you set the program date, Sage will use it as the default date until you change it again or shut down the program. This has no adverse effect on any other programs you may be using and even within Sage, the date will revert to the

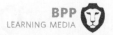

computer clock date the next time you use the program. Note that you will need to set the program date again if you shut down and then restart the program.

Furthermore, when viewing reports or lists within Sage, make sure that you have set the date range correctly otherwise they may not show all the transactions you need to see. We will look at generating reports in Chapter 2.

Task 8

Change the program date to 31 January 2016 and check that you have done so correctly by looking at the foot of the Sage screen.

Then close down the program (**File > Exit**).

---

6 Entering invoices

You may be feeling that you have been working hard but have not actually accomplished much yet! This is one of the few off-putting things about accounting software: it can take quite a while to set everything up properly before you can really get started.

If you are feeling frustrated, just remember that you only have to set all these details up once. In future, the fact that all the data is available at the touch of a button will save you a vast amount of time, so it really is worth the initial effort.

6.1 Purchase invoices using the Batch Invoice function

Purchase invoices are created by your suppliers, whereas sales invoices are documents you create yourself. That means that it is usually simpler to enter purchase invoices, so we'll deal with those first.

Having opened Sage, click on the **Suppliers** button (left of screen), select a supplier, and then click on **Batch Invoice** on the Suppliers toolbar. As always, you can use the **Tab** key to move between different parts of the screen.

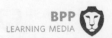

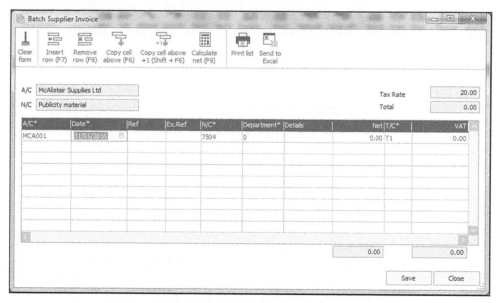

You can enter a number of different invoices from different suppliers on the same screen, and you can also enter each line of an invoice separately, if the invoice is for a variety of items that need to be coded to different nominal accounts.

To repeat the same entry in consecutive lines, just press the **F6** key on your keyboard when you reach the appropriate field.

The following table explains what to do as you tab through each entry field. Pay particular attention to the **Net**, **T/C** and **VAT** fields.

SCREEN ITEM	HOW IT WORKS
A/C column	Select the supplier account from the drop-down list (press the **F4** key to see this, or click on the ⌄ button). The A/C box at the top left of the screen will show the full name of the supplier you select, so you can check to make sure you have the right one.
Date	The program date will be entered by default, but you can change this if you wish. Click on the calendar icon next to this field or press **F4** to see an on-screen calendar.
Ref	Type in the supplier's invoice number.
Ex. Ref	Leave this blank.
N/C	This will show the default code for this supplier (the N/C box at the top left of the screen will show the name of this account). If you need to change it, press **F4** or click the ⌄ button to see a list of nominal ledger accounts.

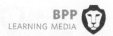

SCREEN ITEM	HOW IT WORKS
Details	Type in a brief but clear description of the item and be sure that your description will be understood by someone other than you. Usually, you will just need to copy the description on the supplier's invoice.
Net	Enter the net amount of the invoice, excluding VAT. If the invoice has several lines, you can enter each line separately but you should use the same Ref for each line.
	The ▣ button in this field will call up an on-screen calculator.
	Alternatively, type in the gross amount and press the **F9** key on your keyboard and Sage will automatically calculate the net amount. You can also calculate the net amount manually. It is equal to the GROSS AMT ÷ (1 + VAT RATE). For example, £10 gross = 10 ÷ (1.20) = £8.33 net (where the VAT rate = 20%).
T/C	The VAT code, as explained earlier. Type in or select the appropriate code for the item.
VAT	This item will be calculated automatically, depending on the tax code selected. Check that it agrees with the VAT shown on the actual invoice. You can overtype the automatic amount, if necessary.

When you have entered all the invoice details, you post them simply by clicking on **Save**. This will post **all** the required accounting entries to the ledgers.

Task 9

Post an invoice from McAlistair Supplies dated 6 January 2016 for 2,000 sheets of A4 paper (net price: £20.35) and a box of 100 blue promotional biros (gross price: £10.00). Post both items to the Publicity material ledger account. The invoice number is PG45783. **Save** and **Close**.

Write down the total amount of VAT, as calculated by the program.

£	

6.2 Nominal Activity

The first time you do this, you will probably not quite believe that double entry to all the ledgers can be so incredibly easy. To check that a purchase invoice has been posted to the individual accounts, click on **Nominal Codes** and select the appropriate accounts.

Depending on which type of transaction you posted, you should then select either the Debtors Ledger Control Account or the Creditors Ledger Control Account by expanding Total Current Assets or Total Current Liabilities using the '+' signs. Having selected the account you want, you should then double click on it. Remember it may be easier to find the accounts by viewing them as a list by selecting the **List** option.

The screenshot below shows the **Nominal Record** for the Trade Creditors Control account.

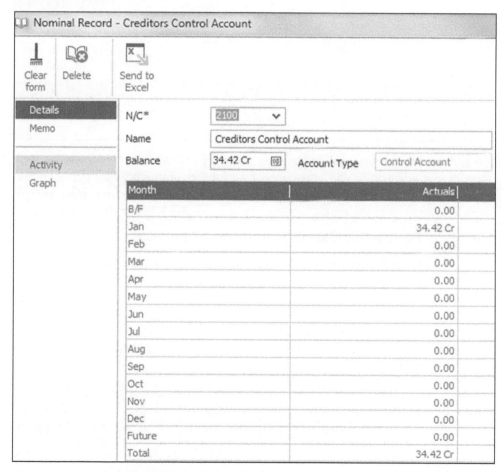

Clicking on **Activity** will show the individual transactions posted to this account, as shown in the screen below.

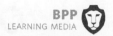

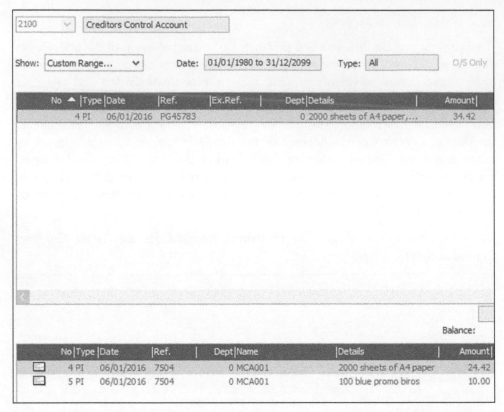

You will see that the transaction has been correctly posted to the Creditors Control Account. But what about the other accounts of the double entry that make up the full transaction? For the invoice from McAlistair Supplies, the double entry should be as follows:

DEBIT   Purchase Tax Control Account (debit VAT amount)

DEBIT   Expenditure account – Publicity Material (debit net amount)

CREDIT   Creditors Control Account (credit gross amount)

You can also check that the transaction has been correctly posted to the Publicity Material account (A/C 7504) and the Purchase Tax Control Account (A/C code 2201) by using the same method as above, ie, checking the **Nominal Record** for these accounts.

Furthermore, to check that the correct amounts have also been posted to the individual supplier account (ie, subsidiary ledger) within the overall Creditors Control Account, select **Suppliers**, then open the record for the relevant supplier and choose the **Activity** section.

BPP
LEARNING MEDIA

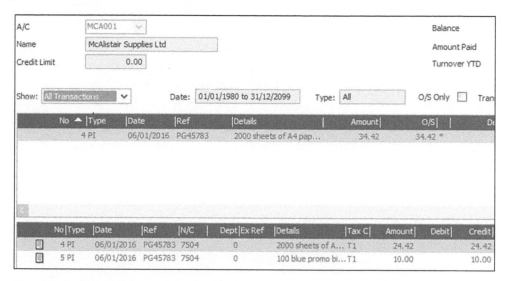

The process for checking individual customer accounts works in the same way.

Finally, if you just want a quick look at the transactions you've posted, click on the **Transactions** from the left side of the screen. This will result in you being shown a list of transactions, numbered in the order in which you posted them. This can be very useful on certain occasions; for instance, if you can't remember the reference number of the last journal you posted, you can quickly check using this screen.

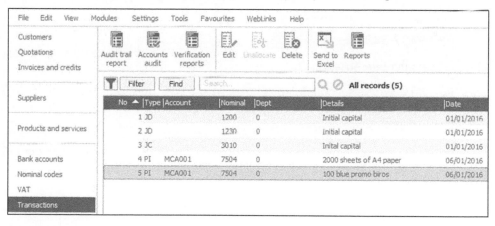

6.3 Sales invoices if no invoice is produced

Some businesses create sales invoices using a different system from their accounts package – for example, using word processing software such as Word. The invoices are then entered into the computerised accounting package.

If that is the case, then sales invoices are entered in exactly the same way as purchase invoices. To do this, click on **Customers** then **Batch Invoice** and enter the invoices in a batch. The batch invoice process works in the same way as for Suppliers described earlier.

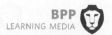

6.4 Sales invoices – if the system creates the invoice

In Sage, you can produce printable invoices that are automatically posted by Sage. If you wanted to do this, you could do so by clicking on **Customers** and then the **New** button. The invoice details can then be entered, saved and an invoice printed.

However, in the assessment you will be given a list of invoices or sample invoices to enter. Therefore, you should only enter invoices using the Batch Invoice method described earlier, rather than creating an invoice.

Task 10

(1) Set up two more **suppliers** with the following details (using the new supplier wizard if you wish).

Widgets Unlimited Ltd
123 High Road
London
W23 2RG
020 8234 2345

Office Products Ltd
321 Low Road
London
E32 2GR
020 8432 5432

(2) Process the purchase of:

(a) 10 widgets (material purchased) from Widgets Unlimited Ltd for a total net cost of £80. Invoice number WU4474, dated 8 January 2016.

(b) A computer (office equipment) from Office Products Ltd for a net cost of £800. Invoice OP1231, dated 10 January 2016.

Both purchases attract VAT at the standard rate.

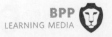

Task 11

(1)   Set up a new **customer** with the following details (using the new customer wizard if you wish).

Alexander Ltd
501 Dart Road
Leeds
LS12 6TC
0113 2454 3241
info@alexander.co.uk

30 days' credit (payment due days)
All other fields can be left blank but tick the terms agreed option.

(2)   Post the following two invoices (remember, you have to use **Save** to post them) to this customer:

(a)   Invoice 001: Product Sale: 10 widgets at a selling price (net) of £20 each. VAT to be charged at standard rate. Date: 15 January 2016.

(b)   Invoice 002: Service Sale: Advice on widgets, at a fee of £50 (net). VAT to be charged at standard rate. Date: 25 January 2016.

(3)   If you have not already done so, change the names of the nominal ledger accounts as necessary to accommodate the different sales types in (2).

Task 12

As you should know from previous studies, a trial balance is a list of balances of all the ledger accounts. Preview a trial balance at this stage. Select **Nominal Codes > Trial Balance > Preview > Run**, and set month period to '1: January 2016'.

Date: 29/02/2016	**SFE Merchandising**		**Page:** 1
Time: 13:04:10	**Period Trial Balance**		

To Period: Month 1, January 2016

N/C	Name	Debit	Credit
0030	Office Equipment	800.00	
1100	Debtors Control Account	300.00	
1200	Bank Current Account	2,750.00	
1230	Petty Cash	250.00	
2100	Creditors Control Account		1,090.42
2200	Sales Tax Control Account		50.00
2201	Purchase Tax Control Account	181.74	
3010	Capital Introduced		3,000.00
4000	Sales - products		200.00
4001	Sales - services		50.00
5000	Materials Purchased	80.00	
7504	Publicity material	28.68	
	Totals:	4,390.42	4,390.42

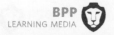

6.5 Credit notes

Supplier credit notes are posted in exactly the same way as supplier invoices, except that you begin by clicking on **Supplier** and then the **Batch Credit** button, instead of the Batch Invoice button. The entries you make will appear in red, as a visual reminder that you are creating a credit note.

Customer credit notes can be posted in this way too.

7 Help!

7.1 Help in Sage

If ever you are unsure about how to perform a task in Sage, take a look through the built-in Help feature. Help is accessed by selecting **Help > F1- In Product Help** or just pressing the **F1** key. Then click on **Search** and type in a word or a phrase on the topic you need help with (eg 'Opening balances') and hit the Enter key. This brings up a number of results of help topics containing the phrase 'Opening balances'. The first result should be the most relevant. There is also an **Ask Sage** option in the Help menu. Selecting this takes you to an online version of Sage help if you are connected to internet.

7.2 Help from your manager and others

Whenever you are unsure about what to do, or are faced with an error message you are unsure about, the golden rule is to **ask for help or advice**.

Don't ignore error messages. If possible, have your manager or someone more senior look at the message immediately and advise you on what action to take. If you need to provide details for someone if they can't get to your screen to view it, take a screenshot for them.

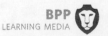

Chapter overview

- Accounting software ranges from simple bookkeeping tools to more complex packages. Sage's products are among the most popular packages in the UK.

- Assessments may involve setting up new customer and supplier accounts, posting journals, invoices, payments and receipts, and generating reports or other types of output.

- It is essential to make sure that you are posting transactions to the correct financial year.

- New nominal ledger accounts can be set up using the accounting package's 'wizard'.

- VAT is dealt with by assigning the correct tax code to a transaction.

- New customer and supplier accounts should be given consistent and meaningful codes.

- Using the keyboard shortcuts may help you when you are entering data into Sage. The Tab key, the Esc key and the function keys (eg F4 and F6) can often speed up your work.

- Familiarise yourself with the Help feature; it could come in handy both in your work and in your assessment.

- Never ignore error messages, ask for help or advice from your manager.

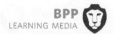

Keywords

- **Activity:** the transactions that have occurred on an account

- **Chart of accounts:** a template that sets out the nominal ledger accounts and how they are organised into different categories

- **Customer:** a person or organisation that buys products or services from your organisation

- **Customer record:** the details relating to the customer account, for example name and address, contact details and credit terms

- **Defaults:** the entries that the accounting package expects to normally be made in a particular field

- **Field:** a box on screen in which you enter data or select from a list (similar to a spreadsheet cell)

- **General ledger:** the ledger containing the statement of profit or loss (income statement) and statement of financial position (balance sheet) accounts

- **Ledger accounts:** accounts in which each transaction is recorded

- **Nominal ledger:** the term Sage uses for the ledger containing the income statement (profit and loss) and statement of financial position (balance sheet) accounts

- **Program date:** the date Sage uses as the default for any transactions that are posted (the default may be overwritten)

- **Supplier:** a person or organisation that your organisation buys products or services from

- **Supplier record:** the details relating to the supplier account, for example name and address, contact details and credit terms

- **Trade creditors ledger:** the collection of supplier accounts, also known as the purchase ledger

- **Trade debtors ledger:** the collection of customer accounts, also known as the sales ledger

- **Tax code:** Sage's term for the code to be used to calculate VAT

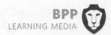

Test your learning

1   What is a 'field' in an accounting package?

2   What do you understand by the term 'default'?

3   What is a chart of accounts?

4   What must be set up before a supplier credit invoice can be posted?

5   How would a supplier invoice be assigned to the correct nominal ledger expenditure account?

6   If you attempt to post a journal that does not balance, the difference will be posted to the suspense account. True or false? Explain your answer.

7   If a purchase invoice has five separate lines, should these be posted individually or is it sufficient just to post the invoice totals?

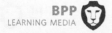

Sage 50 – Part 2

2

Chapter coverage

The topics covered in this chapter follow on from where you should have reached in Chapter 1.

The subjects covered in this chapter are:

- Payments and receipts
- Bank reconciliations
- Reports and other types of output
- Error correction
- Irrecoverable debts
- Month-end procedures

1 Payments and receipts

Your assessment may include details of payments and receipts to enter into the accounts. These could comprise cash, cheques and payments made or received directly from/to the bank account (eg payments made or received by 'BACS' or 'Faster Payments' services).

You need to be able to distinguish between cheques that you have sent to **SUPPLIERS** and cheques received from **customers**. If it is a cheque that you have paid out to a supplier, you may only be shown the cheque stub (that's all you would have in practice, after all), such as illustrated below.

```
Date      ...............................
Payee     ...............................
          ...............................
          ...............................
          ...............................
£         ...............................
          000001
```

If it is a cheque that you have received from a customer, you may be shown the cheque itself.

Lloyds TSB   30-92-10

Benham Branch   Date _____

Pay _____

_____   [   ]

_____

                                    FOR WHITEHILL SUPERSTORES

You can tell that this is a receipt because the name below the signature (here, Whitehill Superstores) will be the name of one of your customers.

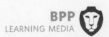

In the assessment, you could also be given details of an electronic payment or receipt, for example, a BACS remittance advice detailing a receipt from a customer.

Alternatively, you may be shown a paying-in slip that may include receipts from several different customers.

Cheques etc.			Brought forward £				£50		
							£20		
							£10		
							£5		
							£2		
							£1		
							50p		
							20p		
							Silver		
			Whitehill	1468	75		Bronze		
			Superstores				Total Cash		
							Cardnet	3818	75
			G T				Cheques		
			Summerfield	2350	00		etc.		
Carried forward £			Carried forward £	3818	75	Total £	3818	75	

Date	23/01/2016	500001	FOR SFE MERCHANDISING	06325143

1.1 Supplier payments

When you pay a supplier, it is important to allocate your payment to invoices shown as outstanding in the purchase ledger. Sage makes this very easy.

There are a number of different payment allocations that can occur in both the sales and purchase ledger. Usually, you will pay most invoices in full or take a credit note in full; however, there may be reasons why an invoice may only be partially paid, due to disputes or cash flow problems. These are unsurprisingly known as 'part payments'. Occasionally, you may not be able to allocate a payment or receipt because it is for an invoice not on the system or the amount does not match with your ledger. In these cases, the payment is recorded against the correct account but not to any particular invoice or credit note and these are known as 'payments on account'.

Discounts can be allowed on payments received from customers (or received on payments made to suppliers), and a discount field is available to make a note of these amounts.

Payments allocated to invoices

To post a payment to a supplier, click on **Bank Accounts** on the left side of the screen and then on the **Supplier Payment** button towards the top of the screen (**not** the **Bank Payments** button, which relates to payments not involving suppliers' accounts).

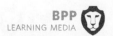

You are presented with a screen that looks a little like a blank cheque with drop-down options which allow you to choose the bank account used for the payment and the supplier who is being paid.

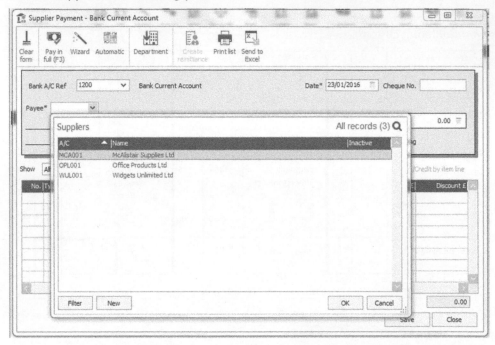

If you choose McAlistair Suppliers Ltd from the drop-down list in the **Payee** field, the next screen completes some of the fields, and the bottom half of the screen shows details of outstanding invoices.

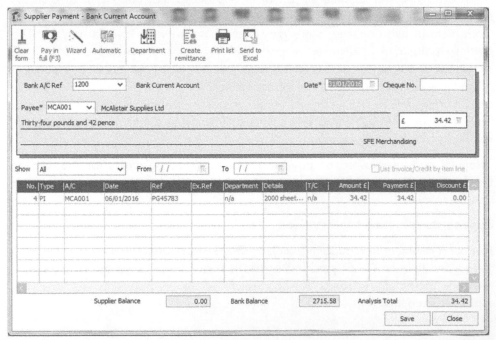

The following table explains the quickest way to post a payment to a supplier. Press **Tab** to move from one field to the next.

SCREEN ITEM	HOW IT WORKS
Payee	Select the code for the supplier you want to pay.
Date	The program date will be entered by default, but you can change this if you wish. Press **F4** to see an on-screen calendar.
Cheque No.	Enter this carefully, as it will help with bank reconciliations. If you are making a payment directly from the bank account such as a BACS payment, you can put the BACS reference in this field.
£ box	Though it might seem odd, leave this at 0.00 when paying an invoice in full, as it will automatically be filled in when we update the Payment £ boxes for the required outstanding invoices to pay.
Payment £	Do not type anything here. Just click on the **Pay in Full** button at the top of the screen. If there are several invoices to pay, ensure you click into the payment field of the required invoice, and click on **Pay in Full**. Using this method, the amount of the payment, shown in the £ box in the top half of the screen, updates each time you click on Pay in Full. The program also writes the amount in words.
Discount	Tab past this if there is no discount. However, if you do need to process a discount, enter the discount amount in the discount field **first,** and Sage will calculate the balance to be paid and enter it automatically into the payment field.
Save	This saves to **all** the ledgers.

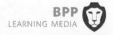

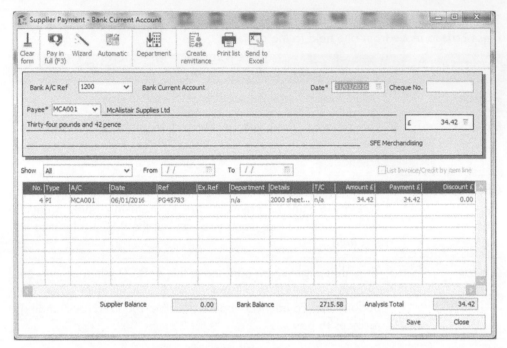

You don't need to pay all the outstanding invoices if you don't want to. You can just click on **Save** when you've paid the ones you want.

This is the quickest way of posting a payment in ordinary circumstances.

Part payments

There may be times when you don't want to pay invoices in full. For instance, you may decide to pay the supplier in the illustration above only £20.00, perhaps because of some problem with the items supplied. In that case, proceed as follows.

SCREEN ITEM	HOW IT WORKS
Payee	As before
Date	As before
Cheque number	As before
£ box	Though it might seem odd, leave this at 0.00
Payment £	Type the amount you want to pay
Discount	Tab past this
Save	This saves to **all** the ledgers

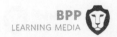

Unallocated payments (payment on account)

There may be times when you need to record a supplier payment but are unable to allocate it to an invoice, either partially or wholly.

For instance, you may decide to pay the supplier in the illustration above only £10.00 but not apply this yet to an invoice(s). In that case, proceed as follows.

SCREEN ITEM	HOW IT WORKS
Payee	As before
Date	As before
Cheque number	As before
£ box	Type the amount you want to pay
Payment £	Leave this at 0.00
Discount	Tab past this
Save	This saves to **all** the ledgers

Click on **Save** and a warning screen comes up asking you to confirm that you want to save the unallocated payment on account. Click **Yes**.

Such payments should be allocated as soon as the relevant information or invoice is available.

Note that VAT is not accounted for on supplier payments. VAT will have already been accounted for when the supplier invoice was posted. Other payments may require VAT to be accounted for when the payment entry is made (see the 'Other payments and receipts' section below).

Applying a credit note to a payment

A further possibility is that there will be a credit note on the account as well as invoices. **Pay in Full** is the answer to this, too. When you reach the credit note line, click on **Pay in Full** and the amount of the cheque will be reduced by the credit amount.

Task 1

Post a payment on 31/01/16 made with cheque 158002 to McAlistair Supplies Ltd for the total of invoice PG45783. Remember to click **'Save'** to effect the posting.

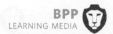

When you make a supplier payment, you also have the option of generating a remittance advice to be sent to the supplier to inform them of the invoices your company is paying. To do this, you use the **Create Remittance** button at the top of the screen, just before you save the payment. You may be asked to generate a remittance during your assessment.

Note. In Sage 50 Accounts Essentials you cannot generate a remittance once you have saved the payment so it must be done just before you click on **Save**. Higher versions of Sage and other programs may allow you to generate remittances retrospectively.

An example is given in the screenshot that follows, where a payment is allocated against an Office Products invoice we created in an earlier task. You can try this for yourself, generating a remittance, but for the purposes of progressing through this Text, you should **not** save the payment.

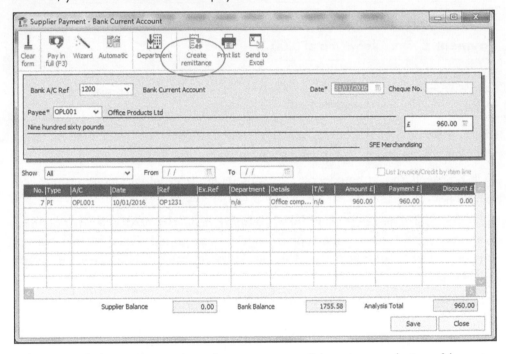

When you click on **Create Remittance,** you will be given a choice of layouts. Selecting the default layout and pressing **Run** should result in a remittance similar to the one shown below.

BPP
LEARNING MEDIA

SFE Merchandising
14a Hapgood House
Dagenham Avenue
Benham
DR6 8LV

Tel :

VAT Reg No. 524376451

Office Products Ltd 321 Low Road London E32 2GR		**REMITTANCE ADVICE**	
		Date	31/01/2016
		Account Ref	OPL001
		Cheque No	

NOTE: All values are shown in Pound Sterling

Date	Ref	Details	Debit	Credit
10/01/2016	OP1231	Office computer		960.00

This can then be exported to a PDF file and saved to your computer by clicking on the **Export** button at the top of the window in which the report is contained. Please refer to the 'Exporting to PDF file' section in Chapter 1 for details of how to do this.

1.2 Customer receipts

When you receive money from your customers, it is important to allocate the payment to sales invoices shown as outstanding in the subsidiary ledger.

To record a receipt from an account customer, click on **Bank Accounts** and then the **Customer Receipt** button towards the top of the screen (**not** the **Bank Receipts** button). Following that, select the customer you have received money from in the **Account** field.

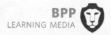

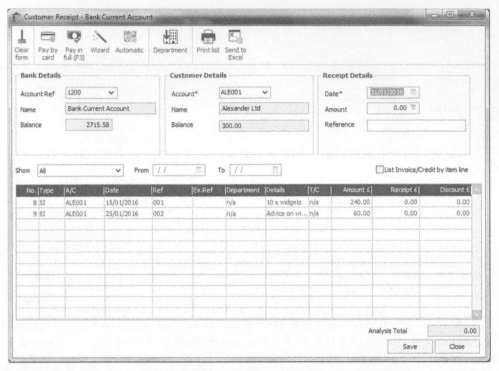

Although this screen looks slightly different from the payment one, it works in exactly the same way, and we recommend that you use it in exactly the same way – in other words, select the **Receipt £** field and click on the **Pay in Full** button, for each invoice you have received payment for. Part payments and unallocated payments (payments on account) are also dealt with in the same way as for suppliers.

One important point to remember when posting receipts is that you should use the paying-in slip number (if you have it) for the **Reference** field. This makes it much easier to complete bank reconciliations, because typically, several cheques will be paid in on a single paying-in slip and the bank statement will only show the total, not the individual amounts.

To recall the details of a payment or receipt that you have already entered, choose **Bank Accounts >** Select the relevant bank account **> Activity**.

Task 2

Post a receipt from Alexander Ltd for £240. This was paid in using paying-in slip 500001 dated 31 January 2016. You should allocate this against Invoice 001.

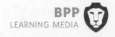

1.3 Other payments and receipts (non-credit transactions)

Some payments and receipts do not need to be allocated to suppliers or customers. Examples include payments like wages and receipts such as cash sales.

If your assessment includes transactions like this, you should post them by clicking on **Bank Accounts and then Bank Receipts** (for receipts), or **Bank Payments** (for payments).

If you click on **Bank receipts**, you are presented with a screen similar to that shown below.

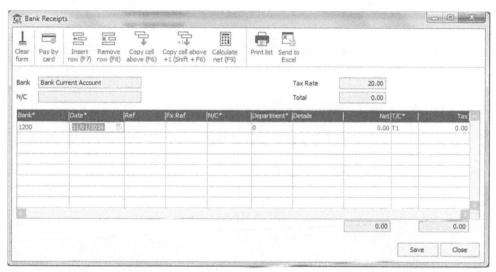

The main differences here to the Customer Receipt screen earlier are that you enter the amount of the receipt directly in the **Net** field; and in the **N/C** field, you select the account where the other side of the double entry for transaction will be posted to. Note that you can split the receipt into different transactions by entering the details in a new line.

VAT on other payments and receipts

Another difference to the customer receipt screen is that you have to specify the VAT treatment of the transaction. VAT is not accounted for on the payment of a sales invoice from a credit customer (a customer receipt) because VAT will already have been accounted for when the sales invoice was posted.

However, for most 'other receipts,' including cash sales[1], the receipt and related transaction are recorded in this one entry. Therefore you must account for any VAT applicable at this point. Refer to the Tax Codes and VAT rates section in Chapter 1 for the **Tax Code** to use.

In this particular program, if the receipt or payment includes VAT, it is the net amount that should appear in the **Net** field. If you are only given the gross amount

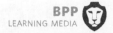

in the Assessment, enter the gross amount in the **Net** field, but press the **F9** Key for the program to calculate the net amount. Alternatively you can calculate the net amount manually by using the formula GROSS AMT /(1+VAT) as covered in Chapter 1.

(1) The term 'cash sale' actually refers to a sale where the sale and receipt of payment occur at the same time. For example, a supermarket sells goods to customers who pay for them immediately – these are cash sales. The payment does not necessarily have to be in cash. Payment can also be by cheque, credit or debit card. Cash sales differ to 'credit sales' in that credit sales allow the customer to pay for the goods or services at a later date (typically 30 days later). Another example of cash sales is sales made online over the internet.

'Other payments' and 'other receipts' that don't involve sales or purchases (eg, wages, loans etc) do not attract VAT, and the **T/C** code to use in these cases is T9.

Example of a non-credit transaction

Here's an example of how online cash sales might be posted to the accounts using the method described above (don't carry out the transaction). Use the **N/C** drop-down to find which nominal code to use.

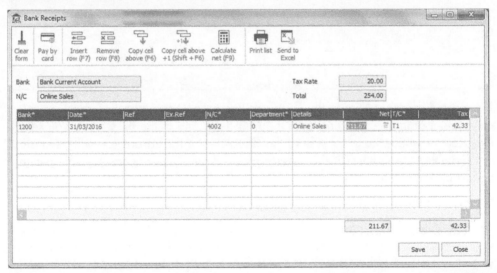

The screen for posting payments such as wages is exactly the same but instead of using the Bank Receipts screen, you access the payments screen through **Bank Payments**.

1.4 Direct debits and standing orders (recurring payments)

Many businesses have regular recurring payments, such as rent and rates, set up by standing order or direct debit. It can be easy to forget to post these – especially as some may be monthly, some quarterly and so on. Sage makes it easy to automate this process. Choosing **Bank accounts > Recurring Items > Add** will produce a screen like the one that follows. It allows you to specify:

- The type of transaction
- Where the debit is to be posted
- Start date
- Frequency
- End date
- Amounts (gross/net/VAT)

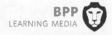

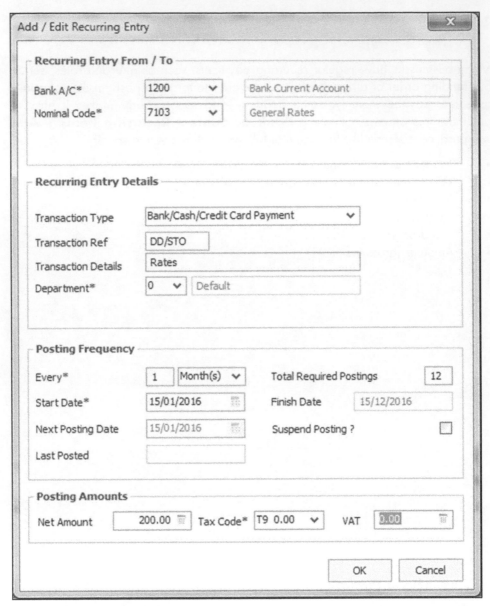

The screen above shows how the details of a regular monthly payment for rates could be entered. Changing the reference can indicate whether it is a standing order or a direct debit. Note that you may be asked to take a screenshot of the screen above during the assessment as evidence of you setting up a recurring entry.

Task 3

Enter and save the recurring rates payment details shown above.

Although the details for recurring payments are now saved, no transactions have been posted. To make the entries, you have to now choose **Bank Accounts > Recurring Items** to bring up the following screen.

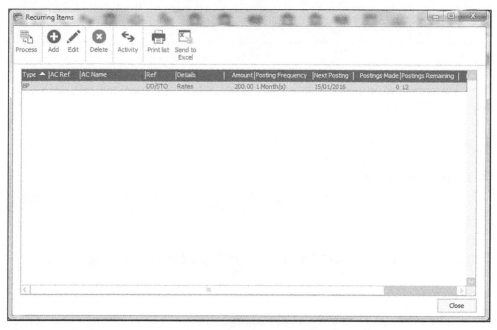

Then you select the relevant series of payments and click on the **Process** button to bring up any recurring payments up to the program date (which was set as 31 January 2016 earlier).

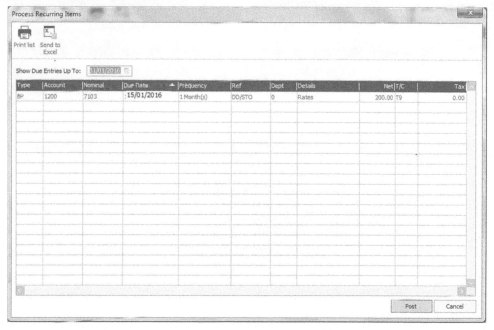

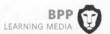

Don't do it now (wait for the next task!), but you can post the payment(s) shown by pressing the **Post** button. You can show all payments due up to a certain date by changing the 'Show Due Entries Up To' date at the top. However, you will only want to post those payments that you expect to go through the bank in the month you are accounting for.

Task 4

Use the recurring payments option to post the rates payment of £200 for **January 2016 only**.

Once you have posted a payment or payments, you should notice that the Recurring Items screen shows a payment or payments have been posted in the 'Postings Made' column.

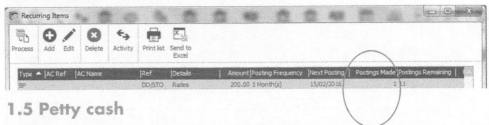

1.5 Petty cash

Petty cash transactions are posted in exactly the same way as non-credit bank payments and receipts (you should refer to the 'Other payments and receipts' section earlier), except that you use the petty cash bank account rather than the bank current account. As with non-credit payments and receipts, VAT is accounted for when entering the transaction for payment or receipt. Therefore take care to use the correct tax code.

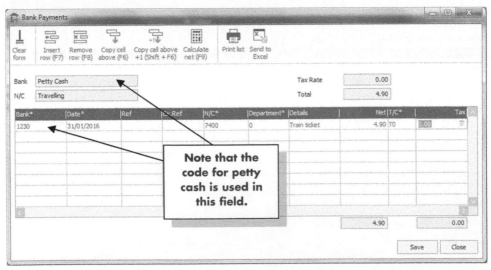

BPP
LEARNING MEDIA

2 Bank reconciliations

As you should know from previous studies a bank reconciliation is a comparison between the bank balance recorded in the accounts and the balance on the bank statement. The differences are called reconciling items and are usually payments and receipts that have not yet cleared the bank account.

To access the bank reconciliation screens, you need to click on **Bank accounts** and then select the account you want to reconcile. In Sage, the default bank current account is account 1200, so you can select this and then click on **Reconcile**. This brings up a statement summary screen.

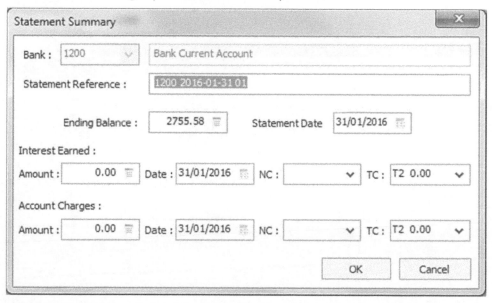

This screen gives you a first opportunity to enter the statement reference, balance and date and to enter any interest or charges appearing on the statement not yet entered in the records. The ending balance that automatically comes up is the balance on the nominal account, so should be updated to the balance shown on the statement.

Say that the closing bank statement balance is £2,790.00. That information would be entered in the **Ending Balance** box of the Statement Summary screen. If the statement is dated 31/01/2016, that can be entered in the **Statement Date** box.

If you forget to update the statement balance or any other details, you can also update them in the next screen (the Bank Reconciliation screen). Adjustments for interest can also be made there.

When you click **OK**, you are taken to the **Bank Reconciliation** screen that follows.

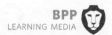

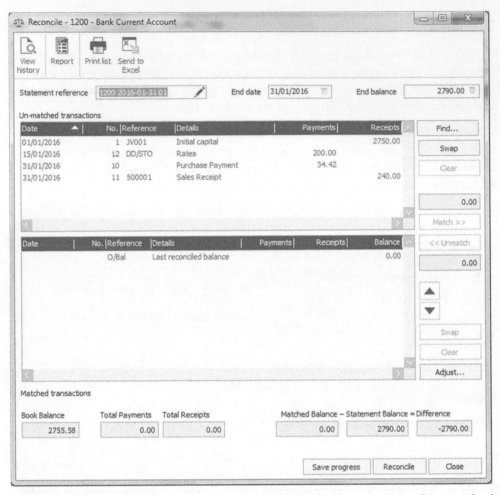

Initially, all cash account amounts are unmatched (you can see the matched balance box at the bottom shows zero) but, by looking at the statement, some will be found to appear there as well. We can match these items. Say that the initial journal of £2,750 into the bank account, the rates payment of £200 and the receipt of £240 from Alexander Ltd are also on the bank statement.

These can be selected and matched by clicking on the transaction and then on **Match >>** (note if you accidentally match the wrong entry, then you can use **<< Unmatch** to go back a step). You can select more than one transaction at a time by holding down the **CTRL** key. The statement screen will then look as follows:

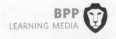

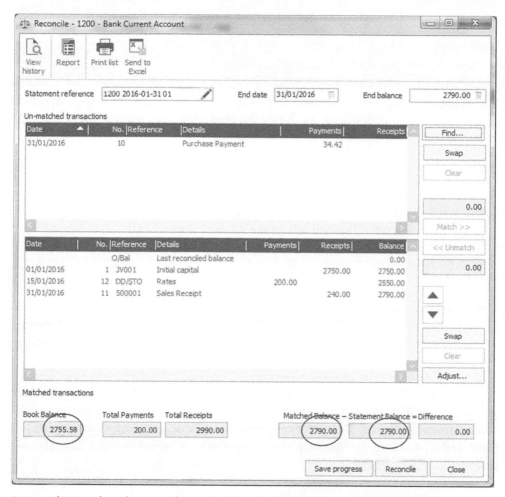

Reconciliation has been achieved! (Matched Balance = Statement Balance) and the unmatched item of £34.42 explains the difference between the statement balance of £2,790.00 and the Sage bank current account balance (Book Balance) of £2,755.58.

(If the book balance does not equal £2,755.58, this might mean that your program date is not set to 31 January 2016. You can check this by selecting **Settings > Change Program Date**)

In order to complete the reconciliation, you must click on the **Reconcile** button; otherwise the reconciliation will not process completely.

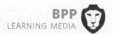

The fields you enter in the Bank Reconciliation screen are as follows:

SCREEN ITEM	HOW IT WORKS
End date	Set this to the same date as the date of the statement received from the bank (probably the date of the last transaction shown on the statement).
End balance	Type in the closing balance on the bank statement, using a minus sign if the account is overdrawn.
Difference	This field is updated by the program as you select transactions on screen. The aim is to make this box show 0.00.

Task 5

Carry out the bank reconciliation explained in this section, assuming that the closing bank statement balance is £2,790. Don't forget to click on **Reconcile** when you have reconciled; otherwise the reconciliation will not process completely.

Although we look at reports in detail later in the chapter, at this stage it is worth pointing out that you can generate a bank reconciliation report (a bank reconciliation statement) from the Bank Reconciliation screen (**Bank accounts > Reconcile**). Clicking on **Report** should generate a report like the one shown below.

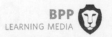

Date: 29/02/2016		SFE Merchandising		Page: 1
Time: 16:28:15		**Bank Reconciliation**		

Bank Ref:	1200		Date To:	31/01/2016
Bank Name:	Bank Current Account		Statement Ref:	1200 2016-01-31 02
Currency:	Pound Sterling			

Balance as per cash book at 31/01/2016:   2,755.58

Add: Unpresented Payments

Tran No	Date	Ref	Details	£
10	31/01/2016		Purchase Payment	34.42

    34.42

Less: Outstanding Receipts

Tran No	Date	Ref	Details	£

    0.00

Reconciled balance :	2,790.00
Balance as per statement :	2,790.00
Difference :	0.00

This can then be exported to a PDF file and saved to your computer by clicking on the **Export** button at the top of the window within which the reconciliation statement is shown. Please refer to the Exporting to PDF file section in Chapter 1 for details of how to do this.

2.1 Adjustments for additional items on bank statement

Even if you have posted all your transactions correctly, there is a good chance that there will be items on the bank statement that you have not included in the accounts. Bank charges and interest are common examples.

For such items, click on the **Adjust** button on the Bank Reconciliation screen, select the type of adjustment to bring up the related adjustment screen (for earlier versions of Sage, you may be taken straight to a general adjustments screen and will not have the option of also posting supplier and customer payments at this stage).

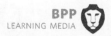

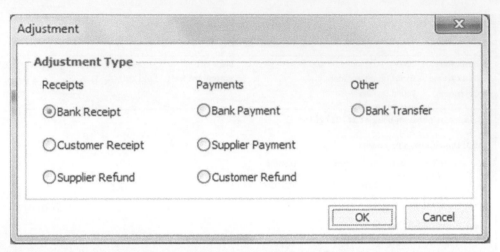

The adjustment screen allows you to enter the amounts and details before saving.

Note. For our purposes, **do not** carry out the following adjustment.

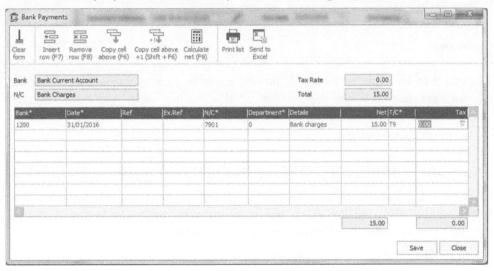

Make sure you use the correct tax code when making adjustments.

Note. On earlier versions of Sage, where you are taken straight to an adjustment screen, you may not be able to use this method to post payments to, or receipts from, credit suppliers or customers because the subsidiary ledgers will not be updated.

2.2 Grouped receipts

As we mentioned earlier, businesses often pay several cheques into the bank on the same paying-in slip and bank statements only show the total of the paying-in slip, not the individual items.

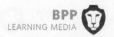

If you use the paying-in slip number as the **Reference** when posting receipts, Sage will allow you to group similar items together when doing a bank reconciliation. This may make it easier to agree them to the bank statement entries.

Within **Bank Defaults** in the **Settings** menu is a tick box called **Group items in Bank Rec**. When this is ticked, consecutive transactions of the same type are combined as one item for display in the Bank Reconciliation screen, if the reference and the date are the same.

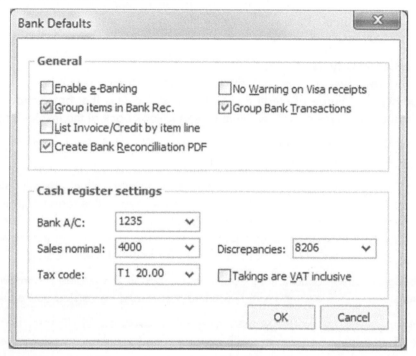

Some versions of Sage have an additional tick box called **Group Bank Transactions**.

If this check box within Bank Defaults is selected, bank transactions (bank payments and bank receipts) with the same reference and transaction date are grouped together within the Bank Activity screen.

To see the individual transactions that make up the grouped transactions, you must use the drill-down facility by clicking on the grouped item.

If you do not want your bank transactions to be grouped together, clear the check boxes related to grouping items. When you clear the check boxes, each bank transaction appears on a separate line of the Bank Activity.

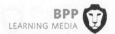

3 Reports and other types of output

3.1 The importance of reports generated by the accounting systems

One of the most important features of an accounting system such as Sage is its ability to provide a range of useful accounting information very quickly. If transactions are entered correctly in the first instance, then accurate summaries or detailed analysis should be available at the click of a button.

To give a simple example of the use of a report by finance staff, the **aged receivables analysis** (or aged debtors analysis) can be generated from Sage (as we will see later) and this will show how old each customer balance is. This will alert staff in charge of credit control to those accounts that are overdue and need chasing for payment, without them having to look back at the invoice dates.

The majority of the reports we will look at are usually produced periodically and used to check on the accuracy of the records.

We look at generating a nominal activity report later, which details all the transactions in a period in each account. A quick review of this report can help to identify errors, for example, transactions posted to the wrong account. The trial balance generated by the accounting system may also highlight errors, for example, if a suspense account has been set up and not yet been cleared.

We looked at bank reconciliations earlier and checking the related report against the bank statements is an important procedure that should be carried out regularly.

The various reports can also be used to gain an overview of different financial areas and as a tool when dealing with customers and suppliers. Areas focused on might include identifying and dealing with overdue customer invoices (aged receivables analysis), seeing which suppliers are due for payment (payables listings) and establishing the cash available to the business to meet its commitments (bank related reports).

3.2 Generating reports

When you have finished entering transactions, the final task in your assessment will be to generate some reports.

Sage offers you a large number of different standard reports. You can also create others of your own if you wish, containing the information you choose. Although the pre-prepared reports that are available in Sage don't all have names that you will immediately recognise from your knowledge of manual accounting systems, rest assured that everything you are likely to be asked to produce in an assessment can easily be found.

One or two reports, such as customer statements, have their own buttons but, in general, to generate a report, you open the part of the program you want a report on and choose the **Reports** button which usually appears on the far right hand side of the menu at the top of the screen:

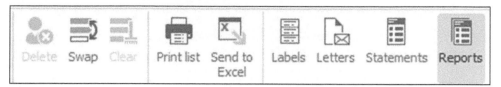

Here's an example of the range of customer reports that you could generate. To get to this screen, click on **Customers,** then **Reports**. By clicking on each folder, you can see the reports available for each category.

Remember Sage uses old UK GAAP terminology.

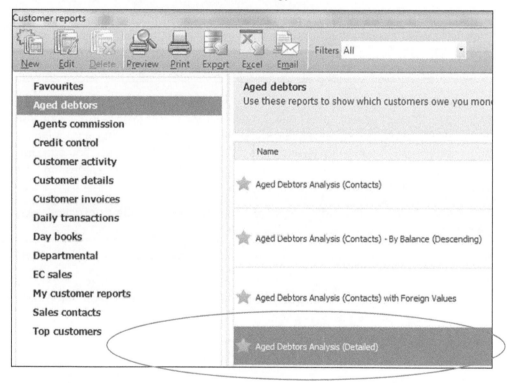

In recent versions of Sage, reports are organised into separate sections by subject, as shown in the illustration. In older versions, this screen is laid out slightly differently, listing reports in folders or individually in alphabetical order. When you have found your report, double click on it or press the **Preview** button.

A screen will appear prompting you to enter the criteria for the report. The screenshot below shows the criteria specification screen that would be displayed if you were producing a supplier activity report (accessed within supplier reports: **Suppliers > Reports > Supplier Activity > Supplier Activity (Detailed)**.

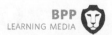
BPP
LEARNING MEDIA

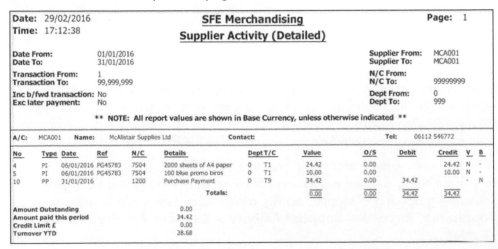

The default settings will produce a report on **all** supplier accounts up until the date specified, unless you have selected a supplier. If you wish, you can specify that you only want a report on a specific account (as in the preceding example), or range of accounts, by making selections in the **Supplier Ref** boxes. You can also restrict your report to cover a specific period by making entries in the **Transaction Date** boxes.

Ensure that the transaction date range you specify covers all the transactions you need to see.

After clicking OK, assuming you selected the **Preview** option, the preview will appear on screen.

Here is the report generated for **supplier** activity based on the information from the screen shown on the previous page.

Date:	29/02/2016			SFE Merchandising					Page:	1	
Time:	17:12:38			**Supplier Activity (Detailed)**							

Date From:	01/01/2016							Supplier From:	MCA001	
Date To:	31/01/2016							Supplier To:	MCA001	
Transaction From:	1							N/C From:		
Transaction To:	99,999,999							N/C To:	99999999	
Inc b/fwd transaction:	No							Dept From:	0	
Exc later payment:	No							Dept To:	999	

** NOTE: All report values are shown in Base Currency, unless otherwise indicated **

| A/C: | MCA001 | **Name:** | McAlistair Supplies Ltd | | | **Contact:** | | | **Tel:** | 06112 546772 | |

No	Type	Date	Ref	N/C	Details	Dept	T/C	Value	O/S	Debit	Credit	V	B
4	PI	06/01/2016	PG45783	7504	2000 sheets of A4 paper	0	T1	24.42	0.00		24.42	N	-
5	PI	06/01/2016	PG45783	7504	100 blue promo biros	0	T1	10.00	0.00		10.00	N	-
10	PP	31/01/2016		1200	Purchase Payment	0	T9	34.42	0.00	34.42		-	N
					Totals:			0.00	0.00	34.42	34.42		

Amount Outstanding	0.00	
Amount paid this period	34.42	
Credit Limit £	0.00	
Turnover YTD	28.68	

Here is an example of a **customer** activity report:

Date: 29/02/201						SFE Merchandising					Page: 1	

Content of the report box:

Date: 29/02/201
Time: 17:14:29

SFE Merchandising
Customer Activity (Detailed)

Page: 1

Date From:	01/01/2016			Customer From:	ALE001	
Date To:	31/01/2016			Customer To:	ALE001	
Transaction From:	1			N/C From:		
Transaction To:	99,999,999			N/C To:	99999999	
Inc b/fwd transaction:	No			Dept From:	0	
Exc later payment:	No			Dept To:	999	

** NOTE: All report values are shown in Base Currency, unless otherwise indicated **

A/C:	ALE001	Name:	Alexander Ltd		Contact:			Tel:	0113 2354 3241

No	Type	Date	Ref	N/C	Details	Dept	T/C	Value	O/S	Debit	Credit	V	B
8	SI	15/01/2016	001	4000	10 x widgets	0	T1	240.00		240.00		N	-
9	SI	25/01/2016	002	4001	Advice on widgets	0	T1	60.00 *	60.00	60.00		N	-
11	SR	31/01/2016	500001	1200	Sales Receipt	0	T9	240.00			240.00	-	R
					Totals:			60.00	60.00	300.00	240.00		

Amount Outstanding	60.00
Amount Paid this period	240.00
Credit Limit £	0.00
Turnover YTD	250.00

These can then be exported to a PDF files and saved to your computer by clicking on the **Export** button at the top of the windows in which the reports are contained. Please refer to the 'Exporting to PDF file' section in Chapter 1 for details of how to do this.

3.3 Invoices and statements

Some reports, such as invoices and statements, may be intended to be printed on pre-printed stationery. Remember that when you preview these documents on screen, you will see words and figures on plain paper. This is obvious if you think about it, but we mention it because it surprises some new users.

To produce a customer statement, select **Customers** from the main menu. Then select the required customer and then click on the **Statements** button within Customers.

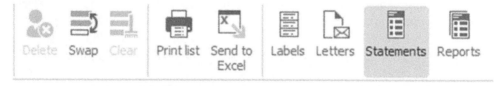

You then click on **Layouts** to bring up a series of different styles of statement.

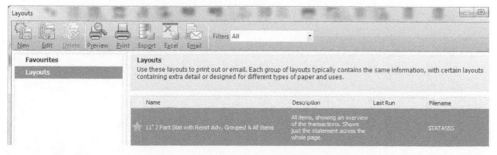

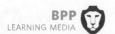

Using the first (default) option, double clicking on it or clicking on **Preview** will bring up a menu where you can specify transaction dates before pressing **OK** to generate a conventional statement similar to the one shown below.

SFE Merchandising
14a Hapgood House
Dagenham Avenue
Benham
DR6 8LV

ALE001

Alexander Ltd   31/01/2016
501 Dart Road

Leeds
LS12 6TC

All values are shown in Pound Sterling

15/01/2016	001	Goods/Services	£	240.00		£	240.00
25/01/2016	002	Goods/Services	£	60.00		£	300.00
31/01/2016	500001	Payment			£ 240.00	£	60.00

This can then be exported to a PDF file and saved to your computer by clicking on the **Export** button at the top of the window in which the report is contained. Please refer to the 'Exporting to PDF file' section in Chapter 1 for details of how to do this.

3.4 Reports in assessments

The following table lists the reports you may be asked for in an assessment, with brief instructions explaining how to obtain them in Sage. Make sure that you select appropriate dates to cover the transactions you have entered. Don't forget to export these reports to PDF files and save them to your computer. Please refer to the 'Exporting to PDF file' section in Chapter 1 for details of how to do this.

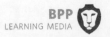

REPORT	HOW TO GET IT	WHICH REPORT TO CHOOSE
Audit trail - a list of every transaction entered into Sage including journal entries in order of entry.	Click on **Transactions**, and then the **Audit Trail Report** button.	**Detailed** type of audit trail with **Landscape Output**. Click on **Run,** then you are asked for **Criteria.** Complete these fields, then click OK, and you will get a list of **all** transactions in the order in which they were posted
Remittance advice – advice of payment to a supplier showing invoice(s) paid	Please refer to the Supplier Payments section earlier in this chapter for details of how to generate and remittance.	Please see details of this earlier in this chapter
Customer statements – statements of account to credit customers	Click on the **Customers** button and then the **Statement** button.	Click on Layouts and then select '11" Stat with Tear Off Remit Adv. Grouped & All Items'
Bank reconciliation – a comparison of bank statement balance to bank nominal ledger account balance	Please refer back to the Bank Reconciliations section of this chapter to see how to generate a bank reconciliation statement. Note that the audit trail will show details of bank reconciled items.	Report within the Bank Reconciliation Screen
Sales and Sales Returns Day Books – a list of customer invoices and credit notes	Click on **Customers**, then **Reports** and then click on **Day books**.	Day Books: Customer Invoices (Detailed) Day Books: Customer Credits (Detailed)
Purchases and Purchases Returns Day Books – a list of supplier invoices and credit notes	Click on **Suppliers**, then **Reports** and then click on **Day books**.	Day Books: Supplier Invoices (Detailed) Day Books: Supplier Credits (Detailed)

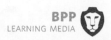

REPORT	HOW TO GET IT	WHICH REPORT TO CHOOSE
Sales ledger accounts (customer accounts) – a list of all transactions with each customer	Click on **Customers**, then **Reports** and then click on **Customer Activity**.	Customer Activity (Detailed)
All purchase ledger (supplier) accounts (showing all transactions within each account) – a list of all transactions with each supplier	Click on **Suppliers**, then **Reports** and then click on **Supplier Activity**.	Supplier Activity (Detailed)
Aged trade receivables/trade payables reports – a list of balances owed from each customer/to each supplier	Click on **Suppliers** or **Customers** as appropriate, and then select **Aged debtors** or **Aged creditors**.	Choose (and preview) the appropriate aged debtor/creditor reports
Bank payments/ receipts – a list of payments and receipts made from the bank account	Click on **Bank accounts**, then **Reports** and choose bank payments, bank receipts etc.	Bank reports > bank payments (Detailed, Base Currency) Bank reports> bank receipts (Detailed)
Nominal ledger accounts – shows all transactions within each account	Click on **Nominal Codes**, then on **Reports** and then on **Nominal Activity**.	Nominal Activity – * See note below
Trial balance – a list of balances all nominal ledger accounts	Click on **Nominal Codes**, then on **Reports**, and then click on the **Trial Balance** button.	Period Trial Balance

* Note. For Nominal Activity reports, you can set the criteria using the screen that follows to include one account, a range of accounts or all accounts. To include all accounts, just leave the Nominal Code fields blank. To generate a report for one account, just enter/select the same account code in both Nominal Code fields, as shown in the following screen print.

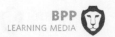

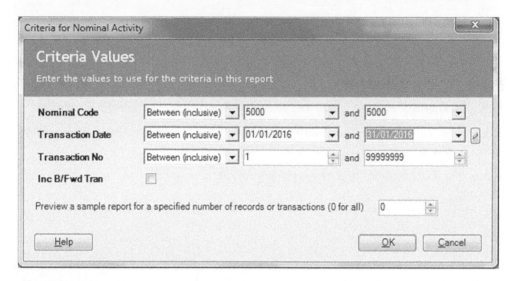

Task 6

Set up another customer as follows:

Springsteen Ltd
223 Home Town
Bradford
BD11 3EE

Process an invoice, Invoice 003, to this customer for £600 (net) for 20 Super-widgets, VAT at standard rate, invoice dated 26 January 2016.

Task 7

You notice that on 15 January, the bank has debited your account £10 for bank charges (no VAT). Enter this transaction to the bank account, debiting the Bank Charges account in the nominal ledger.

On 31 January, the bank credits you with £0.54 interest (no VAT). Rather than net this off against Bank interest charges, you decide to set up a new nominal ledger account: Bank interest received, in the Other sales category, account number 4906. Set up the new account and enter the interest received.

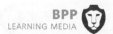

Task 8

Ensure that the program date is set to 31/01/2016. Go to **Customers > Reports > Aged Debtors**.

From the **Aged Debtors** report list, select the Aged Debtors Analysis (Contacts).

Export the report to a specified location on your computer using the default location offered, and a PDF version report will be saved.

Open the PDF version and review your report. It should show all invoices as current.

Transfers

To transfer between bank accounts (including petty cash) choose **Bank accounts > Bank Transfer**. For example, to transfer £100 from the bank current account to the petty cash account, select **Bank** from the menu on the bottom left, then **Bank Transfer** from the task list.

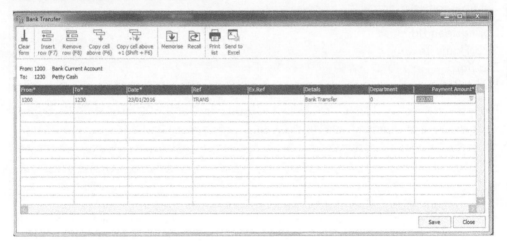

Task 9

On 23 January, you transfer £100 from the bank account into petty cash and immediately spend:

*   £20 on train fares (zero rated for VAT)

*   £10 (gross amount) on coffee mugs for the office (standard rated). The net cost of the cups should be debited to Sundry Expenses

Enter and post the transactions above. Remember, you can use F6 to repeat entries from the previous line.

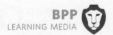

Task 10

Extract a trial balance as at 31/01/2016.

If you wish, you can also preview a statement of financial position (balance sheet) and statement of profit or loss (profit and loss account). You will not have to do this in your assessment, but they are easy documents to produce and it seems a pity not to have a look!

Nominal codes > Reports > Balance Sheet for the balance sheet

Nominal codes > Reports > Profit and Loss for the profit and loss account

Your trial balance in Task 10 should look similar to the one that follows:

Date: 01/03/2016
Time: 15:08:19

SFE Merchandising
Period Trial Balance

Page: 1

To Period: Month 1, January 2016

N/C	Name	Debit	Credit
0030	Office Equipment	800.00	
1100	Debtors Control Account	780.00	
1200	Bank Current Account	2,646.12	
1230	Petty Cash	320.00	
2100	Creditors Control Account		1,056.00
2200	Sales Tax Control Account		170.00
2201	Purchase Tax Control Account	183.41	
3010	Capital Introduced		3,000.00
4000	Sales - products		800.00
4001	Sales - services		50.00
4906	Bank interest received		0.54
5000	Materials Purchased	80.00	
7103	General Rates	200.00	
7400	Travelling	20.00	
7504	Publicity material	28.68	
7901	Bank Charges	10.00	
8250	Sundry Expenses	8.33	
	Totals:	5,076.54	5,076.54

4 Error correction

If you make an error when you are making your entries, it is relatively easy to correct.

Errors made when setting up customer and supplier accounts can be corrected simply by opening the relevant record and changing the data.

Errors made when typing in the details of a transaction (references, descriptions etc) can be corrected by clicking **Transactions**. A list of all the transactions you have posted so far will appear as follows:

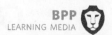

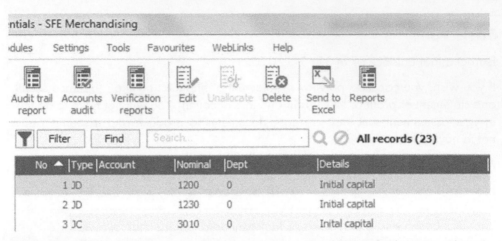

Select the transaction you want to change and click on the **Edit** button at the top of the screen. The following record appears.

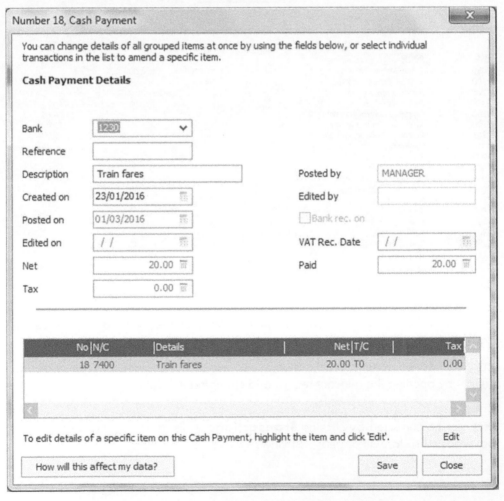

BPP
LEARNING MEDIA

Click on a specific item and click on the **Edit** button (at the bottom of this screen) to change the details as appropriate.

Some corrections that you can make in this way have a bigger effect on the underlying records than others. For example, if you try to change the date or the amounts or account codes for a transaction, the program may let you do so, but to guard against fraud, it will also post a record of what has been changed, and you will be able to see this if you click on **Transactions**: the correction will show up in red.

Some programs do not have the option of correcting transactions by amending the original entry. Therefore, another way is to correct a transaction with another transaction (eg, a credit note, a journal entry), rather than amending the original transaction. In business, this method is also best practice in order to keep a clear audit trail.

Customer invoices

If you have made a mistake on a customer invoice which has been posted, you need to create a credit note, either for the full amount and reissue the invoice, or for the difference. Credit notes are covered in Chapter 1.

Supplier invoices

If a mistake is made by a supplier on an invoice, they will normally send you a credit note, again either for the full amount, with a reissued invoice, or for the difference.

If you have made the mistake yourself, then you need to cancel the invoice, by entering a credit note with the same details. Credit notes are covered in Chapter 1.

Other entries

Other entries should be corrected by journal entry. Students should also be able to post journal entries to correct their own errors that may occur during the assessment. The journal entry is covered in Chapter 1. For a clear audit trail, it is best practice to post a journal entry to reverse the original entry and then post a journal to re-do the transaction correctly.

Task 11

Let's say that the £20 payment entered in petty cash for a train fare should actually have been £15. We could, of course, make adjustments using a journal entry, but here we will use the correction facility.

Click on **Transactions.**

Look down the list of transactions until you find £20 for the train ticket. Double click on that, click Edit, and enter £15 in the net amount. Save the correction.

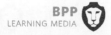

> Now go to **Bank Accounts > Petty Cash** (double click) **> Activity**
>
> You will see that the transaction is now only £15 and the petty cash balance has increased by £5. However, there is a memorandum entry in red stating that £20 has been deleted.

5 Irrecoverable debts

In the assessment you might be required to post a journal to write off an irrecoverable debt.

An irrecoverable debt or 'bad debt' as it is sometimes called, is a balance owing from a customer for invoices that will not be paid, perhaps because the customer has gone bankrupt or due to a dispute. Therefore the original invoice amount(s) needs to be written-off in the accounts.

The journal entry to write off an irrecoverable debt is as follows.

		£	£
DEBIT	Irrecoverable (bad) debts expense	GROSS AMT	
CREDIT	Customer account in trade receivables (debtors) ledger		GROSS AMT

Write off an irrecoverable debt using a credit note

However, in Sage 50 you cannot use the journal function to post this entry, as you cannot post directly to the customer account.

(Remember that each customer account is a subsidiary account of the overall trade receivables ledger account, eg, customer account ALE001 is a subsidiary account of the overall trade receivables account – A/C 1100 – 'Sales Ledger Control Account' in Sage 50),

Instead, you must use the credit note function. This was referred to in Chapter 1. To recap, select the **Batch credit** button in the **Customers module**.

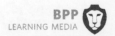

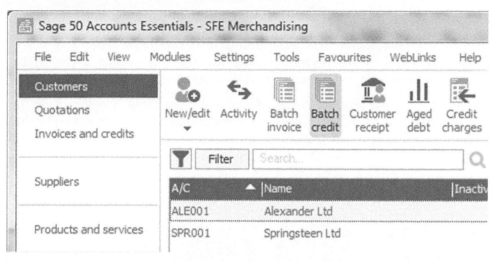

You are presented with the **Batch Customer Credit** screen. The entries you make will be similar to those for entering a sales credit note (ie, selecting **Cr Note** in the **Type** field), but with the following differences.

N/C – select A/C 8100 – 'Bad debt write off'

Net – enter the GROSS amount of the invoice(s) you are writing off

T/C – select T9 as VAT does not apply at this stage.

For example, let's say you received notice that the customer Alexander Ltd has gone bankrupt, and therefore the balance of £60.00 (gross amt) for invoice no. 002 (created in Task 11, Chapter 1) will not be paid. You would enter the following credit note:

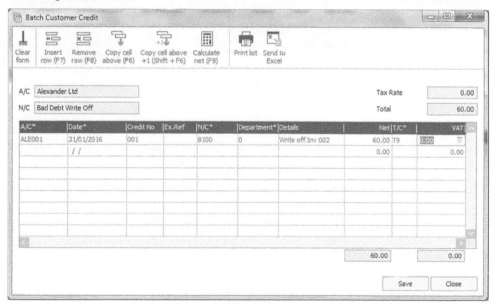

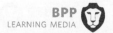

VAT treatment

The VAT treatment above might seem odd at first. You might expect that if you already paid VAT on the original invoice, you can now reclaim the VAT, by entering the net amount, and selecting the tax code as Standard VAT.

However VAT is not reclaimable on all bad debts, as there is a time limit. To comply with current HMRC guidelines, the gross amount is posted to the bad debts account initially, and if VAT is reclaimable, the VAT is separately transferred from the bad debts account to the VAT on purchases account.

6 Month-end procedures

In business there are additional procedures that need to be performed at month-end. The main procedures are:

- Post prepayments
- Post accruals
- Post depreciation
- Close the month to prevent posting of further transactions

You do not have to perform these tasks in the Assessment but it is useful to be aware of these as you will undoubtedly encounter them in the workplace and/or future studies.

6.1 Starting over

All of us can have a bad day sometimes! Occasionally, you may find that you or someone else using the package has made a number of mistakes, perhaps due to a misunderstanding.

If this happens, it may well be better to start again rather than trying to correct all the mistakes, possibly making things worse.

To do so, of course, you need to have made a back-up of the data as it was before all the errors were made. You can then simply restore the correct data and start posting your new entries again.

Back-ups can be made by selecting **File > Back up** and following the on-screen instructions. Restoring data from a back-up can be made by selecting **File > Restore** and following the on-screen instructions.

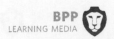

Chapter overview

- Payments and receipts should be allocated to outstanding invoices, as it is important to know which invoices have been paid.

- Bank reconciliations are very important controls in accounting systems and are easily accomplished in Sage.

- All the reports that you are likely to require are available as pre-prepared reports.

- There are various facilities for error correction, but it is best not to make errors in the first place!

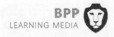

Keywords

- **Bank reconciliation:** a checking process, whereby differences between an organisation's cash book entries, and the bank issued statement are identified. This gives assurance that the cash book is accurate

- **Payment allocations:** matching payments (either received or made) to relevant invoices and credit notes

- **Recurring payments:** payments (or receipts) that are made on a regular, periodic basis. Common examples are standing orders and directy debits

- **Remittance advice:** document that lists all transactions that are being settled by a payment

- **Reports:** form that summarises or analyses data that has been input to a computer system

- **Unallocated payments:** payments or parts of payments that cannot be matched to specific transactions

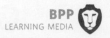

Test your learning

1   When you receive a payment from an account customer this is posted from the Bank menu using the Bank Receipts button. True or false? Explain your answer.

2   Which report would you run to view the transactions posted to a particular ledger account?

3   Why can you not see supplier accounts on the nominal activity report?

4   Which report would you run to view the invoices and payments posted to a particular supplier account?

5   Transfers between bank accounts should always be processed by using the Journal facility. True or false?

6   Assuming VAT is applicable in both cases; why do you need to account for VAT on the receipt of payment for a cash sale, but not the receipt of payment for a credit sale?

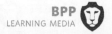

Sage One – Part 1

3

Chapter coverage

You will be required to prove your competence in the use of computerised accounting software by completing an assessment. Assessments are likely to include a series of exercises, for example, entering customer and supplier details, posting transactions such as journals, invoices and credit notes, and generating reports.

This chapter explains how you might complete the hands-on computerised accounts parts of an assessment. It is by no means a comprehensive guide to computerised accounting.

The illustrations in this chapter and the next chapter are from Sage One, which is just one of many accounting software programs that you might use. We use a Sage program because these are popular among small/medium-sized businesses in the UK; and with colleges, for training purposes.

There are a large number of illustrations in this chapter, so don't be put off if it seems long – it should be relatively quick and easy to work through.

The topics covered in this chapter are:

- Accounting software
- Assessments
- Business data and the general (nominal) ledger
- Customer and supplier data
- Journals
- Entering invoices
- Help!

1 Accounting software

Accounting software ranges from simple 'off the shelf' analysed cash book style software to heavy-duty Enterprise Resource Management systems used in large organisations. Very large organisations often have a system that has been built specifically for them, made up of components from a variety of software suppliers, or written for them on a one-off basis.

Obviously, we cannot even begin to cover the vast range of available software programs, but we can illustrate the features of a typical program, and a popular one in the UK among small to medium-sized businesses is Sage.

Sage produces a variety of accounting software products and this book deals with Sage One.

1.1 Hands-on

The illustrations in this Text are taken from Sage One Accounting. This is a 'cloud' based program, which is software that is accessed online through a web browser. All data is stored and backed up online.

Sage One is quite different to traditional Sage products such as Sage 50 or Sage Instant. If you are using Sage 50 or Sage Instant, you should refer to the Sage 50 section of this book.

Sage updates its software regularly and therefore some screens and menus in this book may appear slightly different to the version you are using, but you should be able to work your way through the tasks. A full list of updates to Sage One can be found by visiting the Sage One website:

www.uk.sageone.com

If possible, we strongly recommend that you sit at a computer where you can access Sage One as you read through this chapter. Most of the activities assume that you are doing this and can complete the tasks we describe as you go along.

1.2 Finding your way about : terminology

We'll assume that you know what we mean when we say 'screen' and 'button', but there may be some other terms that you are not sure of, so here is a quick guide. In this chapter, we will use bold text when referring to something that you will see on screen, such as a button or a tab.

We also use arrows to indicate a sequence of actions. For example, we might say 'choose **Settings > Financial Year & VAT**'. This means click on the **Settings** tab and then click on the **Financial Year & VAT** button as shown in the screen below.

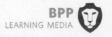

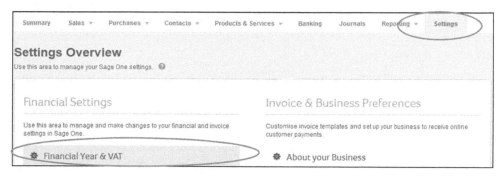

The home screen in Sage is called the **Summary** screen. This can be accessed at any time by clicking on the home 🏠 button at the very top of the screen, or on the Summary tab.

The Summary screen is one of a number of menu 'tabs' in Sage. A 'tab' is so called because it looks like a tab in a paper filing system. Each tab represents a particular module in Sage (eg Sales, Purchases etc). Clicking on a tab brings up the main screen for that module, from which other actions are available.

There are also a number of functions available from the drop-down list of each tab, as shown below for the Purchases tab. A drop-down list is a list of items to select from within a tab. In the screenshot below, the drop-down list is indicated by the downward arrow button next to the tab.

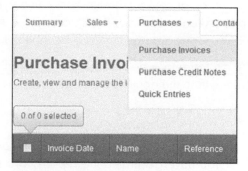

Most of what you do involves making entries or selecting from items in **fields** – for example, the **Ledger Account** field.

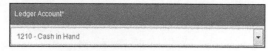

Fields can also contain drop-down lists which can be accessed by clicking on the downward arrow button next to the field.

We also refer to 'check-boxes'. These are boxes which when clicked on, show a tick symbol. When we say something like 'tick the check box', this simply means click on the check-box so that a tick appears in the box.

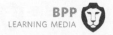

Finally, make sure that you know where the Tab key is on your keyboard (usually above the Caps Lock key). This allows you to move easily between fields and looks something like this.

1.3 Defaults

Computerised software programs make extensive use of **defaults**, which are the most common entries. When you start entering data, you will often find that Sage has done some of the work already, using the default options that would normally be chosen. This saves a great deal of time, but you should always glance at the default entries in case they are not the ones you want. This will become clearer as you start using the program.

1.4 Screenshots

During the assessment, for certain tasks, you will be asked to 'save a screenshot' of a screen to provide evidence that you have completed the task correctly. This means you need to capture and save an image of a particular screen shown on the computer.

To take a screen capture of an entire screen, on your keyboard press **Print Screen** or **PrtScn**. To capture the active window only, press **Alt +Print Screen** or **ALT + PrtScn** (on some keyboards the key may be labelled PrtSc).

The image can then be pasted into a document using an application (using **CTRL + V**) such as **Word** from where the document can be saved as a file (**CTRL + S**).

1.5 Exporting to PDF file

You will also be required to generate various reports from the accounting software. To provide evidence that you have generated the reports, you should export these to PDF (Portable Document Format) files if your accounting software program allows this. If not, you should take screenshots of the full report on screen and paste these to a document. You should save your files to your computer. Reports are covered in Chapter 4.

To export a report to a PDF file, click on the **Export** button shown in the screen of the particular report you have run.

Export

Depending on the type of report, some reports may generate a PDF version on screen directly after clicking on the **Export** button.

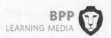

However, for most reports, the following screen will appear when clicking on the Export button (eg, for the Nominal Activity report):

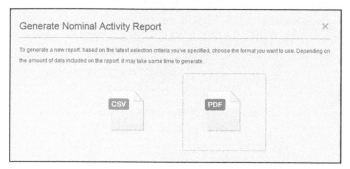

Click on **PDF**; after a short while, the following icon will appear at the top of the screen: 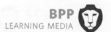.

Click on this icon to reveal a link to the report you have just exported. Click on the link and the report opens in a new window in your internet browser.

Select the save option from your internet browser and this brings up a box (similar to that shown below) that asks you for the location on the computer where you want to save the PDF file to, and the name of the file.

Specify the locaton and name of the file and click on the **Save** button. In the assessment you will be told the location of where to save the file and the type of name to use.

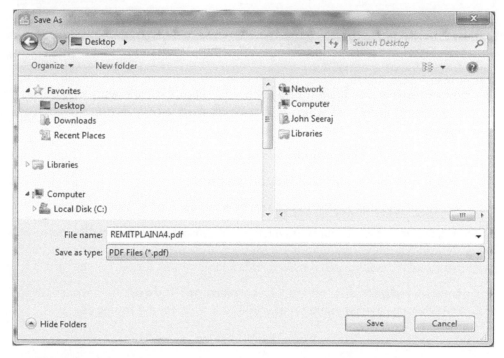

1.6 Uploading files

You will be required to 'upload' the documents or PDF files you have saved. This means that in the assessment, there will be an option on screen to upload files saved in your computer. Selecting this option brings up a box similar to that shown below, which asks you choose the file you wish to upload from your computer.

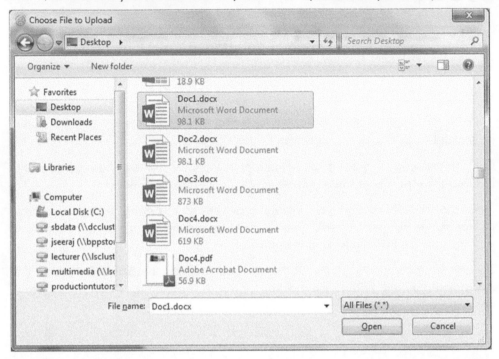

1.7 Accounting entries

This module assumes you have a basic understanding of double entry accounting, the fundamental principle of which is that **each and every transaction has two effects**.

So for every transaction that a business makes, there must be:

- **Debit entries** in particular **ledger accounts**

- An equal and opposite value of **credit entries** in other ledger accounts

Ledger accounts are accounts in which each transaction is recorded – there will be a ledger account for different types of transactions such as sales and purchases, and for every type of asset and liability.

The **general ledger** (also referred to as **nominal ledger**) is the accounting record which forms the complete set of ledger accounts for the business.

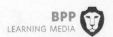

To know when to use debits and credits, use the following general rules:

- An **increase** in an **expense** (eg a purchase of stationery) or an **increase in an asset** (eg a purchase of computer equipment) is a **debit**.

- An **increase** in **revenue** (eg a sale) or an **increase in a liability** (eg buying goods on credit) is a **credit**.

- A **decrease** in an **asset** (eg making a payment from the bank) is a **credit**.

- A **decrease** in a **liability** (eg paying a creditor) is a **debit**.

In this book, we often refer to 'posting' a transaction. This simply means recording the transaction in the ledger accounts.

2 Assessments

Your AAT assessment will involve a number of practical tasks that test your competence in the assessment criteria.

2.1 Before you start ...

Before you start, you should find out from your assessor what the arrangements are for:

- Opening the accounting software and signing in, if necessary
- Changing any overall business details or settings, if required
- Creating new accounts, as necessary
- Posting transactions and completing other assessment tasks
- Saving and exporting your work

Example

The following example is based on a past sample simulation issued by the AAT (simulations were used before assessments).

Situation

SFE Merchandising is a new business that has been set up by Charlize Veron, one of Southfield Electrical's former marketing staff. Charlize is an expert on store layout and management of inventories (stocks) and she intends to sell her skills and knowledge, on a consultancy basis, to medium-sized and large retailers to help them to optimise their sales.

Charlize has started her new venture as a sole trader and has taken on some of the risk herself. However, SFE Merchandising is part-financed by Southfield Electrical, and may well be acquired by them if this new venture is a success. Initial enquiries have been so promising that Charlize has already voluntarily registered for VAT and intends to run the standard VAT accounting scheme. (Assume the standard VAT rate is 20%.)

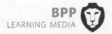

The business commenced trading on 1 January 2016.

Tasks to be completed

It is now 31 January 2016 and you are to complete the tasks in Chapters 3 and 4.

There will be 13 tasks in the real assessment involving setting up data, entering journals, posting sales and purchase transactions, generating reports and so on.

You will be provided with a series of documents such as invoices and cheques. We'll show you how to deal with all of this in the remainder of this Text.

You should now have Sage One open on your computer and follow through the activities.

Task 1

Signing-in

It is assumed at this point that you have already signed up to the Sage One service. (You can sign up either through your college, or if you are an individual student, by visiting http://info.uk.sageone.com/aat-computerised-accounting)

Sign in to Sage One by visiting the following web address:

https://app.sageone.com/login

or through your learning provider's direct login mechanism.

Enter the email address that you used to sign up to Sage One, your password, and click on the **Sign in** button.

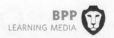

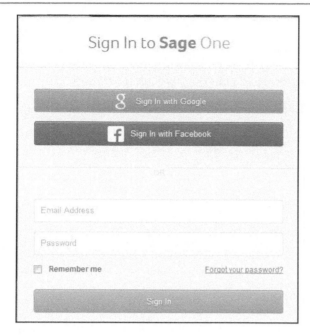

This exercise starts with a new instance of Sage One or a 'clean' business which contains no transactions. At this point, your college should be able to tell you how to start Sage One afresh with a clean business.

If you are studying at home and are using Sage for the first time, you will be presented with a 'business set-up wizard' and will need to enter certain details; go straight to the 'New Set-Up' section below to do this. Otherwise, you will be presented with the **Summary** screen, as shown in the 'Start' section below.

Resetting Data

If you are studying at home and are already using Sage One with existing data, you may start afresh by resetting the data by clicking on the Settings ⚙ button. Then select Service **Settings > Manage Your Data >** Tick the **'I understand'** box to confirm acceptance of resetting your data > Enter the email address you used to sign up **> Reset data**.

Important points to note:

- **You will not be required to set up a new business in your real assessment. We cover this here to enable us to create the same starting point in Sage for all students.**

- **Make sure you don't confuse this Settings button with the Settings tab; which is frequently referred to in these chapters.**

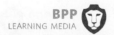

New Set-Up

The first time you sign in to Sage One you are presented with a business set-up wizard. A wizard is a type of software assistant that presents a user with a sequence of boxes that guide the user through a series of steps.

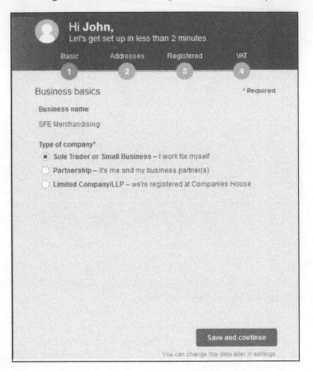

In this series of steps, you should specify/enter the following details, and click on **Save and continue** for each step:

Type of business:	Sole Trader or Small Business
Business Trading Address:	14b Hapgood House, Dagenham Avenue, Benham DR6 8LV United Kingdom
VAT Tax Scheme:	Standard
VAT Number:	524 3764 5 1

Start

At this point it is assumed that you have entered the details required when you first signed up to Sage, and have reset any existing data.

You are presented with the following Summary screen, which is essentially the home screen for this program. This screen can be accessed at any time by clicking on the Summary tab, or on the home 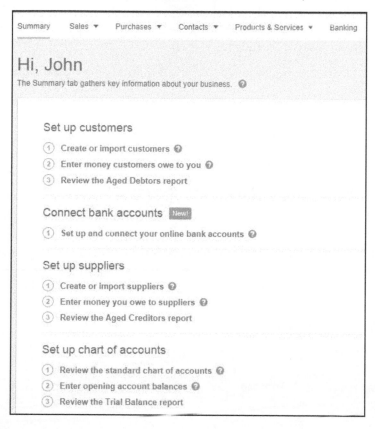 button at the top of the screen. To sign out of the program, click on the sign out button, also at the top of the screen.

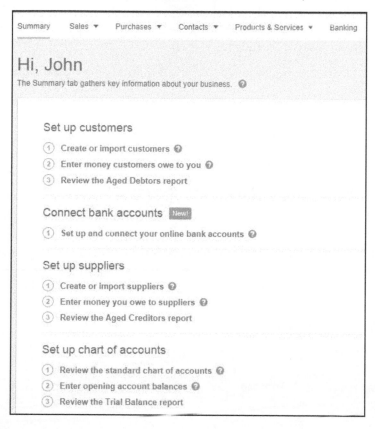

Important note: Sage generally refers to a 'business' in its functions. Such references can encompass sole trader businesses as well as companies.

3 Business data and the general (nominal) ledger

3.1 Business data

If for any reason, you did not enter your full business details using the Business setup wizard described in Task 1, you can do this now by selecting **Settings > About your Business**.

In the **About your business** screen, the **Business name** defaults to the name you registered with Sage One.

At the time of print, this can only be changed by contacting Sage who will do it for you. If this function is still not available when you read this book, it is fine to leave

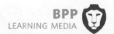

the name as it is, as this will not affect your ability to work through the chapters. Otherwise you can change it to the name below.

The address of the business should also be entered. This information will appear on any documents you produce with the software, such as reports and invoices, so make sure it is accurate and spelled correctly.

Enter or select the following information if you did not already do so when you first signed up to Sage:

Business name: SFE Merchandising

Address: 14b Hapgood House, Dagenham Avenue,

                         Benham, DR6 8LV, United Kingdom

Type of business: Sole trader or Small Business

Use the **Tab** key on your keyboard to move between different lines. Alternatively, click on each line, but this will slow you down, so get into the habit of using the **Tab** key to move from field to field. When you have finished, click on **Save**.

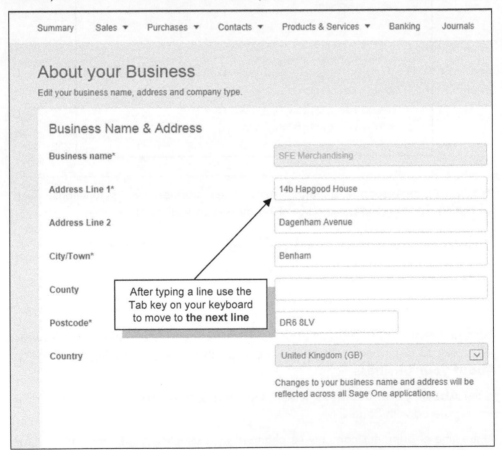

3.2 Financial year & VAT

The Financial Settings screen allows you to enter the financial year and VAT settings. This can be found by clicking on the **Settings** tab and selecting **Financial Year & VAT**.

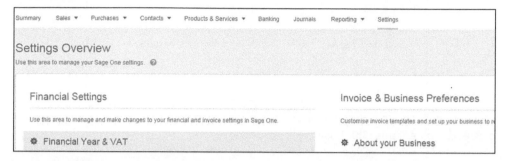

This brings up the **Financial Settings** screen, as shown below. Set the **Year End Date** to 31/12/2016 and the **Accounts Start Date** to 01/01/2016 as shown below. Ignore Year End Lockdown. This function prevents transactions being entered before a specific date.

Financial Settings

Record your financial details such as your VAT scheme details, financial year end an

Year End Date	31/12/2016
Year End Lockdown	
Accounts Start Date	01/01/2016

Our example business is **VAT registered** and is registered for the **Standard** VAT Scheme. If you have not already specified the VAT Scheme and VAT number when you first signed up to Sage, select 'Standard' from the drop-down list in the **VAT Scheme** field, and enter 524 3764 51 as the VAT number, as shown below. Submission Frequency is not relevant for this module; however, you can enter quarterly, as this is a common frequency for most businesses.

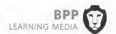

counting transactions. ❓	
VAT Scheme	Standard
Submission Frequency	Quarterly
VAT Number	GB 524376451

Once you have completed this screen, click on **Save**. You are now ready to proceed with entering the business's transactions.

3.3 New accounts and your assessment

In your assessment, you may need to add new nominal ledger accounts to complete your tasks, or you may not. As you work through your assessment, before starting each task, check that the accounts you will need are set up. We recommend you create any new accounts required before starting the task the account is needed in.

If the assessment includes a purchase invoice for stationery, for instance, check that there is already an 'Office stationery' account (in the Overheads category) before you start to post the invoice. The tasks may actually ask you to do this.

To access the **Chart of Accounts** (a list of nominal ledger accounts) screen, click the **Settings** tab. This brings up the **Settings Overview** screen (as shown in the 'Financial year and VAT' section above). Then click on the **Chart of Accounts** button.

You are presented with the default chart of accounts for this program, as shown in the screen below. The list of accounts can be shown in order of the **Nominal Code** heading as show below, but can be ordered by any of the headings in the list by clicking on a particular heading.

The nominal ledger accounts are categorised by account type (eg Fixed Assets, Current Assets). This is shown in the **Category** heading in the screen below. The categories of account types are grouped by asset, liability, income, expenditure or capital account. This is shown in in the **Category Group** heading in the screen below.

 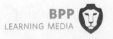

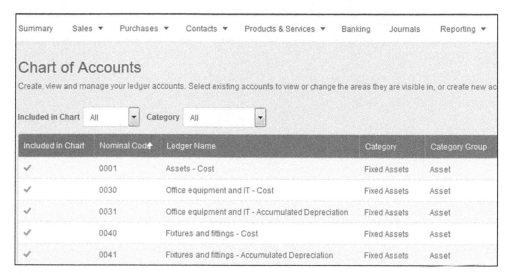

Chart of Accounts

Create, view and manage your ledger accounts. Select existing accounts to view or change the areas they are visible in, or create new ac

Included in Chart	Nominal Code	Ledger Name	Category	Category Group
✓	0001	Assets - Cost	Fixed Assets	Asset
✓	0030	Office equipment and IT - Cost	Fixed Assets	Asset
✓	0031	Office equipment and IT - Accumulated Depreciation	Fixed Assets	Asset
✓	0040	Fixtures and fittings - Cost	Fixed Assets	Asset
✓	0041	Fixtures and fittings - Accumulated Depreciation	Fixed Assets	Asset

You can search for a specific ledger account in the search box by entering the first few digits of the nominal code or first few letters of the ledger name.

For example, if you enter 'Sales Type A' in the search box, the list shows this account only, as shown below.

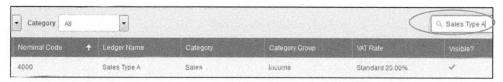

If you search for an account for 'Publicity material', you will see that it is not there, so we will create one.

Task 2

Create a new account for 'Publicity material'.

In the **Chart of Accounts** screen, click on the **New Ledger Account** button:

New Ledger Account

In the **New Ledger Account** box that follows, enter 'Publicity material' in both the **Ledger Name** and **Display Name** fields.

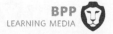

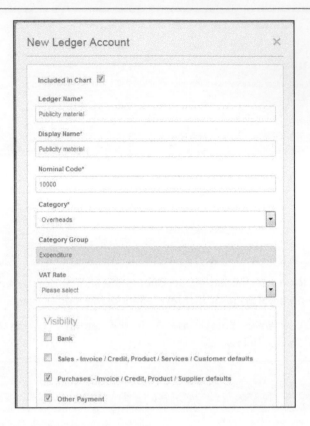

New Ledger Account   ×

Included in Chart ☑

Ledger Name*
Publicity material

Display Name*
Publicity material

Nominal Code*
10000

Category*
Overheads   ▾

Category Group
Expenditure

VAT Rate
Please select   ▾

Visibility
☐ Bank

☐ Sales - Invoice / Credit, Product / Services / Customer defaults

☑ Purchases - Invoice / Credit, Product / Supplier defaults

☑ Other Payment

You can choose a **Nominal Cod**e (account code). It is best practice to group certain types of nominal codes in a particular range within the chart of accounts.

For example, in this program, the nominal codes 4000 to 4999 are available for income accounts. However, when you create a new nominal code, the program will suggest a default code outside these ranges; from 10000 onwards.

You can overwrite this with a code of your choice but, for the purposes of getting through these tasks, we recommend you accept the code given. You don't need to worry about the grouping of nominal codes for this module, but it is important to be aware that in real life, charts of accounts will usually follow a logical structure to facilitate easier reporting and production of accounts. (This is why income accounts are in the range 4000 to 4999 in this program).

You can further refine the **Category** of account (The options available will depend on the type of account you are setting up.)Publicity material is part of overheads, so choose 'Overheads'.

The **Category group** field automatically populates based on the category you have chosen. In this case it is 'Expenditure'.

Ignore the **VAT Rate** for now. In this Text, we will not set a default VAT rate for a ledger account. We will instead select the VAT rate at the time of entering a transaction, since this is required for the assessment. Furthermore, different types of goods or services may have different VAT rates.

The **Visibility** check boxes are automatically populated based on the selections you have made above and you do not need to change anything here at this point. However, if you find that an account is not available to select from in a particular function, this could mean that it is not visible within that function. To make it visible, you should edit the ledger account (described in the section under Task 3 below) and make sure the relevant function is ticked in the **Visibility** section.

After making your selections, click on **Save**. You will now see the account in the **Chart of Accounts** screen (**Settings > Chart of Accounts**).

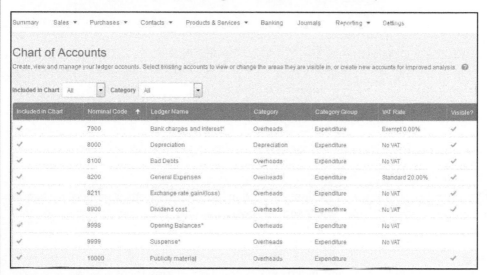

We cover entering opening balances later in the chapter. The options for entering opening balances are also covered in Sage Help. The help page is online and can be accessed by clicking the help button 🔘 at the top of the screen. You can search for a particular topic in the search box, or there are a number of help categories and topics to select from.

Task 3

Vimal was in a hurry to post a transaction and wasn't sure what nominal account to use, so he created a new account named 'L8R'. Why might this cause problems later on?

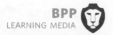

It is also possible to change the name of existing nominal accounts. To do this, you need to select the account you want to change from the **Chart of Accounts** screen. This brings up the **Edit Ledger Account** screen showing details of the selected account. In this screen, you can update the name fields. For example, you could change 'Sales Type A' to something that is more descriptive of the particular sales to be recorded in that account, eg 'Overseas Sales', although don't save anything now.

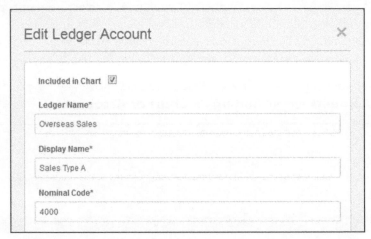

3.4 Entering opening balances in nominal ledger accounts

If you are transferring your business's accounting records from a manual system to a computer system, you will need to post opening balances to your nominal ledger.

Sage One allows you to go directly to the relevant nominal ledger accounts to enter opening balances, and makes the accounting entries for you when you save these. This can be a useful method to use the assessment.

To access the **Nominal Opening Balances** screen, choose **Settings > Nominal Opening Balances**. For example, you may want to post the opening balance for the 'Fixtures and Fittings – Cost' account.

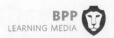

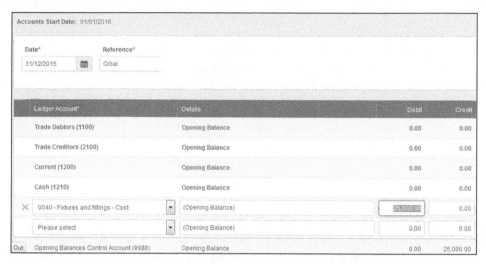

You can enter the opening balance by selecting the Fixtures and Fittings - Cost account from the ledger account field drop-down list and entering the opening balance figure in the appropriate debit or credit field, as shown. This can be posted by clicking on Save (although don't save anything now).

Note. This program requires the opening balances to be created on the date before the accounts start date (see the 'Financial Year & VAT' section to set the accounts start date). This is in order to separate the opening balance from any transactions that occur on the first day of the accounting period. However, this may not be required for other accounting software programs, which may allow opening balances to be created on the accounts start date. The default opening balance date in this program is the day before the accounts start date; in this case, that is 31/12/2015. This should not be changed.

Therefore if you are instructed in the assessment to enter opening balances at, say, 1 January 2016; on Sage One you should enter the opening balance date as 31 December 2015. Other programs may allow you to enter an opening balance of 1 January 2016.

Note that for any entries made using this option, the other side of the double entry will be posted to a suspense account: A/C 9998 - Opening Balances Control Account. However, since opening balances entered should sum to zero (having the same value of debits and credits), entering all opening balances should result in a zero balance overall on the Opening Balances Control Account.

We will look at entering opening balances for customers and suppliers later in this chapter.

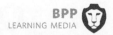

3.5 Tax codes and VAT rates

Other programs may require you to manually set up **tax codes** corresponding to the different VAT rates (eg, zero-rated, standard, reduced and exempt rates). In this program, you do not need to worry about this, as these are automatically set up by Sage.

Occasionally, new VAT rates are introduced or an existing VAT rate percentage is changed. This happened when the UK VAT rate moved from 17.5% to 20% in 2011. In this program, such changes are also automatically updated by Sage. Other programs may require you to manually edit such changes.

At the time of print, the standard VAT rate in the UK is 20%, which is the rate used for this Text. Should there be a change in this rate, the new rate will be automatically updated to the program. However, you will still be able to work through the examples and tasks by selecting the VAT rate as 'Standard'. The only difference will be that the figures for VAT will be calculated using the new rate, rather than 20%, as shown in this Text.

When entering transactions, it is important to use the appropriate VAT rate to ensure the VAT is correctly treated. The VAT rates are summarised below. Note that in the assessment, you do not need to know what the different rates of VAT are used for. You will be told in the assessment if VAT is applicable, and the rate to use.

VAT rate	Used for
Zero-rated	Zero-rated transactions, such as books, magazines and train fares. (Don't confuse this with exempt transactions.)
Standard	Standard rate, currently 20%. Some standard-rated items that catch people out are taxi fares (but only if the taxi driver is VAT registered), restaurant meals, and stationery. You can only reclaim VAT if you have a valid VAT invoice; if not, enter no VAT.
Lower rate	Reduced rate, currently 5% for certain things such as domestic electricity, but this does not normally apply to business expenditure.
Exempt	Exempt transactions such as bank charges and insurance, postage stamps and professional subscriptions.
No VAT*	Transactions not involving VAT, for example wages, charitable donations and internal transfers between accounts (for instance from the bank to the petty cash account). Also used if the supplier is not VAT registered or if you do not have a valid VAT invoice.

* The rate 'No VAT' would also be used for all transactions if your business was not VAT registered. However, in this case study the business is VAT registered.

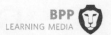

As mentioned above, you will **not** be expected to know the VAT rates for different goods and services. However, you may find the following list of current VAT rates helpful in real life:

www.gov.uk/rates-of-vat-on-different-goods-and-services

3.6 Trade and non-trade receivables

One thing to note is that Sage One does not make a distinction between trade (customers) and non-trade (also known as 'other') receivables. Anyone to whom you grant credit is simply treated as a customer in Sage One.

Another point to note is that Sage uses old UK GAAP (Generally Accepted Accounting Principles) terminology rather than IFRS (International Financial Reporting Standards) and new UK GAAP terminology and therefore uses terms like 'debtors' rather than 'receivables'. Therefore, the receivables control account in Sage is named 'Trade Debtors'.

Note. From now on, we will use the same terminology as Sage uses (ie old UK GAAP terminology) for the purposes of navigating through Sage. However, please be aware of the equivalent terms used in IFRS and new UK GAAP. A list of these is provided at the front of this Text and it is the IFRS/new UK GAAP terminology that will be used in any questions in tasks in your assessment.

4 Customer and supplier data

Before you can post customer and supplier transactions you will also need to set up accounts in the trade debtors ledger (often referred to as the sales ledger) and the trade creditors ledger (often referred to as the purchase ledger).

Note. Customer and supplier accounts are subsidiary accounts of an overall trade debtors ledger account and trade creditors account respectively. Therefore, transactions entered in all customer accounts will be posted to the **one** trade debtors ledger account in the nominal ledger (and the same treatment applies to supplier accounts and the trade creditors ledger).

Once again, we recommend that you set up all the accounts you need before you start posting any transactions.

In an assessment (and in real life) you will find the details you need on the documents you have to hand: the business's own sales invoices and its suppliers' purchase invoices.

4.1 Customer and supplier codes

You will need to decide what kind of codes to use for the customer and supplier accounts. In Sage One, these codes are entered in the Reference field in the New Supplier/New Customer screens (as we will see in the next section). Note although this field is optional in Sage One, you must create a code, as this is a syllabus requirement. Other programs may refer to the code as a supplier/customer code, or account code, and have a mandatory field for this.

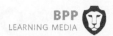

A typical coding system in businesses is to use the first few characters of the supplier/customer name (excluding spaces and punctuation). So, for a customer called 'G.T. Summertown', the code might be GTS. However, this does not allow for customers with similar names. For this reason, many businesses actually introduce numbers into their coding systems. For example, GTS001, GTS002, and so on.

Of course, in your work you would use the coding system prescribed by your organisation. However, in an assessment you will usually be told which code to use. If a task does allow for choice, we recommend an alphanumeric system (a mixture of letters and numbers), as this displays your understanding of the need for understandable but unique codes.

Task 4

Do you think it is possible for a customer and a supplier to have exactly the same code? Explain your answer.

4.2 Entering the account details

We'll now illustrate setting up a supplier account. Please note that the process is identical for customers, apart from the fact that you will be working within the **Customers screens**.

To access the **Suppliers** screen, choose **Contacts > Suppliers**. You are then presented with the following screen.

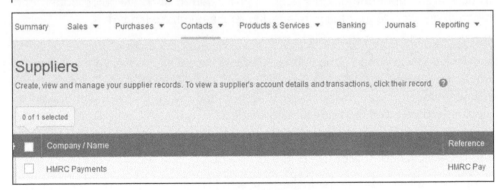

To set up a new account you can click on **New Supplier.**

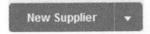

This brings up the following screen.

Create a new supplier ×

Business Name*	Company or Person	Email	
Contact Name		Mobile	
Reference	e.g. Account Number	Telephone	

Account Details   Payment Details   Notes

UK & Ireland ▼

Address 1		VAT Number	
Address 2		Account Default	5000 - Cost of sales - goods ▼
Town / City			
County			
Postcode			
Country	United Kingdom (GB) ▼		

Save

Enter as many details as you have available. The details you need will usually be found on the supplier invoice. If the invoice shows an email address, for instance, be sure to type it in, even though you may not have email addresses for other suppliers. If you cannot find the relevant field, try moving from tab to tab to find the field you want. Take care with typing, as always. Don't forget to enter the **Supplier Code** referred to in the previous section, in the **Reference** field. When you are happy that everything is correct, click on **Save**. Always remember to click **Save** after entering each supplier.

Task 5

Set up a supplier account based on the following details taken from the heading of an invoice.

McAlistair Supplies Ltd
52 Foram Road
Winnesh
DR3 5TP
Tel: 06112 546772 Mobile: 07700 900009
Email: sales@mcalisupps.co.uk
VAT No. 123456788

Leave the Bank Details section blank and don't change the default Purchase Ledger Account or the Payment Terms settings for now. Remember to **Save** the new account.

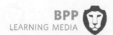

You will see that McAlistair Supplies is now listed as a supplier in the main Suppliers screen (**Contacts > Suppliers**).

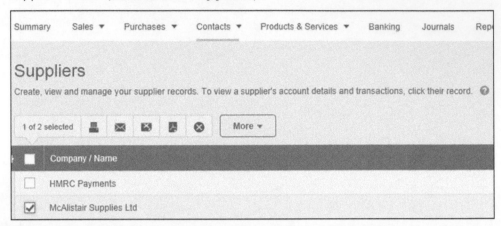

Selecting McAlistair Supplies from the list will bring up the following record.

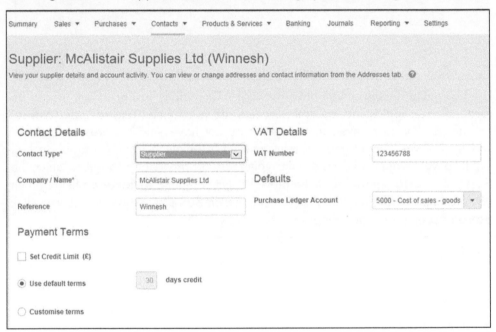

If you make mistake in Task 5 and need to delete the supplier, tick the check-box to the left of the supplier and select the delete icon (circled below) that appears above the **Company Name** heading, as shown in the screen below.

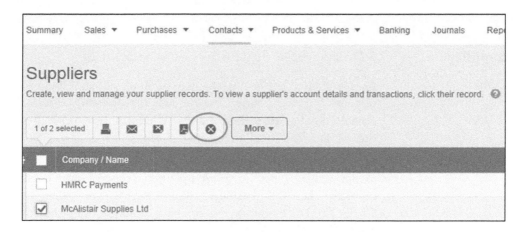

4.3 Entering the opening balance

Earlier in this chapter, we looked at entering an opening balance for a nominal ledger account. The opening balance for the 'Trade creditors' ledger account is made up of the sum of the individual opening supplier balances. The suppliers you are asked to set up in an assessment task may have opening balances. To enter a supplier opening balance, choose the **Settings** tab from the main screen and select **Supplier Opening Balances**. Click on the **New Opening Balance** button and you are presented with the following screen.

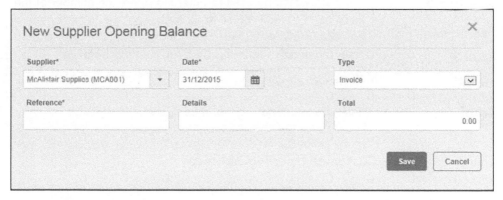

The table below explains what to do as you work through each entry field, in the order in which the Tab key will take you through them.

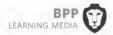

SCREEN ITEM	HOW IT WORKS
Supplier	Select the supplier from the Supplier drop-down list.
Date	As mentioned earlier, when we entered nominal ledger opening balances, Sage One requires the opening balance date to be the **day before** the accounts start date. By default, this field (box) will show this date.
	You should make sure that this is correct; otherwise this means you will not have set up your accounts start date correctly. For this business, the accounts start date is 01/01/2016, therefore the opening balance date should be 31/12/2015.
Type	This program allows you to enter the opening balance as a number of separate entries for individual invoices or credit notes that make up the total balance. This field allows you to specify whether each of these entries is an invoice or credit note. However, this is beyond the scope of this syllabus, as you are only required to enter the total opening balance figure. Therefore, leave this field as Invoice.
Reference	This field would be used to enter the reference number of the invoices or credit notes that make up the total opening balance. However, since this is not applicable, you should enter the initials OB in this field for opening balance.
Details	This field can be left blank.
Total	Enter the total opening balance figure.

Entering customer opening balances is done in the same way, except that you choose **Settings > Customer Opening Balances**.

4.4 Customer and supplier defaults

Ledger account code

In Sage One, when you set up a new customer account, customer invoices you enter will be posted by default to the following account:

DEBIT   Trade debtors account (debit gross amount)

CREDIT   Sales Type A account (credit net amount)

CREDIT   VAT on sales account (credit VAT amount)

For sales, this is probably exactly what you want to happen, unless you are specifically instructed that different types of sales should be posted to different sales accounts in the nominal ledger.

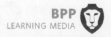

When you set up a new supplier account, the supplier invoices you enter will be posted by default to the following accounts:

DEBIT   VAT on purchases account (debit VAT amount)

DEBIT   Cost of sales account (debit net amount)

CREDIT   Trade creditors account (credit gross amount)

For supplier invoices, however, it would be better to set an appropriate default for the nominal ledger account for each supplier, depending on the type of purchase. For example, you would want to post a stationery supplier's invoices to the stationery account, but an insurance company's invoices to the insurance account.

To change the defaults, just open the supplier record (**Contacts > Suppliers > click on the required supplier**) and click on the box labelled **Purchase Ledger Account**.

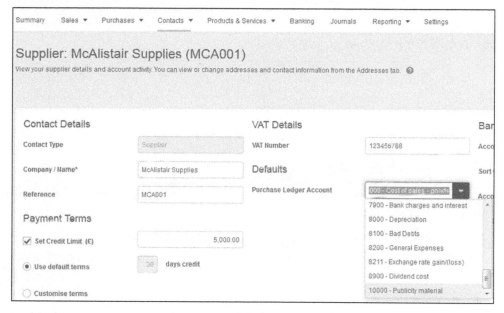

In this box, you can set the nominal ledger expenditure account to which all transactions with this supplier will be posted (unless you specify otherwise when you actually post a transaction). To see a list of all available accounts, click on the arrow at the right of the box. For example, you may wish to set the default for McAlistair Supplies to Publicity materials.

We could scroll down the list to the Publicity materials account created earlier (account 10000). If you need a new nominal account to post to, you can set one up, as mentioned earlier in Task 2.

Note. If you cannot see the account you created in Task 2, this could be for a couple of reasons. Firstly, go into **Edit Ledger Account** (from **Settings > Chart of accounts)** for the particular account and make sure that you have

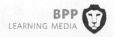

ticked the option: **Purchases – Invoice / Credit, Product / Supplier defaults** in the **Visibility** section.

If the account still does not appear, try using Sage One in a different internet browser. The main internet browsers available are Internet Explorer, Google Chrome, Mozilla Firefox, and Safari (for Mac users).

Payment terms

The default payment terms (ie how long a supplier gives a customer to pay an invoice) is set to 30 days' credit. If in the assessment you are asked to set up a supplier with payment terms of 30 days, make sure the **Use default terms** option is selected in the Supplier record. If you are asked to set up different payment terms, select the **Customise terms** option and enter the required number of days' credit.

The same process also applies for customers.

Also, a credit limit can also be set for each customer/supplier. Tick the box next to **Set Credit Limit (£)** and enter the amount.

Payment Terms		
☑ Set Credit Limit (£)		5,000.00
⦿ Use default terms	30	days credit
○ Customise terms		

Task 6

Open the McAlistair Supplies Ltd supplier record and set the default nominal code to 10000 - Publicity material; the payment terms, to 30 days; and the credit limit, to £5,000.00.

Remember to **Save** this change.

---

5 Journals

If you are setting up a new business, the first entries you are likely to make will be done via a journal; for example, entering the initial capital introduced to a business.

Journals are also used for non-routine transactions, such as the correction of errors and recording drawings from the business. You will be required to enter journals during your assessment.

To post a journal in Sage, click on the **Journals** tab shown on the home screen and click on **New Journal** to bring up the Journal screen as shown below.

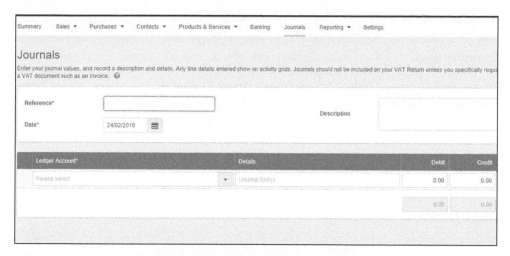

All you need to do is complete the fields and click on **Save**.

Note. Once saved or 'posted' it is not possible to correct a journal and you will need to input another journal to correct any errors, so check carefully before saving.

Let's suppose you want to post the following journal, to enter the initial capital invested in the business.

		£	£
DEBIT	Bank (Current)	2,750.00	
DEBIT	Cash in hand	250.00	
CREDIT	Capital introduced		3,000.00

The table below explains what to do as you work through each entry field in the Journal screen, in the order in which the Tab key will take you through them.

SCREEN ITEM	HOW IT WORKS
Reference	Type in the journal number you are given, if any. Journals should be numbered consecutively, so you may need to check to find out the number of the previous journal. If this is the first ever journal, choose your own coding system and make sure it has room for expansion. For example, 'J001' allows for up to 999 journals in total.
Date	By default, this field (box) will show the PROGRAM DATE, but you should change it to 01/01/16. Clicking the button will make a little calendar appear to select the date from.

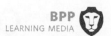

SCREEN ITEM	HOW IT WORKS
Description	Type in the journal narrative, ie the purpose of the journal.
Ledger Account	Enter the nominal ledger code of the account affected, or click the button to the right of this field to select from a drop-down list.
Details	Enter the details for each journal line. This can be the same as the description, or more specific, if required.
Debit/Credit	Type in the amounts in the correct columns. If it is a round sum, such as £250, there is no need to type in the decimal point and the extra zeros.
Include on VAT Return?	This should be left unchecked, as VAT returns are not covered at this level. Sage One gives you the option of choosing whether you want to include the journal on a VAT return.

It is not possible to post a journal if it does not balance, and the following error message is displayed.

> ⚠ • The totals of the debits and credits must match.

Task 7

Enter the journal shown earlier in this section (DEBIT Current 2,750, DEBIT Cash 250, CREDIT Capital Introduced 3,000). Date it 01/01/2016 and give a reference of JVI. Enter 'Initial capital' in the description and details fields. Remember to **Save** the journal.

If you run the **Balance Sheet (Reporting > Balance Sheet Report)** at 31/01/2016, you should see that 3,000 is listed against Total Assets and 3,000 listed against Total Equity.

5.1 The importance of dates

By default, Sage One sets the date of transactions to the current date according to your computer, but this may not be the date you want to use, especially if you are sitting an assessment. You can overwrite the default date in each transaction with the required date.

It is vitally important to enter the correct date when you are using a computerised system, even if you are only doing a practice exercise, because the computer uses

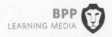

the date you enter in a variety of ways – to generate reports such as aged debtors reports, to reconcile VAT, and so on.

Furthermore, when viewing reports or lists within Sage, make sure that you have set the date range correctly in the particular report or list – otherwise certain transactions might not show up.

Note. In the assessment, you will be asked to set the **system software date** to a specific date as part of the set-up process. This cannot be done in Sage One, as the system software date defaults to the current date. This does not form part of the assessment and will not affect your ability to perform the assessment as you can overwrite the default date within each function.

6 Entering invoices

You may be feeling that you have been working hard but have not actually accomplished much yet! This is one of the few off-putting things about accounting software: it can take quite a while to set everything up properly before you can really get started.

If you are feeling frustrated, just remember that you only have to set all these details up once. In future, the fact that all the data is available at the touch of a button will save you a vast amount of time, so it really is worth the initial effort.

6.1 Purchase invoices using the Batch Invoice function

Purchase invoices are created by your suppliers, whereas sales invoices are documents you create yourself. That means that it is usually simpler to enter purchase invoices, so we'll deal with those first.

At this level, we are entering basic invoice details. Although there is a function to enter invoices individually (**Purchases > Purchase Invoices > New invoice**), for this exercise we will use the Quick Entry function which allows you to enter basic invoice details for a number of suppliers in batches. Choose **Purchases > Quick Entries > New Quick Entry**) which brings up the **Quick Entry** screen as shown below.

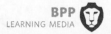

As always, you can use the **Tab** key to move between different parts of the screen.

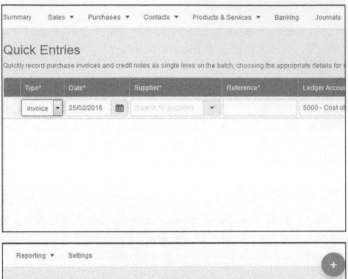

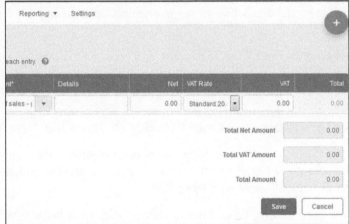

You can enter a number of different invoices from different suppliers on the same screen. You can also enter each line of the same invoice separately, if the invoice is for a variety of items that need to be coded to different nominal accounts. In this case, you should use the same supplier's invoice number in the **Reference** field of each line of the invoice. This will generate a warning message that a similar transaction exists; however, in this instance, this should be ignored and the program will still allow you to save the entries.

The following table explains what to do as you tab through each entry field. Pay particular attention to the **Net**, **VAT rate** and **VAT** fields.

SCREEN ITEM	HOW IT WORKS
Type	Select either Invoice to enter an invoice, or Cr Note to enter a credit note from the drop-down list (click on the button).
Date	The program date will be entered by default, but you can change this if you wish. Clicking the button will make a little calendar appear.
Supplier	Select the supplier account from the drop-down list (click on the button).
Reference	Type in the supplier's invoice number.
Ledger Account	This will show the default ledger expenditure account code associated with this supplier. If you need to change it, click on the button to see a list of nominal ledger accounts.
Details	Type in a brief but clear description of the item and be sure that your description will be understood by someone other than you. Usually, you will just need to copy the description on the supplier's invoice.
Net	Enter the net amount of the invoice, ie excluding VAT. If the invoice has several lines, you can enter each line separately but you should use the same reference for each line.
	If, in the assessment, you are only given the gross amount, (ie, the amount including VAT), the net amount is equal to the gross amount ÷ (1 + VAT rate). For example, £10 gross = 10 ÷ (1.20) = £8.33 net (where the VAT rate = 20%).
VAT Rate	Select the appropriate rate for the item (see 'Tax codes and VAT rates' section earlier). If this field does not appear, check that you have set up your VAT scheme correctly by choosing **Settings > Financial Year & VAT**.
VAT	This item will be calculated automatically, depending on the VAT rate selected. Check that it agrees with the VAT shown on the actual invoice. You can overtype the automatic amount, if necessary.

When you have entered all the invoice details, you post them simply by clicking on **Save**. This will post **all** the required accounting entries to the ledgers.

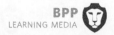

Task 8

Post an invoice from McAlistair Supplies dated 6 January 2016 for 2,000 sheets of A4 paper (net price: £20.35, ledger account: Publicity material) and a box of 100 blue promotional biros (gross price: £10.00, ledger account: Office costs). The invoice number is PG45783 and VAT is applicable on each transaction at the standard rate. **Save** and **Close**.

Write down the total amount of VAT.

£	

6.2 Nominal Activity Report

The first time you do this you will probably not quite believe that double entry to all the ledgers can be so easy. To check that the purchase invoice has been posted you can view the transaction in individual nominal ledger accounts. To check the nominal ledger, choose **Reporting > Nominal Activity**. This brings up a list of each ledger account. Select a date range in the **From** and **To** boxes that is around the transaction date of the invoice, eg 01/01/2016 to 31/01/2016.

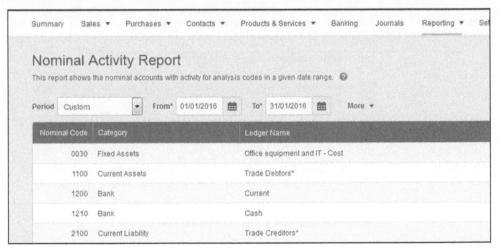

Depending on which type of transaction you posted (ie a customer invoice or supplier invoice) you should then click on either 1100 - Trade Debtors (the debtors ledger control account) or 2100 - Trade Creditors (the creditors ledger control account).

This brings up the **Detailed Nominal Activity** screen for the Trade Creditors account. You will see that the transaction has been correctly posted to the Trade Creditors Account, as shown in the screens below.

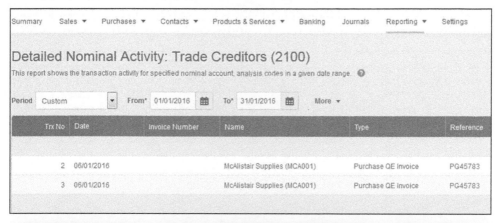

Reference	Description	Debit	Credit
	Opening Balance: 01/01/2016		0.00
PG45783	2000 sheets A4 paper		24.42
PG45783	100 x blue promo biros		10.00
	Closing Balance: 31/01/2016		34.42

What about the other accounts of the double entry that make up the full transaction? For the invoice from McAlistair Supplies, the double entry should be as follows:

DEBIT   VAT on purchases account (debit VAT amount)

DEBIT   Publicity Material (debit net amount)

DEBIT   Office costs (debit net amount)

CREDIT   Trade Creditors (credit gross amount)

You can also check that the transaction has been correctly posted to the Publicity Material account (A/C code 10000), the Office Costs account (A/C code 7500) and the VAT on purchases account (A/C code 2201) by running the Nominal Activity report as described above.

Furthermore, to check that the correct amounts have also been posted to the subsidiary account (ie the individual supplier account within the overall Trade Creditors account), open the supplier record (**Contacts > Suppliers > Click on McAlistair Supplies Ltd**) and click on the **Activity** tab.

This shows a list of all transactions that have been made to the supplier account at the bottom of the screen for a particular date range. If no transactions appear, you may need to change the date range in the **From** and **To** boxes. This list can also

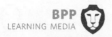

be refined by transaction type and outstanding amounts by clicking on the **Filters** button.

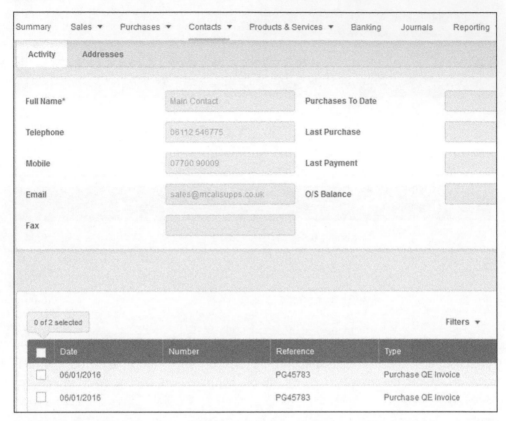

Finally, if you just want a quick look at the transactions you have posted, you can run the **Audit trail**. This shows a list of transactions that have been posted. Choose **Reporting > Audit Trail.** This shows a summary audit trail. Click on **Detailed** to see the detailed version.

Don't forget to ensure the date range is sufficient to include the transactions by selecting **Custom** from the drop-down list in the **Period** field, and specifying the date range in the **From Date** and **To Date** fields. This report can also be exported to a PDF or CSV file by clicking on the **Export** button.

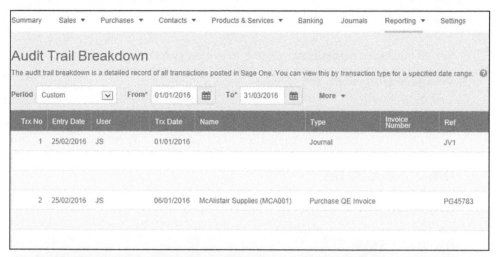

Ref	Ledger Account	Debit	Credit
JV1	Cash (1210)	250.00	0.00
	Capital introduced (3200)	0.00	3,000.00
	Current (1200)	2,750.00	0.00
PG45783	Publicity material (10000)	20.35	0.00
	VAT on Purchases (2201)	4.07	0.00
	Trade Creditors (2100)	0.00	24.42

6.3 Sales invoices – if no invoice is produced

Some businesses create sales invoices using a different system from their accounting software – for example, using word processing software such as Word. The invoices are then entered into the computerised accounting software.

If that is the case, then sales invoices are entered in exactly the same way as purchase invoices. To do this, click on **Sales** then **Quick Entries** and enter the invoices in a batch, in a similar way as you did for the purchase invoice above.

6.4 Sales invoices – if the program creates the invoice

In Sage One, you can produce printable invoices. If you wanted to do this, you could do so by clicking on **Sales > Sales Invoices** and then the **New Invoice** button. The invoice details can then be entered, saved and an invoice printed.

However, in the assessment you will be given a list of invoices or sample invoices to enter. Therefore, you should only enter invoices using the Quick Entry method described earlier, rather than creating an invoice.

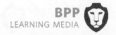

Task 9

(1)   Set up two more **suppliers** with the following details.

Widgets Unlimited Ltd
123 High Road
London
W23 2RG
020 8234 2345

Office Products Ltd
321 Low Road
London
E32 2GR
020 8432 5432

(2)   Process the purchase of:

(a)   10 widgets (Cost of sales - materials) from Widgets Unlimited Ltd for a total net cost of £80. Invoice number WU4474, dated 8 January 2016.

(b)   A computer (Office equipment and IT - Cost*) from Office Products Ltd for a net cost of £800. Invoice OP1231, dated 10 January 2016.

Both purchases attract VAT at the standard rate.

* If the 'Office equipment and IT – Cost' account does not appear in the list of ledger accounts to select from, this means that it is not visible within this particular function of the program. To make it visible choose **Settings > Chart of Accounts > Click on the Office equipment and IT – Cost account**. This brings up the **Edit Ledger Account** screen. To make this account visible in the Purchases function, make sure there is a tick in the check box next to the **Purchases – Invoice/Credit, Product/Supplier defaults** option in the **Visibility** section of this screen as shown below.

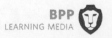

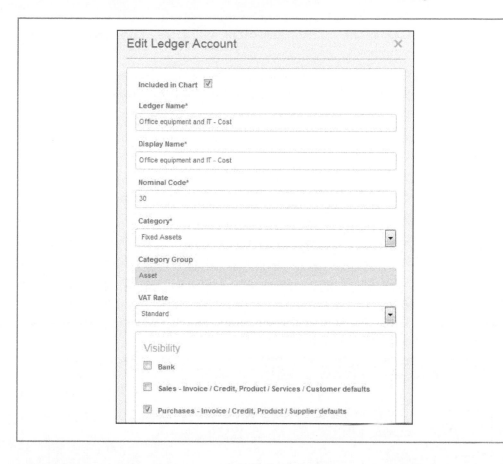

Task 10

(1)   Set up a new **customer** with the following details.

Alexander Ltd
501 Dart Road
Leeds
LS12 6TC
0113 245 3241
info@alexander.co.uk

30 days' credit (payment due days)
All other fields can be left blank.

(2)   Set up a new nominal code called 'Sales Type B'.

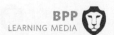

(3) Post the following two invoices (remember, you have to use **Save** to post them) to this customer:

(a) Invoice number 001: Product: 10 widgets at a selling price (net) of £20 each. VAT to be charged at standard rate. Date: 15 January 2016.

(b) Invoice number 002: Service: Advice on widgets, at a fee of £50 (net). VAT to be charged at standard rate. Date: 25 January 2016.

(4) Change the names of the nominal ledger accounts 'Sales Type A' and 'Sales Type B' as necessary to accommodate the different sales types in (3).

Task 11

As you should know from previous studies, a trial balance is a list of balances of all the ledger accounts. Preview a trial balance at this stage. Select **Reporting > Trial Balance**, set the **Period** as **Custom** from the drop-down list, and specify the date range as 01/01/2016 to 31/01/2016.

		Debit	Credit
0030	Office equipment and IT - Cost	800.00	
1100	Trade Debtors	300.00	
1200	Current	2,750.00	
1210	Cash	250.00	
2100	Trade Creditors		1,090.42
2200	VAT on Sales		50.00
2201	VAT on Purchases	181.74	
3200	Capital introduced		3,000.00
4000	Sales - products		200.00
5010	Cost of sales - materials	80.00	
7500	Office costs	8.33	
10000	Publicity material	20.35	
10001	Sales - services		50.00
	TOTAL	£4,390.42	£4,390.42

6.5 Credit notes

If a supplier issues a credit note, for example to account for a return of goods, or to correct an error on their part, a standalone credit note should be entered. This is posted in exactly the same way as a supplier invoice, in the Quick Entries screen, except that you select **Cr Note** instead of **Invoice** in the **Type** field.

Customer credit notes can be posted in this way too.

If you have posted a supplier invoice with errors you made yourself and want to correct it, although the program allows you to amend the original invoice, we recommend that you correct it with a standalone credit note. This provides a clearer audit trail.

7 Help!

7.1 Help in Sage

If ever you are unsure about how to perform a task in Sage, take a look on the online **Help page**. This is accessed by pressing the 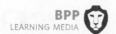 button.

We recommend you explore the options shown below in the Help page. There are a number of useful guides on how to perform common tasks.

To search for help on a specific topic, enter the topic into the search bar and click on the magnifying glass icon in the right of the bar.

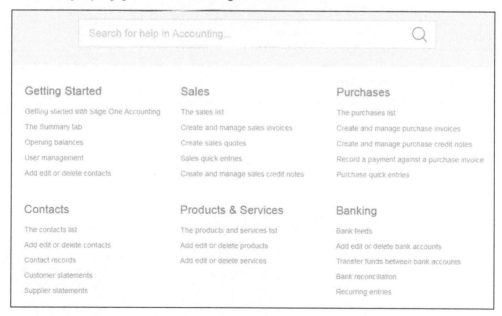

Experiment with this; the ability to find out how to do something yourself could come in handy in your work and in your assessment.

7.2 Help from your manager and others

Whenever you are unsure about what to do, or are faced with an error message you are unsure about, the golden rule is to **ask for help or advice**.

Don't ignore error messages. If possible, have your manager or someone more senior look at the message immediately and advise you on what action to take. If you need to provide details for someone if they can't get to your screen to view it, take a screenshot for them.

Chapter overview

- Accounting software programs range from simple bookkeeping tools to more complex software. Sage's products are among the most popular software programs in the UK.

- Assessments may involve setting up new customer and supplier accounts, posting journals, invoices, payments and receipts, and producing reports or other types of output.

- New nominal ledger accounts can be set up using the accounting software program's chart of accounts.

- VAT is dealt with by assigning the correct VAT rate to a transaction.

- New customer and supplier accounts should be given consistent and meaningful codes.

- Familiarise yourself with the Help feature; it could come in handy both in your work and in your assessment.

- Never ignore error messages – ask for help or advice from your manager.

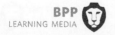

Keywords

- **Activity:** the transactions that have occurred within an account

- **Chart of accounts:** a template that sets out the nominal ledger accounts and how they are organised into different categories

- **Customer:** a person or organisation that buys products or services from your organisation

- **Customer record:** the details relating to the customer account, for example name and address, contact details and credit terms

- **Defaults:** the entries that the accounting software program expects to normally be made in a particular field

- **Field:** a box on screen in which you enter data or select from a list (similar to a spreadsheet cell)

- **General ledger:** the ledger containing the income statement (profit and loss) and statement of financial position (balance sheet) accounts

- **Ledger accounts:** accounts in which each transaction is recorded

- **Nominal ledger:** another term for General Ledger; Sage uses this term for the ledger containing the income statement (profit or loss) and statement of financial position (balance sheet) accounts

- **Supplier:** a person or organisation that your organisation buys products or services from

- **Supplier record:** the details relating to the supplier account, for example name and address, contact details and credit terms

- **Trade creditors ledger:** the collection of supplier accounts, also known as the purchase ledger

- **Trade debtors ledger:** the collection of customer accounts, also known as the sales ledger

- **VAT rate:** the percentage rate of Value Added Tax on a transaction

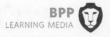

Test your learning

1 What is a 'field' in an accounting software program?

2 What do you understand by the term 'default'?

3 What is a chart of accounts?

4 What must be set up before a supplier invoice can be posted?

5 How would a supplier invoice be assigned to the correct nominal ledger account?

6 If you attempt to post a journal that does not balance, the difference will be posted to a suspense account. True or false? Explain your answer.

7 If a purchase invoice has five separate lines, should these be posted individually or is it sufficient just to post the invoice totals?

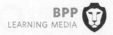

Sage One – Part 2

4

Chapter coverage

The topics covered in this chapter follow on from where you should have reached in Chapter 3.

The subjects covered in this chapter are:

- Payments and receipts
- Bank reconciliations
- Reports and other types of output
- Error correction
- Irrecoverable debts
- Month-end procedures

1 Payments and receipts

Your assessment may include details of payments and receipts to enter into the accounts. These could comprise cash, cheques and automated payments.

You need to be able to distinguish between cheques that you have sent to **suppliers** and cheques received from **customers**. If it is a cheque that you have paid out to a SUPPLIER you may only be shown the cheque stub (that's all you would have in practice, after all), such as illustrated below.

```
┌─────────────────────────────────┐
│                                 │
│   Date      ........................  │
│                                 │
│   Payee     ........................  │
│                                 │
│             ........................  │
│                                 │
│             ........................  │
│                                 │
│             ........................  │
│                                 │
│   £         ........................  │
│                                 │
│             000001              │
└─────────────────────────────────┘
```

If it is a cheque that you have received from a customer, you may be shown the cheque itself.

```
┌──────────────────────────────────────────────┐
│  Lloyds TSB                      30-92-10     │
│                                               │
│  Benham Branch                  Date _____  │
│                                               │
│  Pay _____        │
│                                               │
│  _____   ┌──────────┐     │
│                              │          │     │
│  _____    └──────────┘     │
│                                               │
│                  FOR WHITEHILL SUPERSTORES    │
└──────────────────────────────────────────────┘
```

You can tell that this is a receipt because the name below the signature (here, Whitehill Superstores) will be the name of one of your customers.

In the assessment, you could also be given details of an electronic payment or receipt, for example, a BACS remittance advice detailing a receipt from a customer.

Alternatively, you may be shown a paying-in slip that may include receipts from several different customers.

Cheques etc.			Brought forward £			£50		
						£20		
						£10		
						£5		
						£2		
						£1		
						50p		
						20p		
						Silver		
			Whitehill	1468	75	Bronze		
			Superstores			Total Cash		
						Cardnet		
			G T				3818	75
			Summerfield	2350	00	Cheques etc.		
Carried forward £			Carried forward £	3818	75	Total £	3818	75
Date 23/01/2016		500001	FOR SFE MERCHANDISING			06325143		

1.1 Supplier payments

When you pay a supplier, it is important to allocate your payment to invoices shown as outstanding in the purchase ledger. Sage makes this very easy.

There are a number of different payment allocations that can occur in both the sales and purchase ledger. Usually, you will pay most invoices in full or take a credit note in full; however, there may be reasons why an invoice may only be partially paid, due to disputes or cash flow problems. These are unsurprisingly known as 'part payments'. Occasionally, you may not be able to allocate a payment or receipt because it is for an invoice not on the system or the amount does not match with your ledger. In these cases, the payment is recorded against the correct account but not to any particular invoice or credit note and these are known as 'payments on account'.

Discounts can be allowed on payments received from customers (or received on payments made to suppliers), and a discount field is available to make a note of these amounts.

Payments allocated to invoices

To post a payment to a supplier, click on **Banking** on the main screen and then click on the required bank account. Then select **New Entry > Purchase/Payment > Supplier Payment**.

You are presented with the Supplier Payment screen. If you enter McAlistair Supplies Ltd in the **Supplier** field, the bottom half of the screen shows details of the outstanding invoices, as shown below.

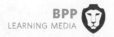

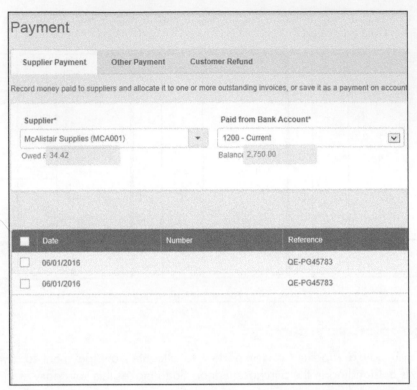

Payment

Supplier Payment	Other Payment	Customer Refund

Record money paid to suppliers and allocate it to one or more outstanding invoices, or save it as a payment on account

Supplier*

McAlistair Supplies (MCA001) ▼

Owed £ 34.42

Paid from Bank Account*

1200 - Current ▼

Balance 2,750.00

☐	Date	Number	Reference
☐	06/01/2016		QE-PG45783
☐	06/01/2016		QE-PG45783

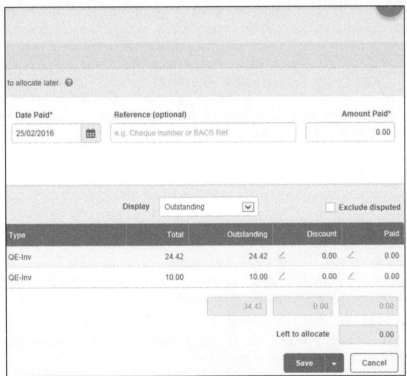

to allocate later. ❷

Date Paid*

25/02/2016 📅

Reference (optional)

e.g. Cheque number or BACS Ref

Amount Paid*

0.00

Display Outstanding ▼   ☐ Exclude disputed

Type	Total	Outstanding		Discount		Paid
QE-Inv	24.42	24.42	∠	0.00	∠	0.00
QE-Inv	10.00	10.00	∠	0.00	∠	0.00
		34.42		0.00		0.00

Left to allocate   0.00

Save ▼   Cancel

The following table explains the quickest way to post a payment and allocate it to supplier invoices. Press **Tab** to move from one field to the next.

SCREEN ITEM	HOW IT WORKS
Supplier	Enter the supplier name or supplier code. Entering the first few characters will bring up a list of suppliers which you can select from.
Paid from Bank Account	Select the bank account from which the payment was made from the drop-down list.
Date Paid	Enter the date the payment was made. The program date will be entered by default, but you can change this by clicking on the 📅 calendar button.
Reference	This is an optional field but can be used to enter a reference to identify the transaction, eg a cheque number. If you are making a payment directly from the bank account such as a BACS payment, you can put the BACS reference in this field. This will help with bank reconciliations.
Amount Paid	Though it might seem odd, leave this at 0.00 when paying an invoice in full, as it will automatically be filled in when you select the invoice.

For the Amount Paid field, the following content appears:

Select the required invoice for payment by ticking the check box next to it.

	Date	Number	Reference
☑	06/01/2016		QE-PG45783
☐	06/01/2016		QE-PG45783

Using this method, the **Amount Paid** field updates each time you select an invoice.

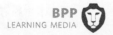

	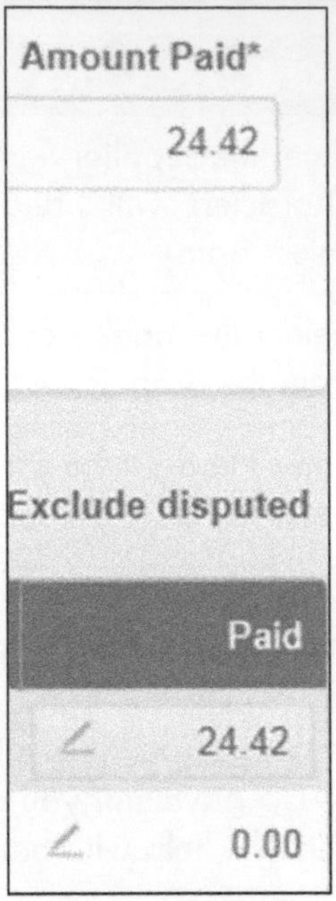 Amount Paid* 24.42 Exclude disputed Paid ∠ 24.42 ∠ 0.00
Discount	Tab past this if there is no discount. However, if you do need to process a discount, this brings up a screen where you should enter the discounted amount in the **Amount to pay** field and the program will calculate the discount. Then click **Apply**.
Save	This saves to all the ledgers.
Owed	This shows the total outstanding balance.
Balance	This shows the current bank balance for the selected bank account.

You don't need to pay all the outstanding invoices if you don't want to. You can just click on **Save** when you've paid the ones you want.

When you click on Save, this will post the transaction to the relevant accounts. Make sure you have all the correct information before you save.

This is the quickest way of posting a payment in ordinary circumstances.

Part payments

There may be times when you don't want to pay invoices in full. For instance, you may decide to pay the supplier in the illustration above only £20.00 for the selected invoice, perhaps because of some problem with the items supplied. In that case, proceed as follows.

BPP
LEARNING MEDIA

SCREEN ITEM	HOW IT WORKS
Supplier	As before
Date Paid	As before
Ref	As before
Amount Paid	Though it might seem odd, leave this at 0.00
Paid	Click in this field and the following screen comes up Part Pay ✕ Enter the amount you want to pay. Reference Outstanding 24.42 Amount to pay 20.00 Discount 0.00 New outstanding amount 4.42 Apply Cancel
Amount to pay	Type in the amount you want to pay
Discount	Tab past this
Apply	This applies the payment to the main payment screen

Applying a credit note to a payment

A further possibility is that there will be a credit note on the account as well as invoices. When you reach the credit note line in the list of outstanding items in the bottom half of the screen, click the check box and the **Amount Paid** field will be reduced by the credit note amount.

Unallocated payments (payment on account)

There may be times when you need to record a supplier payment but are unable to allocate it to an invoice, either partially or wholly.

For instance, you may decide to pay the supplier in the illustration above only £10.00 but not apply this yet to an invoice(s). In that case, proceed as follows.

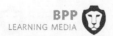

SCREEN ITEM	HOW IT WORKS
Supplier	As before
Date Paid	As before
Ref	As before
Amount Paid	Enter the amount paid

Click on **Save** and a warning screen comes up asking you to confirm that you want to save the unallocated payment on account. Click **Yes**.

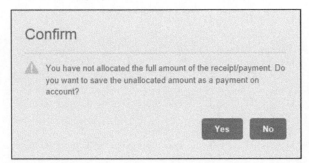

Such payments should be allocated as soon as the relevant information or invoice is available.

Note that VAT is not accounted for on supplier payments. VAT will have already been accounted for when the supplier invoice was posted. Other types of payment may require VAT to be accounted for when the payment entry is made (see 'Other payments and receipts' below).

Task 1

Post a payment on 31/01/16 made with a reference of 158002 to McAlistair Supplies Ltd for the total of invoice PG45783. Remember to click **Save** to effect the posting.

When you post a supplier payment, you also have the option of generating a remittance advice, to be sent to the supplier to inform them of the invoices your business is paying. To do this, you use the **Print Remittance** button available by clicking the down arrow next to the **Save** button. Note that this will save the payment and generate the remittance in one action. You may be asked to generate a remittance during your assessment.

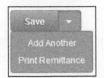

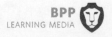

An example is given in the screenshot that follows. You can try this for yourself and generate a remittance.

To recall the payment made in Task 1, click on **Banking,** select **Current,** and then click on the **Activity** tab further down the screen. If you can't see the payment, make sure the **From** and **To** dates are sufficient to include the date of the payment. You can then select the payment from the list.

When you click on **Print Remittance**, this generates the remittance in a new window in your internet browser, similar to that shown below. This can then be saved to your computer as a PDF from your internet browser menu.

SFE Merchandising

SFE Merchandising
14b Hapgood House Dagenham Avenue Benham DR6 8LV

Telephone: VAT Number
07796786718   GB 524376451

McAlistair Supplies (MCA001)

52 Foram Road Winnesh DR3 5TP

Remittance Advice

Reference: 158002   Date Paid: 31/01/2016   Amount Paid: 34.42

Ref	Number	Date	Total Amount	Amount Paid
PG45783		06/01/2016	24.42	24.42
PG45783		06/01/2016	10.00	10.00
			Total Paid:	34.42

1.2 Customer receipts

When you receive money from your customers, it is important to allocate your payment to invoices shown as outstanding.

To record a receipt from an account customer, click on **Banking** on the main menu and then click on the required bank. Then select **New Entry > Sale/Receipt > Customer Receipt**.

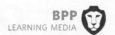

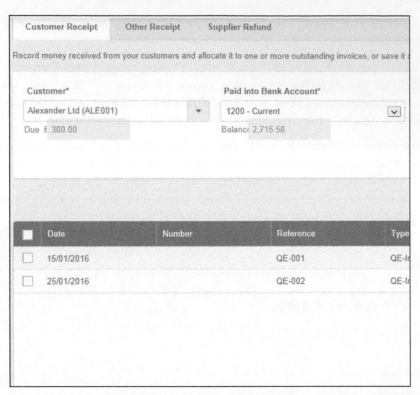

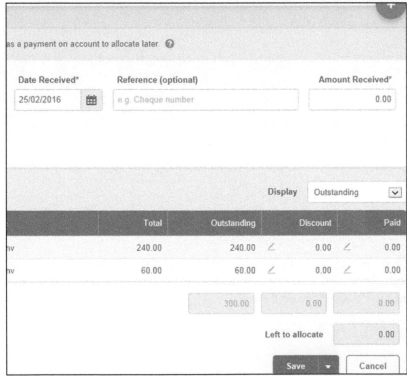

BPP
LEARNING MEDIA

Although this screen looks slightly different from the payment one, it works in exactly the same way, and we recommend that you use it in exactly the same way – in other words, tick the invoices that you have received payment for (which automatically updates the **Amount Received** field), and click on **Save**. If you have unallocated receipts or partial receipts, this works in the same way as described in the 'Supplier payments' section above.

If you are paying in cash and cheques to the bank, one important point to remember when posting receipts is that you should use the paying-in slip number (if you have it) for the **Reference**. This makes it much easier to complete bank reconciliations, because typically, several cheques will be paid in on a single paying-in slip and the bank statement will only show the total, not the individual amounts. If you receive payment electronically, you should use the reference that appears on your bank statement for the receipt, or on the remittance advice from the customer.

Task 2

Post a receipt from Alexander Ltd for £240. This was paid in using paying-in slip 500001 dated 31 January 2016. You should allocate this against Invoice 001. Remember to click **Save** to effect the posting.

1.3 Other payments and receipts (non-credit transactions)

Some payments and receipts do not need to be allocated to customers or suppliers (ie non-credit transactions). Examples include payments like wages and receipts such as cash sales.

If your assessment includes transactions like this, you should post them by clicking the **Banking** tab on the main screen and then clicking on the required bank account.

Then select **New Entry > Sale/Receipt > Other Receipt,** for a receipt (or **New Entry > Purchase/Payment > Other Payment,** for a payment).

You are presented with the **Other Receipt** screen similar to that shown below.

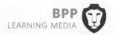

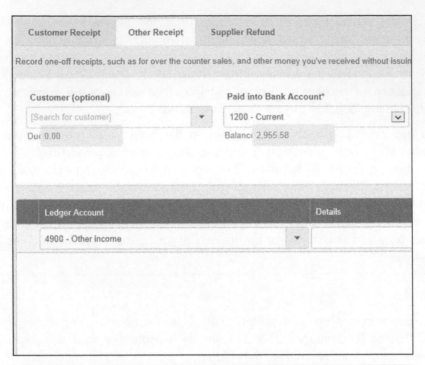

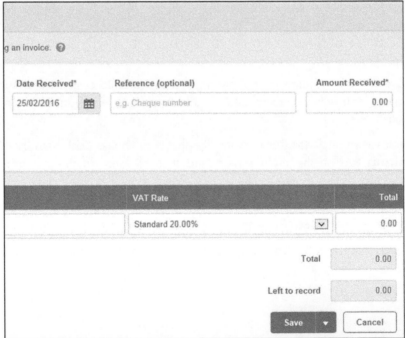

The main differences here to the customer receipt screen earlier are that you enter the amount of the receipt directly in the **Amount Received** field, and that you select the **Ledger Account** where the other side of the double entry for this transaction will be posted to. Note that you can split the receipt into different transactions by entering the details in a new line.

VAT on other payments and receipts

Another difference to the customer receipt screen is that you have to specify the VAT treatment of the transaction. VAT is not accounted for on a receipt of payment of a sales invoice from a credit customer (a customer receipt). This is because VAT will already have been accounted for when the sales invoice was posted.

However, for most 'other receipts,' including cash sales[1], the receipt and related sales transaction are recorded in this one transaction. Therefore you must account for any VAT applicable at this stage. Refer to the Tax Codes and VAT rates section in Chapter 3 for the VAT rates to use.

If the receipt or payment includes VAT, in this program, you should enter the **gross amount** of the receipt or payment. The program then automatically calculates the VAT, and posts it to the correct VAT ledger account when you save the entry.

(1)   The term 'cash sale' actually refers to a sale where the sale and receipt of payment occur at the same time. For example, a supermarket sells goods to customers who pay for them immediately – these are cash sales. The payment does not necessarily have to be in cash. Payment can also be by cheque, credit or debit card. Cash sales differ to 'credit sales' in that credit sales allow the customer to pay for the goods or services at a later date (typically 30 days later). Another example of cash sales is sales made online over the internet.

'Other payments' and 'other receipts' that don't involve sales or purchases (eg, wages, loans etc) do not attract VAT, and the VAT code to use in these cases is 'No VAT'.

Example of a non-credit transaction

The screen that follows shows an example of how online cash sales might be posted to the accounts using the method described above (don't carry out the transaction). Use the **Ledger Account** drop-down to find which ledger account to use (create a new one if there is not already an appropriate account, using the method described in Task 2 in Chapter 3 – remember to ensure the correct check-boxes are ticked in the Visibility section when creating the account to ensure that the account appears).

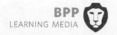

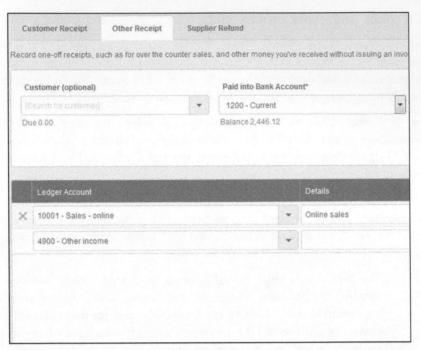

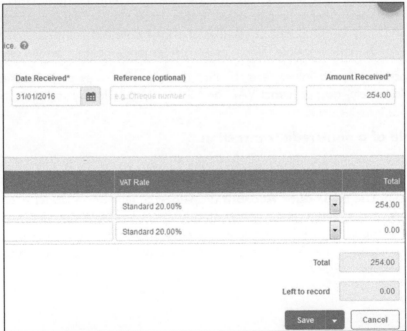

The screen for posting 'other payments' such as wages is exactly the same but instead of using the Other Receipts screen, you access the payments screen through **Other Payments**.

1.4 Direct debits and standing orders (recurring payments)

Many businesses have regular recurring payments, such as rent and rates, set up by standing order or direct debit. It can be easy to forget to post these – especially as some may be monthly, some quarterly and so on. Sage One makes it easy to automate this process.

The process is described as follows but don't carry this out until Tasks 3 and 4. Firstly, you need to create and save the first payment using the 'Other Payments' function, as described above. Enter the reference as 'DD' if it is a direct debit, or 'STO' if it is a standing order. This will help identify the transaction when doing the bank reconciliation.

Then choose **Banking** and click on the bank account where the initial payment was created.

Go to the **Activity** screen and you will see the payment. Make sure that the date range is sufficient to include the payment by entering dates in the **From** and **To** fields.

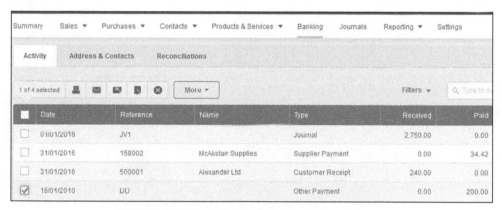

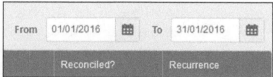

Click on the payment which brings up the details of the payment.

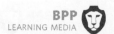

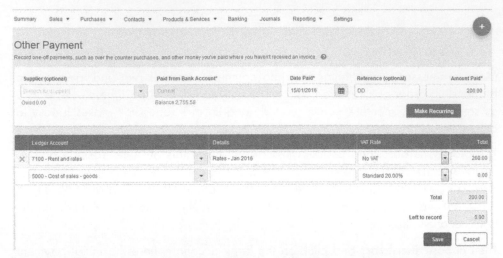

On this screen, click on the **Make Recurring** button; this will bring up a screen like the one that follows. It allows you to specify the frequency and end date of the recurring payment. Clicking on **Save** will activate the recurring payment. The program will then automatically post each payment on the specified date each month.

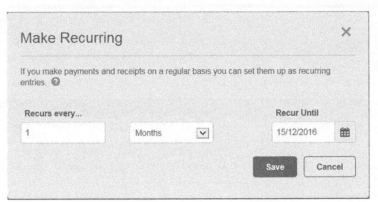

The recurring payment will be identifiable on the **Activity** screen within the banking screen with a ⇄ button next to it under the **Recurrence** heading.

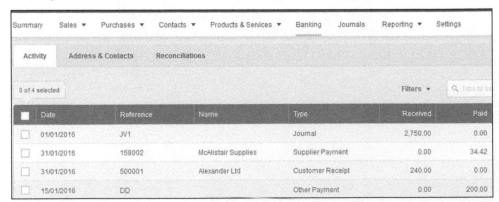

BPP
LEARNING MEDIA

Paid	Cleared	Reconciled?	Recurrence
0.00			
34.42			
0.00			
200.00			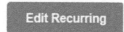

To view the details of the recurrence, click on the recurring payment shown in the **Activity** screen above, which brings up a screen showing the details of the payment. Then click on the **Edit Recurring** button in this screen.

Edit Recurring

This brings up the following screen which shows the details of the recurrence.

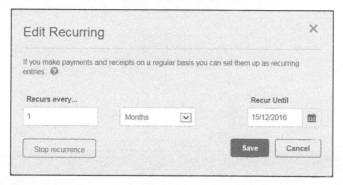

The example above shows how the details of a regular monthly payment for rates could be entered. Note that you may be asked to take screenshots of the screens shown above during the assessment as evidence of you setting up a recurring entry.

Note. In the assessment, as well as being asked to set up a recurring payment, you may be asked to process the first payment. Creating and posting the first payment, as described above, will cover the requirement of processing the first payment.

Task 3

Post the first rates payment shown in the example above, ie £200 for **January 2016 only**, starting on 15 January 2016.

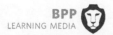

Task 4

Enter and save the recurring rates payment details shown in the example above, ie £200 per month for a further 11 months after the initial payment.

1.5 Petty cash

Petty cash transactions are posted in exactly the same way as non-credit bank payment and receipts (you should refer to the 'Other payments and receipts' section earlier), except that you use the petty cash ('Cash') bank account rather than the bank current account. As with non-credit payments and receipts, VAT is accounted for when entering the transaction for payment or receipt. Therefore, take care to use the correct VAT rate.

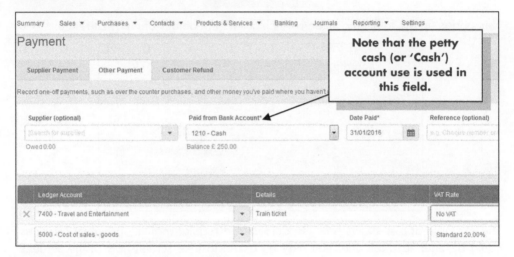

2 Bank reconciliations

As you should know from previous studies a bank reconciliation is a comparison between the bank balance recorded in the accounts and the balance on the bank statement. The differences are called reconciling items and are usually payments and receipts that have not yet cleared the bank account.

To access the bank reconciliation screens, you need to click on **Banking** and then click on the account you want to reconcile. In Sage, the default bank current account is account 1200 – Current. Select this and then click on the arrow next to the **Connect to Bank** button, and select **Reconcile**.

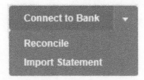

This brings up the **Bank Reconciliation** screen. The first part of this screen gives you the opportunity to enter the bank statement date and balance:

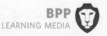

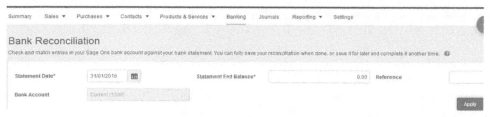

Bank Reconciliation

Check and match entries in your Sage One bank account against your bank statement. You can fully save your reconciliation when done, or save it for later and complete it another time.

Statement Date*	31/01/2016 📅	Statement End Balance*	0.00	Reference	
Bank Account	Current (1200)				Apply

Say that the closing bank statement balance is £2,790.00. That figure would be entered in the **Statement End Balance** box. If the statement is dated 31/01/2016 that can be entered in the **Statement Date** box. The reference field is optional but it is advisable to enter a reference such as the bank statement page number or the date of the reconciliation. Once you have entered these, click **Apply** to start reconciling.

In the main part of the **Bank Reconciliation** screen you will see that initially, all amounts are unmatched, as they do not have a tick in the **'Reconciled'** column:

Date	Reference	Name	Category	Received	Paid	Cleared	Reconciled?
01/01/2016	JV1		Journal	2,750.00	0.00		☐
31/01/2016	150002	McAlistair Supplies	Supplier Payment	0.00	34.42		☐
31/01/2016	500001	Alexander Ltd	Customer Receipt	240.00	0.00		☐
15/01/2016	DD		Other Payment	0.00	200.00		☐

This is also evident as the **Reconciled Balance** box at the bottom shows 0.00:

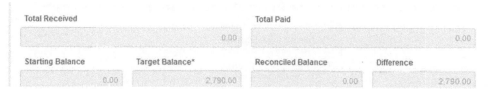

Total Received		Total Paid	
	0.00		0.00

Starting Balance	Target Balance*	Reconciled Balance	Difference
0.00	2,790.00	0.00	2,790.00

However, by looking at the bank statement, some of these transactions will be found to appear there. We can match these items. Say that the initial journal of £2,750 into the bank account, the rates payment of £200 and the receipt of £240 from Alexander Ltd are also on the bank statement. These can be selected and matched by ticking the check box next to the transaction in the **Reconciled?** column (note that if you accidentally match the wrong entry, then you can untick these).

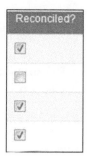

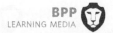

The bottom part of the **Bank Reconciliation** screen will then look as follows:

Total Received		Total Paid	
	2,990.00		200.00

Starting Balance	Target Balance*	Reconciled Balance	Difference
0.00	2,790.00	2,790.00	0.00

Reconciliation has been achieved! The target balance, ie Statement End Balance = Reconciled Balance. The unmatched item of £34.42 explains the difference between the statement balance of £2,790.00 and the Sage bank current account ledger balance of £2,755.58 at 31 January 2016.

Click on the **Finish** button to complete the bank reconciliation. If you have not finished, you can save the reconciliation for later by clicking on the **Save for later** button.

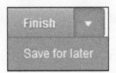

When you go back into the **Bank Reconciliation** screen, the incomplete reconciliation will be there. If you need to start again, you can select **Unreconcile all entries** from the **Interest and Charges** drop-down menu.

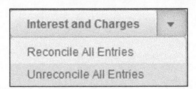

Task 5

Carry out the bank reconciliation explained in this section, as at 31 January 2016, assuming that the closing bank statement balance is £2,790.

Although we look at reports in detail later in the chapter, at this stage it is worth pointing out that you can generate a bank reconciliation report (a bank reconciliation statement) from the **Bank Reconciliation** screen.

You can see completed reconciliations by choosing **Banking,** clicking on required bank account, selecting the **Reconciliations** tab in the bottom half of the screen, and selecting a bank reconciliation.

Clicking on **Print** generates the bank reconciliation report in a new window in your internet browser, similar to that shown below. This can be saved to your computer as a PDF file from your internet browser menu.

SFE Merchandising

SFE Merchandising
14b Hapgood House , Dagenham Avenue, Benham, DR6 8LV,
United Kingdom

Telephone: 07796786718   **VAT Number** GB 524376451

Bank Account	Current (1200)			**Statement Date**	31/01/2016
Reference				**Reconciled By**	John See

Date	Reference	Name	Category	Paid	Received
01/01/2016	JV1		Journal	0.00	2,750.00
31/01/2016	500001	Alexander Ltd	Customer Receipt	0.00	240.00
15/01/2016	DD		Other Payment	200.00	0.00

Total Received	2,990.00
Total Paid	200.00
Starting Balance	0.00
Statement End Balance	2,790.00
Reconciled Balance	2,790.00
Difference	0.00

2.1 Adjustments for additional items on the bank statement

Even if you have posted all your transactions correctly, there is a good chance that there will still be items on the bank statement that you have not included in the accounts. Bank charges and interest are common examples.

Unrecorded bank transactions such as bank charges and interest paid or received should be entered using the method described in the **Other payments and receipts** section. Make sure you select the appropriate VAT rate and the appropriate nominal ledger code: 7900 - Bank charges and interest.

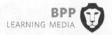

3 Reports and other types of output

3.1 The importance of reports generated by the accounting systems

One of the most important features of an accounting system such as Sage One is its ability to provide a range of useful accounting information very quickly. If transactions are entered correctly in the first instance, then accurate summaries or detailed analysis should be available at the click of a button.

To give a simple example of the use of a report by finance staff: **the aged debtors report** can be generated from Sage One (as we will see later) and this will show how old each customer balance is. This will alert staff in charge of credit control to those accounts that are overdue and need chasing for payment, without them having to look back at the invoice dates.

The majority of the reports we will look at are usually produced periodically and used to check on the accuracy of the records.

We will look at generating a **nominal activity report**, which details all the transactions in a period in each account. A quick review of this report can help to identify errors, for example, transactions posted to the wrong account. The trial balance generated by the accounting system may also highlight errors, for example, if a suspense account has been set up and not yet been cleared.

We looked at bank reconciliations earlier and checking the related report against the bank statements is an important procedure that should be carried out regularly.

The various reports can also be used to gain an overview of different financial areas and as a tool when dealing with customers and suppliers. Areas focused on might include identifying and dealing with overdue customer invoices (aged debtors), seeing which suppliers are due for payment (aged creditors) and establishing the cash available to the business to meet its commitments (bank related reports).

3.2 Generating reports

When you have finished entering transactions, the final task in your assessment will be to generate some reports.

Sage One offers you a large number of different standard reports. Although the pre-prepared reports that are available in Sage don't all have names that you will immediately recognise from your knowledge of manual accounting systems, rest assured that everything you are likely to be asked to produce in an assessment can easily be found.

One or two reports, such as customer statements, have their own buttons within the functions they relate to but, in general, to generate most other reports, click on **Reporting** and you are presented with a suite of reports.

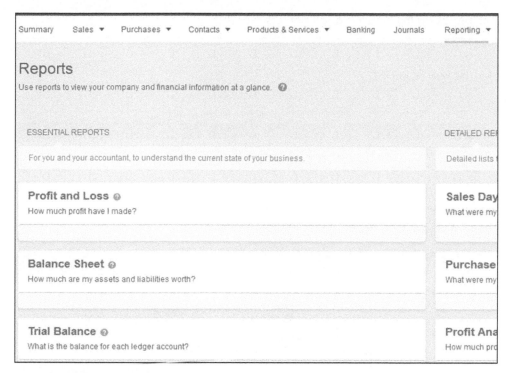

Aged Debtors Report

Click on **Aged Debtors** to generate a summary aged debtors report. Clicking on calendar icon next to the **To** field allows you to select the date you want to report the aged debtors up to.

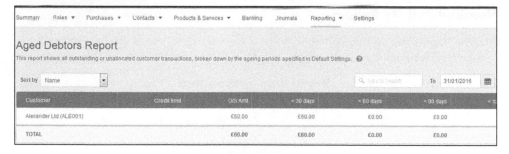

To view a detailed report, click on the **Detailed** button.

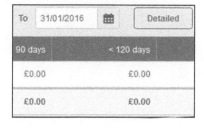

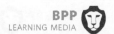

This brings up the detailed aged debtors report:

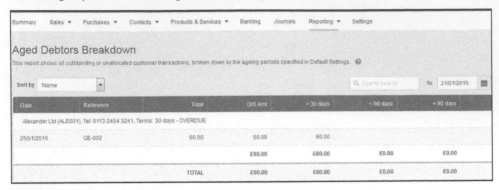

The next step is to select the type of output you require.

Use the **Export** button to export the report as a PDF file and save it to your computer. Please refer to the 'Exporting to PDF file' section in Chapter 3 for details on how to do this.

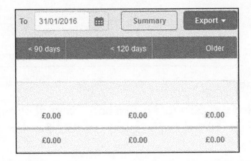

Nominal Activity Report

Another key report is the Nominal Activity Report. This details all the transactions in a period for each account.

To run this report, choose **Reporting > Nominal** Activity. You are initially presented with a screen similar to that shown below which shows a summary of the debits and credits posted to each nominal ledger account for the specified period.

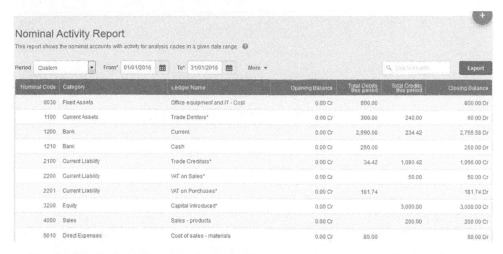

Select the **Period** as **Custom** from the drop-down list, and specify the date range as 01/01/2016 to 31/01/2016 in the **From** and **To** date fields.

The **More** button allows you to refine the report by category, or by a specific ledger account. You can select the ledger account from the drop-down list in the **Ledger Account** field.

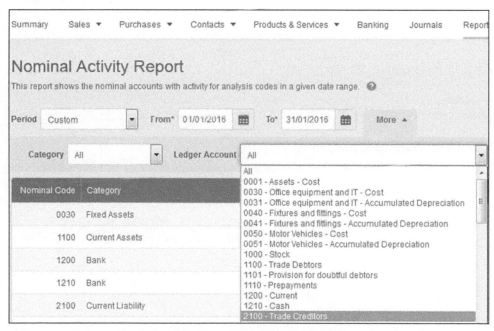

To see each transaction in the selected nominal ledger account, click on the summary line for that account to view the detailed activity.

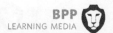

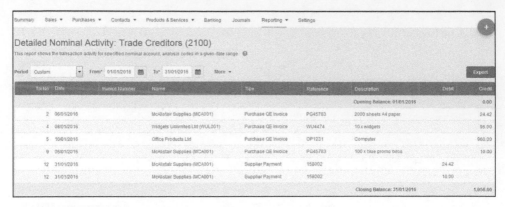

Use the **Export** button to export the report as a PDF file and save it to your computer. Please refer to the 'Exporting to PDF file' section in Chapter 3 for details on how to do this.

Audit Trail

The **Audit Trail** report provides a detailed breakdown of all transactions posted to Sage One. This can be accessed by choosing **Reporting > Audit Trail.** This brings up a summary report. Click on the **Detailed** button to get the detailed report.

Detailed

The detailed report looks similar to this:

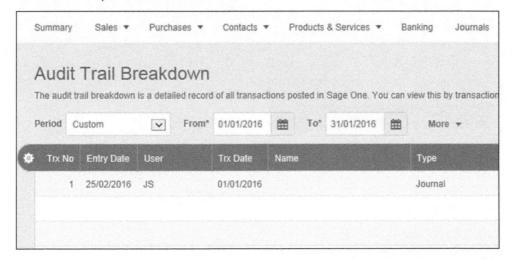

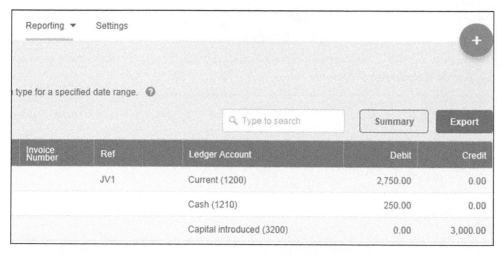

You should ensure that the date range covers every transaction you have entered. To specify the date range, select **Custom** from the **Period** drop-down list and specify the date range in the **From** Date and **To** Date fields.

This will generate a list of all the transactions, numbered in the order in which you posted them. If you need to, you are also able to refine the report by a particular type of transaction, eg journals, by clicking on the **More** button and then selecting **Journal** from the drop-down list in the **Type** field, as shown below.

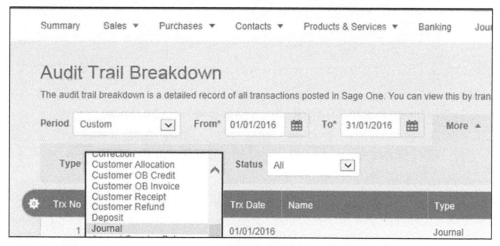

You can search for a particular transaction by entering the amount of the transaction or, more specifically, the transaction reference in the search box.

Generating an Audit Trail report is also a syllabus requirement, and part of this requirement is for the report to show bank reconciled transactions. This can be done on the Audit Trail report by adding a specific column for bank reconciled transactions. To do this, click the button that looks like a cog at the left end of the menu bar as shown below.

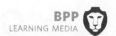

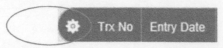

This brings up the following selection of columns. Click on the check-box next to the **Bank Reconciled** option.

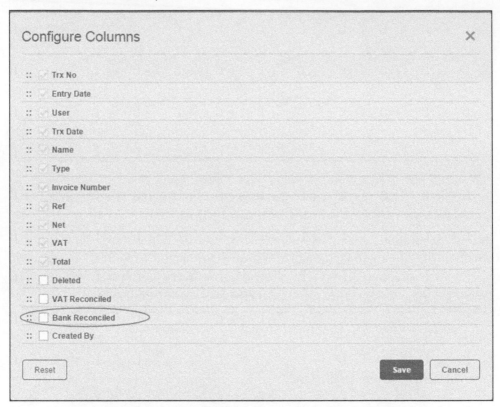

A column entitled **Bank Reconciled** is now included in the report.

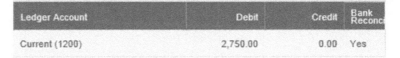

Ledger Account	Debit	Credit	Bank Reconc...
Current (1200)	2,750.00	0.00	Yes

Note. If you cannot see the **Bank Reconciled** column at this stage, you may need to reduce the size of the screen by holding the **Ctrl** and **–** keys at the same time.

Use the **Export** button to export the report as a PDF file and save it to your computer. Please refer to the 'Exporting to PDF file' section in Chapter 3 for details on how to do this.

3.3 Invoices and statements

Some reports, such as invoices and statements, may be intended to be printed on pre-printed stationery. Remember that when you preview these documents on

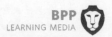

screen, you will see words and figures on plain paper. This is obvious if you think about it, but we mention it because it surprises some new users.

To produce a customer statement, choose the customer by **Contacts >** **Customers >** click on the customer **> Manage > Statements**.

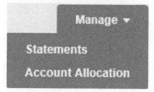

Select the date you want the statement up to in the **To** field and the statement appears on screen.

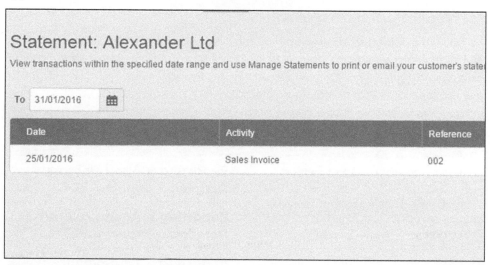

Clicking on **Manage Statement** gives you options for the output of the statement.

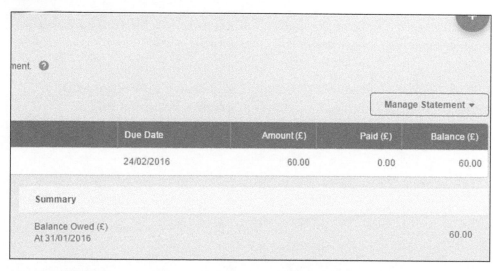

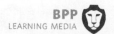

You should select **Print** and this will generate the statement in a new window in your internet browser. You can then save the statement as a PDF file to your computer using the menu in your internet browser.

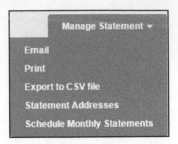

3.4 Reports in assessments

The following table lists the reports you may be asked for in an assessment, with brief instructions explaining how to obtain them in Sage One. Make sure that you select appropriate dates for your reports in the **Period** field and don't forget to save the reports as PDF files to your computer.

REPORT DESCRIPTION	REPORT NAME (Sage One)	WHERE TO FIND IT
Balance owed from each customer	Aged Debtors	**Reporting > Aged Debtors > Detailed > Export > PDF**
Balance owed to each supplier	Aged Creditors	**Reporting > Aged Creditors > Detailed > Export > PDF**
A list of balances all nominal ledger accounts	Trial Balance	**Reporting > Trial Balance > Export > PDF**
A list of customer invoices and credit notes	Sales Day Book (includes Sales Returns)	**Reporting > Sales Day Book > Export > PDF**
A list of supplier invoices and credit notes	Purchase Day Book (includes Purchases returns)	**Reporting > Purchases Day Book > Export > PDF**

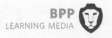

REPORT DESCRIPTION	REPORT NAME (Sage One)	WHERE TO FIND IT
All transactions with each customer	Customer Activity	**Contacts > Customers >** click on the check box next to the required customer **> More > Activity Report > Generate** To select all customers, click on the check box on the menu bar next to 'Company/Name'. Note that receipts allocated to transactions in the customer accounts are identifiable as they have 0.00 in the 'Outstanding' column.
All transactions with each supplier	Supplier Activity	**Contacts > Suppliers >** click on the check box next to the required supplier **> More > Activity Report > Generate** To select all suppliers, click on the check box on the menu bar next to 'Company/Name'. Note that payments allocated to items in the supplier accounts are identifiable as they have 0.00 in the 'Outstanding' column.
Statements of account to credit customers	Customer Statements	**Contacts > Customers >** click on the required customer **> Manage > Statements > Manage Statement > Print**
Advice of payment to a supplier showing invoice(s) paid	Remittance Advice	**Banking >** click on the required bank account **> Activity > click on the required payment > Print remittance (drop down next to Save button)**

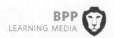

REPORT DESCRIPTION	REPORT NAME (Sage One)	WHERE TO FIND IT
Audit trail – a list of every transaction entered into Sage including journal entries in order of entry.	Audit trail	**Reporting > Audit Trail > Detailed > Export > PDF** If you can only see the 'Summary' button, this means you are already in the detailed report. Make sure that you configure the columns in this report to include 'Bank Reconciled' transactions as described earlier in the Audit Trail Report section earlier.
All transactions within nominal ledger accounts	Nominal Activity	**Reporting > Nominal Activity > Export > PDF** This will generate a report for all Nominal ledger codes. To generate a report for one account, click on **More** and select the required ledger code from the **Ledger account** field.
Comparison of bank statement balance to bank nominal ledger account balance	Bank reconciliation	**Banking >** click on the required account > **Reconciliations >** click on the required reconciliation > **Print**
List of payments and receipts made from the bank account	Receipts & Payments Day Book	**Reporting > Receipts & Payments Day Book > More>** select required bank account > **Receipt/Payment > Export> PDF**

* **Note.** The syllabus requires you to generate an Audit Trail report to include details of all transactions, including details of items in the bank account that have been reconciled, and details of receipts/payments allocated to items in customer/supplier accounts. The Audit Trail report on Sage One does not indicate that receipts/payments have been allocated to items in the customer/supplier accounts. To get around this, you can run the **Customer/Supplier Activity** report, as described in the table above. Receipts/payments allocated to items in the customer/supplier accounts are identifiable, as they have 0.00 in the **Outstanding** column.

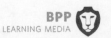

Task 6

Set up another customer as follows:

Springsteen Ltd
223 Home Town
Bradford
BD11 3EE

Process a sales invoice, Invoice no. 003, to this customer for £600 (net) for 20 Super-widgets, VAT at standard rate, invoice dated 26 January 2016.

Task 7

You notice that on 15 January the bank has debited your current account £10 for bank charges (no VAT). Enter this transaction.

On 31 January the bank credits you with £0.54 interest (no VAT). Rather than net this off against the Bank charges and interest account, you decide to set up a new nominal ledger account: Bank interest received, in the Other income category. Set up the new account and enter the transaction for the interest received.

Task 8

Go to **Reporting > Aged Debtors > Detailed**. Run the report up to 31/01/2016.

Export the report to a PDF and save it to your computer.

Open the PDF version and review your report. It should show all invoices as current.

3.5 Transfers

To transfer between bank accounts, including petty cash (cash in hand), you use the **Bank Transfer** option. For example, to transfer £100 from the bank current account to the cash in hand account, select **Banking > New Entry > Bank Transfer**. Select the **Paid from** bank account as the current account, and the **Paid into** bank account as the cash in hand account. Enter the date that the money was transferred in the **Amount Transferred** field. You may find it helpful to enter TRANS in the **Reference** field.

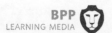

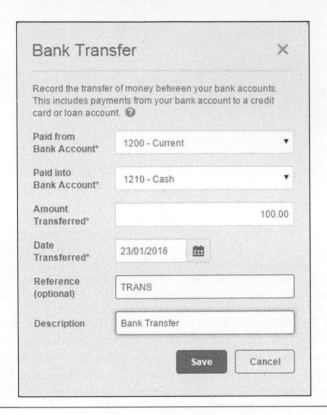

Bank Transfer ✕

Record the transfer of money between your bank accounts. This includes payments from your bank account to a credit card or loan account. ❓

Paid from Bank Account*	1200 - Current ▼
Paid into Bank Account*	1210 - Cash ▼
Amount Transferred*	100.00
Date Transferred*	23/01/2016 📅
Reference (optional)	TRANS
Description	Bank Transfer

Save Cancel

Task 9

On 23 January, you transfer £100 from the bank account into petty cash and immediately spend:

- £20 on train fares (zero rated for VAT)

- £10 (gross amount) on coffee mugs for the office (standard rated). The net cost of the mugs should be debited to General Expenses

Enter the above transactions.

Task 10

Extract a trial balance for all transactions up to 31/01/2016. If you wish, you can also preview a statement of financial position (balance sheet) and statement of profit or loss (profit and loss account). You will not have to do this in your case study, but they are easy documents to produce and it seems a pity not to have a look!

Reporting > Balance Sheet Report for the balance sheet

Reporting > Profit & Loss for the profit and loss account

 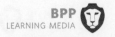

Your trial balance in Task 10 should look similar to the one that follows:

Nominal Code	Name	Selected Period	
		Debit	Credit
0030	Office equipment and IT - Cost	800.00	
1100	Trade Debtors	780.00	
1200	Current	2,646.12	
1210	Cash	320.00	
2100	Trade Creditors		1,056.00
2200	VAT on Sales		170.00
2201	VAT on Purchases	183.41	
3200	Capital introduced		3,000.00
4000	Sales - products		800.00
5010	Cost of sales - materials	80.00	
7100	Rent and rates	200.00	
7400	Travel and Entertainment	20.00	
7500	Office costs	8.33	
7900	Bank charges and interest	10.00	
8200	General Expenses	8.33	
10000	Publicity material	20.35	
10001	Sales - services		50.00
10003	Bank interest received		0.54
	TOTAL	£5,076.54	£5,076.54

4 Error correction

If you make an error when you are making your entries, it is relatively easy to correct.

Errors made when setting up customer and supplier accounts can be corrected simply by opening the relevant record and changing the data.

For transaction errors, some accounting software programs have the option of correcting transactions by amending the original entry. In Sage One, this option is available but cannot be done in certain circumstances, eg if an invoice has been allocated to a payment. Therefore, as a standard approach, we recommend correcting transactions with another transaction (eg a credit note, journal entry), rather than amending the original transaction. Besides, this is best practice in order to keep a clear audit trail.

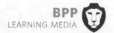

Customer invoices

If you have made a mistake on a customer invoice which has been posted, you need to create a credit note, either for the full amount and reissue the invoice, or for the difference. Credit notes are covered in Chapter 3.

Supplier invoices

If a mistake is made by a supplier on an invoice, they will normally send you a credit note, again either for the full amount, with a reissued invoice, or for the difference.

If you have made the mistake yourself, then you need to cancel the invoice, by entering a credit note with the same details.

Credit notes are covered in Chapter 3.

Other entries

Other entries should be corrected by journal entry. Students should also be able to post journal entries to correct their own errors that may occur during the assessment. The journal entry is covered in Chapter 3. For a clear audit trail, it is best practice to post a journal entry to reverse the original entry and then post a journal to re-do the transaction correctly.

Task 11

Let's say that the £20 payment entered in petty cash for a train fare should actually have been £15.

Correct this using a journal entry.

---

5 Irrecoverable debts

In the assessment you might be required to post a journal to write off an irrecoverable debt.

An irrecoverable debt or 'bad debt' as it is sometimes called, is a balance owing from a customer for invoices that will not be paid, perhaps because the customer has gone bankrupt or due to a dispute. Therefore the original invoice amount(s) needs to be written-off in the accounts.

The journal entry to write off an irrecoverable debt is as follows.

		£	£
DEBIT	Irrecoverable (bad) debt expense	GROSS AMT	
CREDIT	Customer account in trade receivables (debtors) ledger		GROSS AMT

Write-off an irrecoverable debt using a credit note

However, in Sage One you cannot use the journal function to post the entry above, as you cannot post directly to the customer account.

(Remember that each customer account is a subsidiary account of the overall trade debtors account, eg, customer account ALE001 is a subsidiary account of the overall trade debtors account – A/C 1100: 'Trade debtors' in Sage One).

Instead, you must use the credit note function. This was referred to in Chapter 3. To recap, select **Sales > Quick Entries > New Quick Entry.**

You are presented with the **Quick entries** screen. The entries you make will be similar to those for entering a sales credit note (ie, selecting **Cr Note** in the **Type** field), but with the following differences.

Ledger Account – select A/C 8100: 'Bad debts' (If this account is not available, ensure you tick the option: **Sales – Invoice / Credit, Product / Services / Customer defaults** in the **Visibility** section of the Edit Ledger Account function, described in the section under Task 3 in Chapter 3).

Net – enter the GROSS amount of the invoice(s) you are writing off

VAT Rate – select 'No VAT' as VAT does not apply at this stage.

For example, let's say you received notification that the customer Alexander Ltd has gone bankrupt, and therefore the balance of £60.00 (gross amt) for invoice no. 002 (created in Task 10, Chapter 3) will not be paid. You would enter the following transaction.

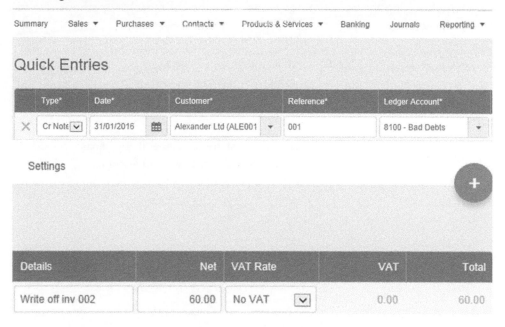

VAT treatment

The VAT treatment above might seem odd at first. You might expect that if you already paid VAT on the original invoice, you can now reclaim that VAT, by entering the net amount, and selecting the VAT Rate as Standard.

However VAT is not reclaimable on all bad debts, as there is a time limit. To comply with current HMRC guidelines, the gross amount is initially posted to the bad debts account, and if VAT is reclaimable, the VAT is separately transferred from the bad debts account to the VAT on purchases account.

6 Month-end procedures

In business there additional procedures that need to be performed at month-end. The main procedures are:

- Post prepayments
- Post accruals
- Post depreciation
- Close the month to prevent posting of further transactions

You do not have to perform these tasks in the Assessment but it is useful to be aware of these as you will undoubtedly encounter them in the workplace and/or future studies.

6.1 Starting over

All of us can have a bad day sometimes! Occasionally, you may find that you or someone else using the software has made a number of mistakes, perhaps due to a misunderstanding.

If this happens, it may well be better to start again rather than trying to correct all the mistakes, possibly making things worse. This can be done by resetting the data, as described in the Assessments section in Chapter 3. This is not normal practice in business of course; however, this function is purely for the Education market.

Note. This option should be taken as a last resort since it will erase all data, including any customers, suppliers and nominal codes you have set up.

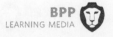

Chapter overview

- Payments and receipts should be allocated to outstanding invoices, as it is important to know which invoices have been paid.

- Bank reconciliations are very important controls in accounting systems and are easily accomplished in Sage One.

- All the reports that you are likely to require are available as pre-prepared reports.

- There are facilities for error correction, but it is best not to make errors in the first place!

Keywords

- **Bank reconciliation:** a checking process, whereby differences between an organisation's cash book entries, and the bank issued statement are identified. This gives assurance that the cash book is accurate

- **Customer:** a person or organisation that buys products or services from your organisation

- **Customer record:** the details relating to the customer account, for example name and address, contact details and credit terms

- **Payment allocations:** matching payments (either received or made) to relevant invoices and credit notes

- **Remittance advice:** document that lists all transactions that are being settled by a payment

- **Recurring payments:** payments (or receipts) that are made on a regular, periodic basis. Common examples are standing orders and directy debits

- **Reports:** form that summarises or analyses data that has been input to a computer system

- **Supplier:** a person or organisation that your organisation buys products or services from

- **Supplier record:** the details relating to the supplier account, for example name and address, contact details and credit terms

- **Trade creditors ledger:** the collection of supplier accounts, also known as the purchase ledger

- **Trade debtors ledger:** the collection of customer accounts, also known as the sales ledger

- **Unallocated payments:** payments or parts of payments that cannot be matched to specific transactions

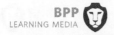

Test your learning

1   When you receive a payment from an account customer, this is posted using the Other Receipts button. True or false? Explain your answer.

2   Which report would you run to view the transactions posted to a particular ledger account?

3   Why can you not see supplier accounts on the nominal activity report?

4   Which report would you run to view the invoices and payments posted to a particular supplier account?

5   Transfers between bank accounts should always be processed by using the Journal facility. True or false?

6   Assuming VAT is applicable in both cases; why do you need to account for VAT on the receipt of payment for a cash sale, but not the receipt of payment for a credit sale?

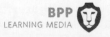

Answers to chapter tasks

Chapter 1 Sage 50 – Part 1

Task 1

This is a hands-on activity. You need to start either with a new instance of Sage, or a blank company.

Task 2

This is a hands-on activity. The Name should be Publicity material, the Type is Overheads, the Category is Printing and Stationery. Sage will suggest a Ref (account number) such as 7504 or 7506, and you should accept this. There is no opening balance to enter.

Task 3

Vimal could easily forget to give the account a proper name next time he uses the package and in future, he may not have any idea what sort of expense should be recorded in that account. Nobody else who uses the system will have a clue either. The moral of the story is, don't use abbreviations that others might not understand, and take care with spelling too. A bit of care will save time in the long run.

Task 4

It is possible for a customer and a supplier to have the same code, because it is quite possible that a business will both sell and buy goods from the same person. Although the accounts would use the same code, the accounts would be held in different ledgers.

Task 5

This is a hands-on activity. Use the **New** button or the **Wizard** button in the **Suppliers** function and fill in as much detail as possible. When you have finished, open your record and check the details on screen against those given. The illustration in the Task shows the code MCA001 (consistent with the alphanumeric format recommended earlier in the chapter).

Task 6

This is a hands-on activity. You can check that you have performed this action correctly by reviewing the supplier record; the defaults tab should show the nominal code for Publicity Material.

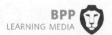

Task 7

This is a hands-on activity. Make sure that your journal has an appropriate reference and that each line has a description (use the F6 key for the second two lines).

You can check your journal by clicking the **Transactions** button or by looking at the activity of the nominal ledger accounts affected (**Nominal Codes >** select the nominal code **> Activity**.

Task 8

This is a hands-on activity. If you exit the program as suggested, remember to reset the date to 31/1/16 when you relaunch Sage.

Task 9

This is a hands-on activity. (Use the F6 key when entering the second line of the invoice, to save typing.) The total VAT is £5.74 (£4.07 on the first item, which was given **net**, and £1.67 on the second, where we told you the **gross** amount). Don't forget that you can use the F9 button to calculate the net amount.

Task 10

This is a hands-on activity. You should have set up the two suppliers, remembering to tick the 'terms agreed' box in the credit control tab (or in the wizard). You could also have changed the default nominal code for Office Products Ltd to Office Equipment (0030), as this is the type of purchase we have made from them. After setting up the two suppliers, you should have clicked on 'batch invoice' and entered these two transactions as per Task 9. After the task is complete, you should see a balance of £1,090.42 on your creditors control account.

Task 11

This is a hands-on activity. You should have decided to post the different types of sales (one was products, one was a service) to different sales accounts. You should have renamed the standard sales accounts in Sage to suit your particular business.

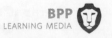

Chapter 2 Sage 50 – Part 2

Task 1

This is a credit transaction so use the 'supplier payment' option, <u>not</u> the 'bank payment' option.

Choose: Bank Accounts > Supplier Payments.

Task 2

This is a credit transaction so use the 'customer receipt' option, <u>not</u> the 'bank receipt' option.

Choose: Bank Accounts > Customer Receipts.

Task 3

Choose: Bank accounts > Recurring Items > Add.

The details you enter should match those shown in the Add/Edit Recurring Entry screen shot above Task 3 in Chapter 2 of the Text.

Task 4

Choose: Bank Accounts > Recurring Items, select the recurring payment and click on Process. Before you click on Process, the Postings Made column should show 0. Once you have processed the payment, the Postings Made column should show 1.

Task 5

To access the bank reconciliation screen choose: Bank Accounts > Select current account > Reconcile.

Follow the steps outlined in the Bank Reconciliation section of the Text, and check that your reconciliation matches that shown in the screen shot.

The only reconciling item between the bank statement balance (£2,790.00) and the ledger balance (£2,755.58) should be the payment to McAlistair Supplies of £34.42. The other bank transactions should be as reconciled.

Task 6

A new customer can be set up by choosing: Customers > New/Edit.

Task 7

Make sure you set up the new ledger account first. This can be done in the same way as in Task 2 in Chapter 1 (ie, click on Nominal Codes from the left side of the screen, and then click on the Wizard button).

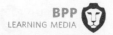
BPP LEARNING MEDIA

Task 8

Run the aged debtors report as instructed in the task, ie, Customers > Reports > Aged Debtors. You can export to a PDF file by clicking on the Export button, and saving to your computer.

Task 9

Firstly, use the bank transfer function to transfer £100 from the current account to the petty cash account. Choose: Bank Accounts > Bank Transfer.

The 'from' account' is 1200: Bank Current Account, and the 'to' account is 1230: Petty Cash.

Secondly, use the 'bank payment' function in the same way as in Task 1 above. Remember to select the correct tax code.

Note that you are given the gross amount for the coffee mugs. In Sage 50, you can enter the gross amount, and then press F9; the program will automatically calculate the VAT (of £1.67).

Task 10

Choose: Nominal Codes, > Reports > Trial Balance.

Select the period as Month 1, January 2016.

Check that your Trial Balance matches that shown in the Text. If there are differences, go back and work out where you were wrong. You can correct your errors using the methods described in the Error Correction section in Chapter 2 of the Text.

Task 11

Choose: Nominal Codes > Journal Entry. It is best practice to post a journal to reverse the incorrect entry, and then post another journal for the correct entry.

The reversal of the original entry is:

DEBIT	1230 – Petty Cash	20.00	
CREDIT	7400 – Travelling		20.00

The correct entry is:

DEBIT	7400 – Travelling	15.00	
CREDIT	1230 – Petty Cash		15.00

Chapter 3 Sage One – Part 1

Task 1

This is a hands-on activity. You need to start either with a new instance of Sage, or a blank company.

Task 2

This is a hands-on activity. The Ledger Name and Display Name should be Publicity material, the Category is Overheads. Sage will suggest a Nominal Code (account number) such as 10000 or 10001, and you should accept this. The opening balance is not entered at this stage.

Task 3

Vimal could easily forget to give the account a proper name next time he uses the package and in future, he may not have any idea what sort of expense should be recorded in that account. Nobody else who uses the system will have a clue either. The moral of the story is, don't use abbreviations that others might not understand, and take care with spelling too. A bit of care will save time in the long run.

Task 4

It is possible for a customer and a supplier to have the same code, because it is quite possible that a business will both sell and buy goods from the same person. Although the accounts would use the same code, the accounts would be held in different ledgers.

Task 5

This is a hands-on activity. Use New Supplier button and fill in as much detail as possible. When you have finished, open your record and check the details on screen against those given. The illustration in the Task shows the code MCA001 (consistent with the alphanumeric format recommended earlier in the chapter).

Task 6

This is a hands-on activity. The following fields should read as follows if you have performed this correctly: 'Set Credit Limit (£)': 5,000.00; 'Purchase Ledger Account': 10000 – Publicity material; and the 'Use default terms' field should be selected.

Task 7

This is a hands-on activity. Make sure that your journal has an appropriate reference and that each line has a description.

You can check your journal by generating the Audit trail report, or by generating the Nominal Activity report and looking at the detail of the nominal ledger accounts affected, if you wish.

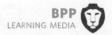

Task 8

This is a hands-on activity. The total VAT is £5.74 (£4.07 on the first item, which was given **net**, and £1.67 on the second, where we told you the **gross** amount). You can calculate the net amount by dividing the gross amount by (1 + VAT rate), ie £10.00 / 1.20.

Task 9

This is a hands-on activity. You should have set up the two suppliers, remembering to tick the 'terms agreed' box in the credit control tab (or in the wizard). You could also have changed the default nominal code for Office Products Ltd to 'Office Equipment and IT – Cost' (0030), as this is the type of purchase we have made from them. After setting up the two suppliers, you should have clicked on 'batch invoice' and entered these two transactions as per Task 9. After the task is complete, you should see a balance of £1,090.42 on your creditors control account.

Task 10

This is a hands-on activity. You should have decided to post the different types of sales (one was products, one was a service) to different sales accounts. You should have renamed the standard sales accounts in Sage to suit your particular business.

Task 11

This is a hands-on activity. Check your final balance to the one shown at the activity.

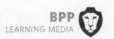

Chapter 4 Sage One – Part 2

Task 1

This is a credit transaction so use the 'supplier payment' option, <u>not</u> the 'other payment' option.

Choose: Banking > Select current account > New Entry > Purchase/Payment > Supplier Payment.

Task 2

This is a credit transaction so use the 'customer receipt' option, <u>not</u> the 'other receipt' option.

Choose: Banking > Select current account > New Entry > Sale/Receipt > Customer Receipt.

Task 3

You can create the first payment using the 'other payment function'.

Task 4

You can find the payment you made in Task 3 in the Activity screen within Banking.

Choose: Banking > Select current account > Activity.

Make sure that the dates in the From and To boxes are around the time of payment (15 January 2016), otherwise it will not show.

Clicking on the payment will show the details of the payment, including a 'Make Recurring' button. Click on this button to enter and save the details of the recurrence.

Task 5

To access the bank reconciliation screen choose: Banking > Select current account > Click on the drop-down arrow next to Connect to Bank > Reconcile.

Follow the steps outlined in the Bank Reconciliation section in the Text, and check that your reconciliation matches that shown in the screen shot.

The only reconciling item between the bank statement balance (£2,790.00) and the ledger balance (£2,755.58) should be the payment to McAlistair Supplies of £34.42. The other bank transactions should be as reconciled.

Task 6

A new customer can be set up by choosing: Contacts > Customer > New Customer.

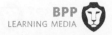

Task 7

Make sure you set up the new ledger account first. This can be done in the same way as in Task 2 in Chapter 3 (ie, choose: Settings > Chart of Accounts > New Ledger Account).

Task 8

Run the aged debtors report as instructed in the task, ie, Reporting > Aged Debtors > Detailed. You can export to a PDF file by choosing: Export > PDF, which will generate a PDF version which you can save to your computer.

Task 9

Firstly, use the bank transfer function to transfer £100 from the current account to the petty cash account. Choose: Banking > Select Current account > New Entry > Bank Transfer. The 'paid from account' is 1200: Current, and the 'paid to account' is 1210: Cash.

Secondly, use the 'other payment' function in the same way as in Task 1 above. Remember to select the correct VAT rates.

Note that you are given the gross amount for the coffee mugs. In Sage One, you should enter the gross amount, as the program will automatically calculate the VAT (of £1.67) and post it to the VAT on purchases account.

Task 10

Choose: Reporting > Trial Balance.

Select the Period as Custom and enter From: 01/01/2016 To: 31/01/2016.

Check that your Trial Balance matches that shown in the Text. If there are differences, go back and work out where you wrong. You can correct your errors using the methods described in the Error Correction section in Chapter 4 of the Text.

Task 11

Choose: Journals > New Journal. It is best practice to post a journal to reverse the incorrect entry, and then post another journal for the correct entry.

The reversal of the original entry is:

DEBIT	1210 – Cash	20.00	
CREDIT	7400 – Travel and entertainment		20.00

The correct entry is:

DEBIT	7400 – Travel and entertainment	15.00	
CREDIT	1210 – Cash		15.00

Test your learning: answers

Chapter 1 Sage 50 – Part 1

1   A field is a box on screen in which you enter data or select from a list (similar to a spreadsheet cell).

2   A default is the entry that the accounting package knows will normally be made in a particular field – for example, today's date or the nominal code that a purchase from a certain supplier would normally be posted to.

3   The chart of accounts is a kind of template setting out the structure of the nominal ledger – which accounts are classed as non-current (fixed) assets, which are current assets, which are current liabilities, which are expenses in the statement of profit or loss (income statement), and so on.

4   You must set up an account for the supplier in the purchase ledger before you can post an invoice received from the supplier.

5   You can either set a default nominal ledger expenditure account when you set up the supplier account, or you can choose the nominal ledger account at the time that you post the invoice.

6   This is false. The system will not allow you to post a journal that does not balance.

7   It is usually better to post the invoice lines individually. It is essential to do so if the individual expenses need to be posted to different nominal ledger codes.

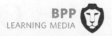

1   This is false. Receipts from customers with accounts need to be allocated to outstanding invoices. From the **Bank accounts** menu, these receipts are processed using the **Customer Receipt** button.

2   The **Nominal Activity report** shows the transactions that have been posted to each nominal ledger account.

3   Supplier accounts are subsidiary accounts of the **Trade Creditors account**. Therefore, supplier **transactions** are posted to this one account.

4   The **Supplier Activity report** shows the transactions that have been posted to each supplier account.

5   False. The transfer should be processed by selecting **Bank accounts**, selecting the required bank account and then selecting **Bank Transfer**.

6   For a credit sale, VAT is accounted for on the sales invoice sent to the customer, and not the subsequent receipt of payment by the customer. For a cash sale, the sale and receipt of payment occur at the same time in one transaction; therefore, VAT must be accounted for at this point.

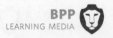

Chapter 3 Sage One – Part 1

1   A field is a box on screen in which you enter data or select from a list (similar to a spreadsheet cell).

2   A default is the entry that the accounting package knows will normally be made in a particular field, for example, today's date or the nominal code that a purchase from a certain supplier would normally be posted to.

3   The chart of accounts is a kind of template setting out the structure of the nominal ledger – which accounts are classed as non-current (fixed) assets, which are current assets, which are current liabilities, which are expenses in the statement of profit or loss (income statement), and so on.

4   You must set up an account for the supplier in the purchase ledger before you can post an invoice received from the supplier.

5   You can either set a default nominal ledger account when you set up the supplier account, or you can choose the nominal ledger account at the time that you post the invoice.

6   This is false. The system will not allow you to post a journal that does not balance.

7   It is usually better to post the invoice lines individually. It is essential to do so if the individual expenses need to be posted to different nominal ledger codes.

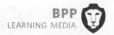

1   This is false. Receipts from customers with accounts need to be allocated to outstanding invoices using the **Customer Receipt** function. This is accessed from **Banking > Clicking on the required bank account > New Entry > Sale/Receipt > Customer Receipt**.

2   The **Nominal Activity report** shows the transactions that have been posted to each nominal ledger account.

3   Supplier accounts are subsidiary accounts of the **Trade Creditors account**. Therefore, supplier **transactions** are posted to this one account.

4   The **Supplier Activity report** shows the transactions that have been posted to each supplier account.

5   False. The transfer should be processed by selecting **Banking**, clicking on the required bank account and then selecting **Bank Transfer** from the **New Entry** drop-down list. Note that the transfer option is also available from the **New Entry** drop down list in the main **banking** screen

6   For a credit sale, VAT is accounted for on the sales invoice sent to the customer, and not the subsequent receipt of payment by the customer. For a cash sale, the sale and receipt of payment occur at the same time in one transaction; therefore, VAT must be accounted for at this point.

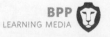

AAT AQ2016 SAMPLE ASSESSMENT USING ACCOUNTING SOFTWARE

Time allowed: 2 hours

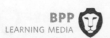

Using Accounting Software
AAT sample assessment

Assessment information:

The time allowed to complete this assessment is **2 hours.**

This assessment consists of **13 tasks** and it is important that you attempt them all.

- You will be asked to produce documents and reports to demonstrate your competence.

- You must then upload these documents so they can be marked by AAT.

All documents must be uploaded within the **total time** available. It is important that you upload **all** reports and documents specified in the tasks so your work can be assessed.

You will be able to attach and remove files throughout the duration of this assessment until you click on 'Finish', which will submit your assessment.

All uploaded documents should be saved and titled with the following information:

- evidence number
- your name
- your AAT membership number.

The evidence number to use for each document is stated in the table in Task 13.

Example

Your name is Simon White, and your AAT membership number is: 12345678

Evidence 1

A document showing all of the purchase invoices and credit notes (by purchase type) posted in June 20XX.

This document would be saved and uploaded as: Evidence 1 – Simon White – 12345678

If multiple documents are uploaded to show competency in an individual task, name these Evidence 1A and Evidence 1B and so on.

Unless the assessment asks for a specific format, you can choose the format which will best enable the marker to review and assess your work.

During the assessment, you will only make entries to the nominal ledger accounts you created in Task 3. You will not be required to make any entries to any accounts other than those you have already created.

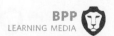

Information

The Graze Office Store is a UK furniture business. The business sells a mix of new and second-hand office furniture and has been trading successfully for five years. The owner, Kate Allen, has always used spreadsheets to carry out routine bookkeeping tasks. However the business has grown significantly over the last 12 months and Kate has decided to start using an accounting software package from 1 June 20XX onwards

Information relating to the business:

Business name:	The Graze Office Store
Business address:	1 Hope Street Cathertown Lumley LM61 2RT
Business owner:	Kate Allen
Accounting period end:	31 May (each year)
VAT Number:	781163367 (standard scheme)
VAT rate:	Standard rate VAT of 20% charged on all sales

Sales

Most of The Graze Office Store's income is generated from online sales where customers pay through an online payment system. The business also sells its items to other business in the north and south of the United Kingdom.

Kate likes to keep a record of the different sales made by the business, by sales type:

- online sales
- sales to shops - North
- sales to shops - South

You have been asked to carry out the bookkeeping tasks for June 20XX **only**, the first month that the business will be using computerised accounting software and the start of the new accounting period.

All documents have been checked for accuracy and have been authorised by Kate Allen.

Before you start the assessment you should:

- Set the system software date as 30 June of the current year.
- Set the financial year to start on 1 June of the current year.

Task 1 (3 marks)

Refer to the customer listing below and set up customer records to open sales ledger accounts for each customer, entering opening balances at 1 June 20XX.

Customer listing

Customer name and address	Customer account code	Customer account details at 1 June 20XX
Giffall Recruitment 3 High Street Meadowville ME2 6US	GIF001	Opening balance: £844.26 Payment term: 30 days
Happy Engineers Ltd 27 The Grange Totton TT21 2SA	HAP001	Opening balance: £1,425.65 Payment term: 30 days
Perry Cars 25 Edge Avenue Jeanpurt JE3 8TY	PER001	Opening balance: £4,680.00 Payment term: 45 days

Task 2 (3 marks)

Refer to the supplier listing below and set up supplier records to open purchase ledger accounts for each supplier, entering opening balances at 1 June 20XX.

Supplier listing

Supplier name and address	Supplier account code	Supplier account details at 1 June 20XX
Fabrics Delight Unit 3, The Dome Centre Whittingham Greater Whitt GW2 3TX	FAB001	Opening balance: £1,320.11 Payment term: 60 days

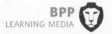
BPP
LEARNING MEDIA

Supplier name and address	Supplier account code	Supplier account details at 1 June 20XX
QC Exclusive Ocean House London NW2 9GY	QCE001	Opening balance: £920.46 Payment term: 30 days
Totally Wood 35 Montpellier Street Great Lowe Georgemarnier GM3 8LD	TOT001	Opening balance: £135.56 Payment term: 30 days

Task 3 (19 marks)

Refer to the list of nominal ledger accounts below taken from the spreadsheet that the business has been using.

Set up nominal ledger records for each account, entering opening balances (if applicable) at 1 June 20XX, ensuring you select, amend or create appropriate nominal ledger account codes.

Opening Trial Balance as at 1 June 20XX

Account names	Note	Debit balance £	Credit balance £
Computer equipment – cost		4,600.00	
Computer equipment – accumulated depreciation			1,200.00
Delivery vehicles – cost		22,800.00	
Delivery vehicles – accumulated depreciation			5,000.00
Fixtures and fittings – cost		6,445.00	
Fixtures and fittings – accumulated depreciation			1,625.00
Bank current account		13,984.24	
Petty cash		75.00	
Sales ledger control account	1	6,949.91	

Account names	Note	Debit balance £	Credit balance £
Purchase ledger control account	1		2,376.13
Sales tax control account	2		12,100.00
Purchase tax control account	2	7,540.00	
Capital			40,093.02
Online sales	3		NIL
Sales to shops – North	3		NIL
Sales to shops – South	3		NIL
Purchases – completed units	3	NIL	
Purchases – raw materials	3	NIL	
Wages	3	NIL	
Rent and rates	3	NIL	
Electricity	3	NIL	
Delivery vehicle expenses	3	NIL	
Bank charges	3	NIL	
Stationery	3	NIL	
Travel and subsistence	3	NIL	
		62,394.15	**62,394.15**

Notes

1   As the individual customer and supplier balances have already been posted, the accounting software you are using may require you to make a separate adjustment for these.

2   The software you are using may not require you to post these balances individually. The opening balance on the account is £4,560 (credit) if posting as a single brought forward balance.

3   These nominal accounts are needed for transactions taking place in June 20XX.

In the rest of the assessment, you will only make entries to the nominal ledger accounts you created in Task 3. You will not be required to make any entries to any accounts other than those you have already created.

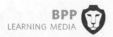

Task 4 (15 marks)

Refer to the following summary of sales invoices and summary of sales credit notes. Enter these transactions into the accounting software, ensuring you enter all the information below and select the correct sales code.

Summary of sales invoices

Date	Customer	Invoice number	Gross £	VAT £	Net £	Sales analysis £ Shop sales – North	Shop sales – South
6 June	Happy Engineers Ltd	HAP001/IN24	960.00	160.00	800.00	800.00	
12 June	Giffall Recruitment	GIF001/IN17	510.00	85.00	425.00	425.00	
24 June	Perry Cars	PER001/IN4	2,460.00	410.00	2,050.00		2,050.00
28 June	Happy Engineers Ltd	HAP001/IN25	2,237.94	372.99	1,864.95	1,864.95	
Totals			**6,167.94**	**1,027.99**	**5,139.95**	**3,089.95**	**2,050.00**

Summary of sales credit notes

Date	Customer	Invoice number	Gross £	VAT £	Net £	Sales analysis £ Shop sales – North	Shop sales – South
26 June	Happy Engineers Ltd	HAP001/C6*	186.00	31.00	155.00	155.00	
Totals			**186.00**	**31.00**	**155.00**	**155.00**	

* The credit note relates to some items on invoice HAP001/IN24.

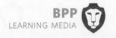

Task 5 (9 marks)

Refer to the following purchase invoices and the purchase credit note and enter these transactions into the accounting software, ensuring you enter all the information below and select the correct purchases code.

Purchase invoices

QC Exclusive	**Date: 1 June 20XX**
Ocean House	
London	
NW2 9GY	
VAT Registration No 554 222 657 14	

Invoice No: 365

To:
The Graze Office Store
1 Hope Street
Cathertown
Lumley
LM61 2RT

	£
150 plastic chairs (Net)	**1,500.00**
VAT @ 20%	**300.00**
Total	**1,800.00**

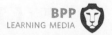

Totally Wood   **Date: 12 June 20XX**
35 Montpellier Street
Great Lowe
Georgemarnier
GM3 8LD

Invoice No: PRE/14

To:
The Graze Office Store
1 Hope Street
Cathertown
Lumley
LM61 2RT

	£
40 metres of 2 inch plywood (Net)	**340.00**
VAT @ 20%	**68.00**
Total	**408.00**

Purchase credit note

Totally Wood	**Date: 18 June 20XX**
35 Montpellier Street	
Great Lowe	
Georgemarnier	
GM3 8LD	

Credit Note No:
PRE/CN3
Linked to Invoice No: PRE/14

To:
The Graze Office Store
1 Hope Street
Cathertown
Lumley
LM61 2RT

	£
12 metres of 2 inch plywood (Net)	**102.00**
VAT @ 20%	**20.40**
Total	**122.40**
Detail: Inferior quality plywood	

The Graze Office Store sells to most of its customers online. All payments made by customers are done through a secure online payment system called CashChum.

CashChum make payments to The Graze Office Store at the end of each week using 'Faster Payments'.

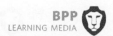

Task 6a (6 marks)

Refer to the following 'Online cash sales listing' and enter these receipts into the accounting software.

Online cash sales listing for June (Bank receipts)

Week ending	Amount received from CashChum* £
9 June 20XX	4,255.66
16 June 20XX	3,854.25
23 June 20XX	3,614.22
30 June 20XX	1,996.99

*All online sales include VAT at the standard rate.

Task 6b (3 marks)

Refer to the following email from Kate Allen and enter this transaction into the accounting software.

Email	
From:	Kate Allen
To:	Accounting Technician
Date:	16 June 20XX
Subject:	Delivery Drivers Wages

Hi,

Wages for the month are £6,200 and this will be paid today by BACS.

Thanks,

Kate

Task 7 (6 marks)

Refer to the following BACS remittance advices received from customers and enter these transactions into the accounting software, ensuring you allocate all amounts as stated on each remittance advice note.

BACS remittance advices

Happy Engineers

BACS Remittance Advice

To: The Graze Office Store

Date: 22 June 20XX

Amount: £1,425.65

Detail: Payment of balance owed as at 1 June 20XX.

Giffall Recruitment

BACS Remittance Advice

To: The Graze Office Store

Date: 30 June 20XX

Amount: £1,265.00

Detail: Payment of balance owed as at 1 June 20XX plus part payment of invoice number GIF001/IN17.

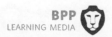

Task 8 (9 marks)

Refer to the following summary of cheque payments made to credit and cash suppliers. Enter these transactions into the accounting software, ensuring you allocate (where applicable) all amounts as shown in the details column.

Cheques paid listing

Date	Cheque number	Supplier	£	Details
16 June	000294	Fabrics Delight	1,320.11	Payment of opening balance
29 June	000295	Totally Wood	421.16	Payment of opening balance plus Invoice No: PRE/14 and Credit Note No: PRE/CN3
30 June	000296	Mick's Motors*	450.00 (including £75 VAT)	Repair of delivery van and new tyres

*Mick's Motors is not a credit supplier and does not have an account with the business.

Task 9 (4 marks)

Refer to the following standing order schedule below and:

(a) set up the recurring entry for rent

(b) save a screenshot of the screen setting up the recurring entry prior to processing. You will be provided with the required evidence number for this in Task 13.

(c) process the first payment.

Standing order schedule

Details	Amount £	Frequency of payment	Payment start date
Monthly rent	600	Each month	01 June 20XX

Detail:

The owner of the unit block increases the monthly rent charge annually on 1 June.

The recurring payment is set up each year on 1 June and is set up for 12 months. VAT is not applicable.

Task 10 (3 marks)

Refer to the following petty cash vouchers and enter these into the accounting software.

Petty cash vouchers

Date: 9 June 20XX
Name: Jim Murfin
Authorised by: **Kate Allen**
Voucher: 124

	£
Stationery	6.00
VAT	1.20
Total amount	7.20

Date: 9 June 20XX
Name: Sandra Owen
Authorised by: **Kate Allen**
Voucher: 125

	£
Travel for course	14.00 (No VAT)

Date: 14 June 20XX
Name: Suki Joshi
Authorised by: **Kate Allen**
Voucher: 126

	£
Train fare	4.75 (No VAT)

Task 11 (4 marks)

Refer to the following journal entries and enter them into the accounting software.

Journals

Date	Account	Debit £	Credit £
30 June 20XX	Computer equipment – cost	95.00	
30 June 20XX	Fixtures and fittings – cost		95.00
Narrative: Being the correction of an incorrectly coded non-current asset purchase invoice from May.			
30 June 20XX	Wages	25.95	
30 June 20XX	Bank current account		25.95
Narrative: Being an error in the wages figure shown in the email on 16 June 20XX.			

Task 12 (11 marks)

Refer to the following bank statement. Using the accounting software and the transactions you have already posted:

(a) Enter any additional items on the bank statement that have yet to be recorded, into the accounting software (ignore VAT on any of these transactions).

(b) Reconcile the bank statement. If the bank statement does not reconcile, check your work and make the necessary corrections.

(c) Save a screenshot of the bank reconciliation screen. You will be provided with the required evidence number for this in Task 13.

Bank of Markham
201 Manor Road
Lumley
LM61 2RT

The Graze Office Store
1 Hope Street
Cathertown
Lumley
LM61 2RT

Sort code: 44 - 21 - 09

Account Number: 01872249

Statement date: 30 June 20XX

Statement of account

Date 20XX	Details	Money In £	Money Out £	Balance £
01 June	Opening balance			13,984.24
01 June	SO – Rent		600.00	13,384.24
09 June	FP – CashChum	4,255.66		17,639.90
16 June	Cheque 294		1,320.11	16,319.79
16 June	FP – CashChum	3,854.25		20,174.04
16 June	BACS – Wages		6,225.95	13,948.09
22 June	BACS – Happy Engineers	1,425.65		15,373.74
23 June	FP – CashChum	3,614.22		18,987.96
27 June	DD – Electricity		101.00	18,886.96
28 June	Bank charges		14.00	18,872.96
29 June	Cheque 295		421.16	18,451.80
30 June	BACS – Giffall Recruitment	1,265.00		19,716.80
30 June	FP – CashChum	1,996.99		21,713.79
30 June	Cheque 296		450.00	21,263.79

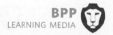

Task 13 (5 marks)

Documentation of evidence

You are now required to generate the following documents to demonstrate your competence:

Document and reports	Save / upload as:
A document showing all transactions with each customer during June 20XX.	**Evidence 1a** – Name – AAT Number
A document showing the balance owed by each customer as at 30 June 20XX.	**Evidence 1b** – Name – AAT Number
The following information must be evidenced within these documents: • *Customer name* • *Account code* • *Payment terms*	*Depending on your software, you may need to upload one or more documents.*
A document showing all transactions with each supplier during June 20XX.	**Evidence 2a** – Name – AAT Number
A document showing the balance owed to each supplier as at 30 June 20XX.	**Evidence 2b** – Name – AAT Number
The following information must be evidenced within these documents: • *Supplier name* • *Account code* • *Payment terms*	*Depending on your software, you may need to upload one or more documents.*
Audit trail, showing full details of all transactions, including details of receipts/payments allocated to items in customer/supplier accounts and details in the bank account that have been reconciled.	**Evidence 3** – Name – AAT Number
Trial balance as at 30 June 20XX.	**Evidence 4** – Name – AAT Number
A screenshot of the recurring entry screen including all relevant input details.	**Evidence 5** – Name – AAT Number
A screenshot of the bank reconciliation screen showing reconciled items.	**Evidence 6** – Name – AAT Number

AAT AQ2016 SAMPLE ASSESSMENT USING ACCOUNTING SOFTWARE

ANSWERS

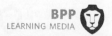

Using Accounting Software
AAT sample assessment

Answers

The model answers here are not exhaustive. The actual format of the document will be dependent on the accounting software used. Candidates may upload more than once piece of documentary evidence per task.

Evidence 1a/1b

The answer provided below shows all of the information required. The candidate may upload more than one piece of evidence.

Customer: Giffall Recruitment

Account: GIF001

Terms: 30 days

Date	Detail	Debit £	Credit £	Balance £
1 June 20XX	Opening balance	844.26		844.26
12 June 20XX	GIF001/IN17	510.00		1,354.26
30 June 20XX	BACS Payment of OB and IN17		1,265.00	89.26
Balance at 30 June 20XX				89.26

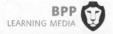

Customer: Happy Engineers
Account: HAP001
Terms: 30 days

Date	Detail	Debit £	Credit £	Balance £
1 June 20XX	Opening balance	1,425.65		1,425.65
6 June 20XX	HAP001/IN24	960.00		2,385.65
22 June 20XX	BACS payment		1,425.65	960.00
26 June 20XX	HAP001/C6: IN24		186.00	774.00
28 June 20XX	HAP001/IN25	2,237.94		3,011.94
Balance at 30 June 20XX				3,011.94

Customer: Perry Cars
Account: PER001
Terms: 45 days

Date	Detail	Debit £	Credit £	Balance £
1 June 20XX	Opening balance	4,680.00		4,680.00
24 June 20XX	PER001/IN4	2,460.00		7,140.00
Balance at 30 June 20XX				7,140.00

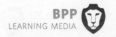

Evidence 2a/2b

The answer provided below shows all of the information required. The candidate may upload more than one piece of evidence.

Supplier: Fabrics Delight
Account: FAB001
Terms: 60 days

Date	Detail	Debit £	Credit £	Balance £
1 June 20XX	Opening balance		1,320.11	1,320.11
16 June 20XX	Chq No:294	1,320.11		-
Balance at 30 June 20XX				NIL

Supplier: QC Exclusive
Account: QCE001
Terms: 30 days

Date	Detail	Debit £	Credit £	Balance £
1 June 20XX	Opening balance		920.46	920.46
1 June 20XX	Inv 365		1,800.00	2,720.46
Balance at 30 June 20XX				2,720.46

Supplier: Totally Wood Account: TOT001 Terms: 30 days		Debit £	Credit £	Balance £
Date	**Detail**			
1 June 20XX	Opening balance		135.56	135.56
12 June 20XX	PRE/14		408.00	543.56
18 June 20XX	PRE/CN3	122.40		421.16
29 June 20XX	Chq No:295	421.16		-
Balance at 30 June 20XX				NIL

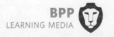

Evidence 3

Audit trial

Task	Transaction Type	Account(s)	Date 20XX	Invoice/ credit note number	Net Amount £	VAT £	Allocated Against receipt/ payment	Reconciled with bank statement	Notes
1	Customer O/bal	GIF001	01 Jun		844.26		✓		
	Customer O/bal	HAP001	01 Jun		1425.65		✓		
	Customer O/bal	PER001	01 Jun		4,680.00				
2	Supplier O/bal	FAB001	01 Jun		1,320.11		✓		
	Supplier O/bal	QCE001	01 Jun		920.46		✓		
	Supplier O/bal	TOT001	01 Jun		135.56				

Task	Transaction Type	Account(s)	Date 20XX	Invoice/credit note number	Net Amount £	VAT £	Allocated Against receipt/payment	Reconciled with bank statement	Notes
3	Dr	Computer equipment – cost	01 Jun		4,600.00				
	Cr	Computer equipment – acc depn	01 Jun		1,200.00				
	Dr	Delivery vehicles – cost	01 Jun		22,800.00				
	Cr	Delivery vehicles – acc depn	01 Jun		5,000.00				
	Dr	Fixtures fittings – cost	01 Jun		6,445.00				
	Cr	Fixtures fittings – acc depn	01 Jun		1,625.00				
	Dr	Bank current account	01 Jun		13,984.24			✓	
	Dr	Petty cash	01 Jun		75.00				
	Cr	Sales tax control account	01 Jun		12,100.00				
	Dr	Purchases tax control account	01 Jun		7,540.00				
	Dr	Capital	01 Jun		40,093.02				
	Cr	Sales ledger control*	01 Jun		6,949.91				
	Cr	Purchases ledger control*	01 Jun		2,376.13				
		*If appropriate							

Task	Transaction Type	Account(s)	Account(s)	Date 20XX	Invoice/ credit note number	Net Amount £	VAT £	Allocated Against receipt/ payment	Reconciled with bank statement	Notes
4	Sales inv	HAP001	Sales – North	06 Jun	HAP001/ IN24	800.00	160.00			
	Sales inv	GIF001	Sales – North	12 Jun	GIF001/ IN17	425.00	85.00	✓		
	Sales inv	PER001	Sales – South	24 Jun	PER001/ IN4	2,050.00	410.00			
	Sales inv	HAP001	Sales – North	28 Jun	HAP001/ IN25	1,864.95	372.99			
	Sales CN	HAP001	Sales – North	26 Jun	HAP001/ C6	155.00	31.00			
5	Purchases inv	QCE001	Completed units	01 Jun	365	1,500.00	300.00			
	Purchases inv	TOT001	Raw materials	12 Jun	PRE/14	340.00	68.00	✓		
	Purchases CN	TOT001	Raw materials	18 Jun	PRE/CN3	102.00	20.40	✓		

Task	Transaction Type	Account(s)	Date 20XX	Invoice/ credit note number	Net Amount £	VAT £	Allocated Against receipt/ payment	Reconciled with bank statement	Notes
6	Bank receipt	Bank	09 Jun		3,546.38	709.28		✓	Accept Net and VAT amounts of + or − 1 penny for online sales due to software rounding
	Bank receipt	Bank	16 Jun		3,211.88	642.37		✓	
	Bank receipt	Bank	23 Jun		3,011.85	602.37		✓	
	Bank receipt	Bank	30 Jun		1,664.16	332.83		✓	
	Bank payment	Bank	16 Jun		6,200.00			✓	
7	Customer receipt	HAP001	22 Jun		1,425.65			✓	
	Customer receipt	GIF001	30 Jun		1,265.00			✓	
8	Supplier payment	FAB001	16 Jun		1,320.11			✓	
	Supplier payment	TOT001	29 Jun		421.16	75.00		✓	
	Bank payment	Bank	30 Jun		375.00			✓	

Note on Account(s) column: Online sales (rows 1-4 of Task 6), Wages (Task 6 bank payment), Bank (Task 7 both rows), Bank (Task 8 FAB001 and TOT001), Delivery expenses (Task 8 bank payment).

Task	Transaction Type	Account(s)	Date 20XX	Invoice/ credit note number	Net Amount £	VAT £	Allocated Against receipt/ payment	Reconciled with bank statement	Notes
9	Bank payment	Bank	Rent – SO	01 Jun		600.00			✓	
10	Cash payment	Petty cash	Stationery	09 Jun		6.00	1.20			
	Cash payment	Petty cash	Travel	09 Jun		14.00				
	Cash payment	Petty cash	Travel	14 Jun		4.75				
11	Journal debit	Computer equipment – cost		30 Jun		95.00				
	Journal credit	Fixtures and fittings – cost		30 Jun		95.00				
	Journal debit	Wages		30 Jun		25.95				
	Journal credit	Bank		30 Jun		25.95			✓	
12	Bank payment	Bank	Electricity	27 Jun		101.00			✓	
	Bank payment	Bank	Bank charges	28 Jun		14.00			✓	

Evidence 4

Trial balance

Account Names	Debit Balance	Credit Balance
Computer equipment – Cost	4,695.00	
Computer equipment – Accumulated depreciation		1,200.00
Delivery vehicles – Cost	22,800.00	
Delivery vehicles – Accumulated depreciation		5,000.00
Fixtures and Fittings – Cost	6,350.00	
Fixtures and Fittings – Accumulated depreciation		1,625.00
Bank Current Account	21,263.79	
Petty cash	49.05	
Sales Ledger Control Account	10,241.20	
Purchase Ledger Control Account		2,720.46
Sales Tax Control Account		15,383.84
Purchase Tax Control Account	7,963.80	
Capital		40,093.02
Online sales		11,434.27
Sales to shops – North		2,934.95
Sales to Shops – South		2,050.00
Purchases – Completed units	1,500.00	
Purchases – Raw materials	238.00	
Wages	6,225.95	
Rent and rates	600.00	
Electricity	101.00	

Account Names	Debit Balance	Credit Balance
Delivery vehicle expenses	375.00	
Bank charges	14.00	
Stationery	6.00	
Travelling	18.75	
	82,441.54	82,441.54

Evidence 5 and 6 are dependent on software used.

Additional guidance for individual tasks

If you struggled with the assessment, we suggest you read the guidance that follows and attempt the assessment again. Note that when we refer to 'Sage' in this section, this covers both Sage 50 and Sage One, unless otherwise stated.

Task 1 (3 marks)

Make sure you set up all **customers** listed and be careful to set them up as customers, rather than suppliers. Enter the dates and opening balances carefully and check that all of your entries match the information you have been given.

Note that if you are using Sage One, you need to enter the opening balance date as **31 May 20XX** as the program requires it to be one day before the accounts start date. Other programs, including Sage 50, may allow you to enter the opening balance date as 1 June 20XX.

Task 2 (3 marks)

Make sure you set up all **suppliers** listed and be careful to set them up as suppliers, rather than customers. Enter the dates and opening balances carefully and check that all of your entries match the information you have been given.

Note that if you are using Sage One, you need to enter the opening balance date as **31 May 20XX** as the program requires it to be one day before the accounts start date. Other programs, including Sage 50, may allow you to enter the opening balance date as 1 June 20XX.

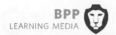

Task 3 (19 marks)

Most of these accounts will already be on Sage, so you just need to enter the opening balances for these. However, for some accounts, you will need to either create new accounts or amend the names of existing accounts.

To help reduce the chance of error, be careful and methodical when entering the balances and selecting the appropriate nominal accounts. When finished, check you have not missed any accounts – you can do this by previewing a trial balance. Assuming you entered Task 1 and 2 data correctly, if you are using Sage, you will not need to enter opening balances for the sales ledger and purchase ledger control accounts.

Note that if you are using Sage One, you need to enter the opening balance date as **31 May 20XX** as the program requires it to be one day before the accounts start date. Other programs, including Sage 50, may allow you to enter the opening balance date as 1 June 20XX.

Task 4 (15 marks)

Enter the invoices and the credit note carefully, ensuring you don't enter the credit note as an invoice or vice-versa. Remember that it is very important to select the correct income account in the nominal ledger. It is clear from the invoices which type of sale each invoice relates to. Always check you have entered **all** of the transactions.

Task 5 (9 marks)

When posting purchase invoices/credit notes, make sure you select the right supplier and an appropriate nominal account. VAT should be correctly accounted for and if you select the correct tax code in Sage 50 (VAT rate in Sage One), this will be calculated automatically – all you need to do then is check it matches the VAT per the invoice. Always check you have entered **all** of the transactions.

Task 6a and 6b (9 marks)

This task requires you to process payments and receipts that are not related to credit transactions with customers or suppliers. You should use the Other Payment/Other Receipt function in Sage One or the Bank Payment/Bank Receipt function in Sage 50.

Ensure you use the right way of accounting for VAT for cash sales. You are only given the gross amount. Therefore, in Sage One, you should enter the gross amount, and the program will automatically calculate and post the VAT. In Sage 50, although it may seem odd, firstly enter the gross amount in the Net field. Then press F9 and the program will automatically calculate the net amount.

As always, the choice of nominal account is important. Depending on your software, you will probably need to create a new account or rename an existing account (as described in Task 2, Chapter 1/3). Be careful not to omit any payments or receipts.

Tasks 7 and 8 (15 marks)

When entering supplier payments or customer receipts using Sage, you should use the **Supplier Payment** or **Customer Receipt** functions (not the Bank Payment or Bank Receipt functions (Other Payment/Other Receipt functions in Sage One) as demonstrated earlier in this Text. You should find this makes it easy to allocate the payment/receipt to the correct supplier/ customer account. Don't miss out any transactions.

Task 9 (4 marks)

Recurring payments are a bit tricky in Sage 50 – when you first enter the details, they do not impact on the nominal ledger. When you go back into Recurring items in Sage 50 to process the payment, remember **you only need to process the first payment.**

For Sage One however, the process is a bit different. You create and post the first payment using the **Other Payment** function. You then go back into the payment to set up the recurrence.

Details on how to do this were covered in Chapter 2/Chapter 4 of this Text.

Note that you are required to take a screen print in this task and you can do this by pressing **Print Screen** or **PrtScn (or PrtSc)**.

In Sage One, take a screenshot of both the 'Other Payment' screen with the details of the first payment, and the 'Make Recurring' screen with details of the recurrence.

In Sage 50 take a screenshot of the Add/Edit recurring entry screen with details of the first payment and recurrence.

Task 10 (3 marks)

Remember to change the **nominal code** in Sage 50 to the **Petty Cash** ('Cash' in Sage One) nominal code when entering the payments in this task.

You can use the **Bank Transfer** function in Sage for the payment from the Bank account to the Petty cash account.

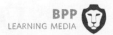

Task 11 (4 marks)

Journals should be entered carefully to ensure you debit and credit the correct accounts. Don't get the debits and credits mixed up.

....

Task 12 (11 marks)

Having entered the bank charges and bank interest (using the 'Other Payment' function in Sage One or the 'Bank Payment' function in Sage 50), you should reconcile the bank using the method covered in Chapter 2/Chapter 4.

In the answer provided, you can see which items you should have reconciled as they appear in the 'Matched transactions' section in the bottom half of the bank reconciliation screen in Sage 50. In Sage One, the reconciled items have a tick in 'Reconciled' column in the bank reconciliation screen.

Take a screenshot of the bank reconciliation screen just before you save the reconciliation (ie, before you click on Save button in Sage One, or the 'Reconcile' button in Sage 50).

....

Task 13 (5 marks)

This task tests your ability to generate the reports specified. You will get the marks available for this particular task by **generating the correct report**. You will receive these marks, even if some of the transactions within the report are incorrect, because you entered them incorrectly in earlier tasks.

There is a comprehensive section on generating reports in Chapter 2/Chapter 4 of this Text. You should look back at this if you were unable to generate and save as PDF files, any reports. **Make sure you check that you have saved all the reports.**

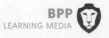

Specific guidance for each document/report is given below in **bold**.

Document and reports	Save/upload as:
Ensure you specify the correct date/date range for all reports:	**For the purpose of this sample assessment, save the documents to your desktop on your computer. In a real assessment you would also be required to upload these documents, but ignore the step of uploading for this sample assessment.**
A document showing all transactions with each customer during June 20XX **Run the 'Customer Activity' report. Run the 'Detailed' report in Sage 50. In Sage One, select all customers to obtain one report for all.**	File name = Evidence 1a – Name – AAT Number
A document showing the balance owed by each customer as at 30 June 20XX **Run the 'Aged Debtors Analysis – Detailed' report in Sage 50, or the 'Aged Debtors' report in Sage One and click the 'Detailed' button.**	File name = Evidence 1b – Name – AAT Number
The following information must be evidenced within these documents: • *Customer name* • *Account code* • *Payment terms* **You need a separate document for payment terms – a screenshot of the Customer Record screen for each customer in Sage One. For Sage 50, you need the Credit Control screen within each Customer Record.**	Depending on your software you may need to save one or more documents. **Name these in the same way as above, continuing the sequence, eg, Evidence 1c...**

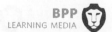

Document and reports	Save/upload as:
A document showing all transactions with each supplier during June 20XX **Run the 'Supplier Activity' report. Run the 'Detailed' report in Sage 50. In Sage One, select all suppliers to obtain one report for all.**	File name = **Evidence 2a – Name – AAT Number**
A document showing the balance owed to each supplier as at 30 June 20XX **Run the 'Aged Creditors Analysis – Detailed' report in Sage 50, or the 'Aged Creditors' report in Sage One and click the 'Detailed' button.**	File name = Evidence 2b – Name – AAT Number
The following information must be evidenced within these documents: • *Supplier name* • *Account code* • *Payment terms* You need a separate document for payment terms – a screenshot of the Supplier Record screen for each supplier in Sage One. For Sage 50, you need the Credit Control screen within each Supplier Record)	Depending on your software you may need to save one or more documents.
Audit trail, showing full details of all transactions, including details of receipts/payments allocated to items in customer/supplier accounts and details in the bank account that have been reconciled **Run the 'Audit Trail – Detailed' report.** **To show bank reconciled items:** *Sage 50 - reconciled items have an 'R' in the 'B' column of the report.*	File name = **Evidence 3 – Name – AAT Number**

Document and reports	Save/upload as:
Sage One - ensure the report is configured to include 'Bank Reconciled' column. Reconciled items have a tick in this column. **To show receipts/payments allocated to items in customer/supplier accounts:** *Sage 50 - the report indicates the invoices that receipts/payments are allocated to, eg, '24.42 to PI 4' shows that a payment of 24.42 is allocated to purchase invoice no. 4.* *Sage One - use the Customer/Supplier Activity reports generated in 1a and 2a above. Allocated items are identified by having 0.00 in the 'Outstanding' column)*	
Trial Balance as at 30 June 20XX **Run the 'Trial balance' report**	File name = **Evidence 4 – Name – AAT Number**
A screenshot of the recurring entry screen including all relevant input details. **From Task 9b** **In Sage One, take a screenshot of both the 'Other Payment' screen with the details of the first payment, and the 'Create Recurring Payment' screen with details of the recurrence.** **In Sage 50 take a screenshot of the Add/Edit recurring entry screen with details of the first payment and recurrence.**	File name – **Evidence 5 – Name – AAT Number**

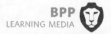

Document and reports	Save/upload as:
A screenshot of the bank reconciliation screen showing the reconciled items. **From Task 12b** **Take a screenshot of the bank reconciliation screen just before you save the reconciliation (ie, before you click on Save button in Sage One and Reconcile button in Sage 50)**	File name = **Evidence 6 – Name – AAT Number**

BPP PRACTICE ASSESSMENT 1
Using Accounting Software

Time allowed: 2 hours

- You are now ready to attempt the BPP practice assessment for Using Accounting Software.

- This practice assessment uses a standard rate of VAT of 20%.

- It requires you to input data into a computerised accounting package and produce documents and reports.

- Answers are provided at the end of the assessment.

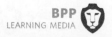

Using Accounting Software
BPP practice assessment 1

Assessment information (taken from AAT Sample Assessment)

The time allowed to complete this assessment is **2 hours.**

This assessment consists of **13 tasks** and it is important that you attempt them all.

- You will be asked to produce documents and reports to demonstrate your competence.

- You must then upload these documents so they can be marked by AAT.

All documents must be uploaded within the **total time** available. It is important that you upload **all** reports and documents specified in the tasks so your work can be assessed.

You will be able to attach and remove files throughout the duration of this assessment until you click on 'Finish', which will submit your assessment.

All uploaded documents should be saved and titled with the following information:

- Evidence number
- Your name
- Your AAT membership number

The evidence number to use for each document is stated in the table in Task 13.

Example

Your name is Simon White, and your AAT membership number is: 12345678

Evidence 1

A document showing all of the purchase invoices and credit notes (by purchase type) posted in January 20XX.

This document would be saved and uploaded as: Evidence 1 – Simon White – 12345678

If multiple documents are uploaded to show competency in an individual task, name these Evidence 1A and Evidence 1B and so on.

Unless the assessment asks for a specific format, you can choose the format which will best enable the marker to review and assess your work.

During the assessment, you will only make entries to the nominal ledger accounts you created in Task 3. You will not be required to make any entries to any accounts other than those you have already created.

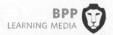

Information

This assessment is based on an existing business, **Steadman Computer Solutions (SCS)**, a UK business that supplies computers to local businesses. It also offers a computer repair service. The owner of the business is **James Steadman,** who operates as a sole trader. James is changing from a manual book-keeping system to a computerised one from **1 January 20XX**. You are employed as an accounting technician.

Information relating to the business:

Business name:	Steadman Computer Solutions
Business address:	50 George Street Cheltenham GL50 1XR
Business owner:	James Steadman
Accounting period end:	31 December (each year)
VAT Number:	123456789 (standard scheme)
VAT rate:	Standard rate VAT of 20% charged on all sales

Sales

James likes to keep a record of the different sales made by the business, by sales type:

- Desktop computers
- Laptop computers
- Computer repairs

You have been asked to carry out the bookkeeping tasks for January 20XX **only**, the first month that the business will be using computerised accounting software and the start of the new accounting period.

All documents have been checked for accuracy and have been authorised by James Steadman.

Before you start the assessment you should:

- Set the system software date as **31st January of the current year**.
- Set the financial year to start on **1st January of the current year**.

Task 1

Refer to the customer listing below and set up customer records to open sales ledger accounts for each customer, entering opening balances at 1 January 20XX.

Customer Listing

CUSTOMER NAME, ADDRESS AND CONTACT DETAILS	CUSTOMER ACCOUNT CODE	CUSTOMER ACCOUNT DETAILS AT 1 JANUARY 20XX
Always Insurance plc 26 High Road Cheltenham GL52 8KK	ALW01	Payment terms: 30 days Opening balance: £1,821.70
Local Bank Ltd 56 Long Lane Gloucester GL10 8BN	LOC01	Payment terms: 30 days Opening balance: £1,300.00
Large Firm LLP 1 Main Road Swindon SN3 1PP	LAR01	Payment terms: 30 days Opening balance: £800.80

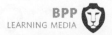

Task 2

Refer to the supplier listing below and set up supplier records to open purchases ledger accounts for each supplier, entering opening balances at 1 January 20XX.

Supplier Listing

SUPPLIER NAME, ADDRESS AND CONTACT DETAILS	SUPPLIER ACCOUNT CODE	SUPPLIER ACCOUNT DETAILS AT 1 JANUARY 20XX
Bell Computers Ltd 15 Queen Street London W12 9ZZ	BEL01	Payment terms: 30 days Opening balance: £1,400.00
Discount IT Supplies 50 Banner Place Gloucester GL10 4GG	DIS01	Payment terms: 30 days Opening balance: £790.40
Anderson Garages 19 Anderson Road Cheltenham GL51 5JR	AND01	Payment terms: 30 days Opening balance: £178.80

Task 3

Refer to the list of nominal ledger balances below:

Set up nominal ledger records for each account, entering opening balances (if applicable) at 1 January 20XX, ensuring you select, amend or create appropriate nominal ledger account codes.

Opening Trial Balance as at 01.01.20XX

ACCOUNT NAMES	Debit balance £	Credit balance £
Office Equipment	3,567.00	
Motor Vehicles	12,750.00	
Bank	3101.80	
Petty Cash	200.00	
Sales ledger control* (see note below)	3,922.50	
Purchases ledger control* (see note below)		2,369.20
Sales tax control account		1,540.60
Purchase tax control account	1,080.20	
Capital		20,000.00
Drawings	4,660.10	
Sales – Desktops		8,780.00
Sales – Laptops		5,920.00
Sales – Computer repairs		620.80
Computers for resale – purchases	8,880.20	
Rent and rates	810.00	
Bank interest paid	NIL	
Bank charges	NIL	
Motor vehicle expenses	258.80	
	39,230.60	**39,230.60**

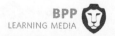

* **Note.** As you have already entered opening balances for customers and suppliers, the software package you are using may not require you to enter these balances.

In the rest of the assessment, you will only make entries to the nominal ledger accounts you created in Task 3. You will not be required to make any entries to any accounts other than those you have already created.

Task 4

Refer to the following summary of purchase invoices and purchase credit notes and enter these transactions into the accounting software, ensuring you enter all the information below and select the correct purchases code.

Summary of purchase invoices

Date 20XX	Supplier Name	Invoice Number	Gross £	VAT £	Net £	Computers for resale £	Motor expenses £
03.01.XX	Bell Computers	SC2040	2,520.00	420.00	2,100.00	2,100.00	
09.01.XX	Anderson Garages	R2168	192.00	32.00	160.00		160.00
21.01.XX	Discount IT Supplies	1806	2,493.60	415.60	2,078.00	2,078.00	
28.01.XX	Bell Computers	SC2349	600.00	100.00	500.00	500.00	
	Totals		5,805.60	967.60	4,838.00	4,678.00	160.00

Summary of purchase credit notes

Date 20XX	Supplier Name	Invoice Number	Gross £	VAT £	Net £	Computers for resale £	Motor expenses £
23.01.XX	Bell Computers	CR0358*	480.00	80.00	400.00	400.00	
	Totals		480.00	80.00	400.00	400.00	

* The credit note relates to some items on invoice SC2040.

Task 5

Refer to the following sales invoices and sales credit notes and enter these transactions into the accounting software, ensuring you enter all the information below and select the correct sales code.

Steadman Computer Solutions
50 George Street, Cheltenham, GL50 1XR
VAT Registration No 478 3164 00

Telephone: 01242 866 5128
Email: J.Steadman@SCS.co.uk

SALES INVOICE NO 0100

Date: 01 January 20XX

Local Bank Ltd
56 Long Lane
Gloucester
GL10 8BN

	£
2 new laptops	800.00
VAT @ 20%	160.00
Total for payment	960.00
Terms: 30 days	

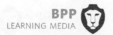

Steadman Computer Solutions
50 George Street, Cheltenham, GL50 1XR
VAT Registration No 478 3164 00

Telephone: 01242 866 5128
Email: J.Steadman@SCS.co.uk

SALES INVOICE NO 0101

Date: 15 January 20XX

Large Firm LLP
1 Main Road
Swindon
SN3 1PP

	£
5 new desktop PCs	2,520.50
VAT @ 20%	504.10
Total for payment	3,024.60
Terms: 30 days	

Steadman Computer Solutions
50 George Street, Cheltenham, GL50 1XR
VAT Registration No 478 3164 00

Telephone: 01242 866 5128
Email: J.Steadman@SCS.co.uk

S A L E S   CREDIT NOTE N O   0020
Linked to INVOICE NO 0100
Date: 18 January 20XX

Local Bank Ltd
56 Long Lane
Gloucester
GL10 8BN

	£
Return of unwanted laptop	400.00
VAT @ 20%	80.00
Total for payment	480.00

Terms: 30 days

Task 6a

Refer to the following receipt issued for cash sales and enter these transactions into the accounting software.

Date	Payment method	Details	Amount
7 January 20XX	Cheque	Minor repair to a laptop computer	£60.00 including VAT
15 January 20XX	Cash	Repair to desktop PC computer	£120.00 including VAT
23 January 20XX	Cheque	Sales of used laptop computer	£200.00 including VAT
27 January 20XX	Cash	Sale of used desktop PC computer	£150.00 including VAT

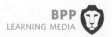

Task 6b

Refer to the following email below from James Steadman and enter this transaction into the accounting software.

Email
From: James Steadman **To:** Accounting Technician **Date:** 12 January 20XX **Subject:** Drawings

Hello

I have withdrawn £180 in cash from the business bank for my personal use.

Please record this transaction.

Thanks

James

Task 7

Refer to the following summary of payments received from customers and enter these transactions into the accounting software, making sure you allocate all amounts, as shown in the details column.

Receipts listing

Date	Receipt type	Customer	£	Details
14.01.XX	BACS	Always Insurance plc	1,821.70	Payment of opening balance
28.01.XX	Faster Payment	Local Bank Ltd	480.00	Payment of invoice 0100 including credit note 0020

Task 8

Refer to the following summary of payments made to suppliers and enter these transactions into the accounting software, making sure you allocate (where applicable) all amounts, as shown in the details column.

Cheques paid listing

Date	Cheque number	Supplier	£	Details
11.01.XX	003241	Bell Computers Ltd	1,000.00	Payment on account
20.01.XX	003242	Anderson Garages	192.00	Payment of invoice R2168
23.01.XX	003243	Discount IT Supplies	790.40	Payment of opening balance

Task 9

Refer to the following direct debit details:

(a) Set up a recurring entry, as shown in the table below.

(b) Save a screen shot of the screen, setting up the recurring entry prior to processing. You will be provided with the required evidence number for this in Task 13.

(c) Process the first payment.

Direct debit details

Details	Amount	First payment	Number of monthly payments
Rates (VAT not applicable)	£300	24 January 20XX	12

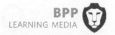

Task 10

(a) **Refer to the following petty cash vouchers and enter the petty cash payments into the accounting software.**

Petty Cash Voucher	
Date 16 January 20XX	**No** PC042
Train ticket for business travel – VAT not applicable Receipt attached	£ 38.00

Petty Cash Voucher	
Date 20 January 20XX	**No** PC043
A4 pads, folders and ball point pens VAT Total Receipt attached	£ 31.60 6.32 37.92

(b) **Refer to the following petty cash reimbursement slip and enter this transaction into the accounting software.**

Petty Cash Reimbursement PCR No 03	
Date: 31 January 20XX Cash from the bank account to restore the petty cash account to £200.00.	£75.92

Task 11

Refer to the following journal entries and enter them into the accounting software.

JOURNAL ENTRIES TO BE MADE 15.01.XX	£	£
Drawings	85.00	
Motor expenses		85.00
Being journal to reflect personal motor expenses posted as business expenses		

JOURNAL ENTRIES TO BE MADE 30.01.XX	£	£
Sales - Desktops	400.00	
Sales - Laptops		400.00
Being correction of an error in where a Laptop sale was originally incorrectly recorded as a Desktop sale		

Task 12

Refer to the following bank statement. Using the accounting software and the transactions you have already posted:

(a) Enter any additional items on the bank statement that have yet to be recorded, into the accounting software (ignore VAT on any of these transactions).

(b) Reconcile the bank statement. If the bank statement does not reconcile, check your work and make the necessary corrections.

(c) Save a screenshot of the bank reconciliation screen. You will be provided with the required evidence number for this in Task 13.

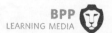

South Bank plc
60 Broad Street
Cheltenham
GL51 9YY

Steadman Computer Solutions
50 George Street
Cheltenham
GL50 1XR
Account number 00698435

31 January 20XX

STATEMENT OF ACCOUNT

Date 20XX	Details	Paid out £	Paid in £	Balance £
01 Jan	Opening balance			3,101.80C
09 Jan	Counter credit		60.00	3,161.80C
12 Jan	Cash withdrawal	180.00		2,981.80C
14 Jan	BACS: Always Insurance plc		1,821.70	4,803.50C
14 Jan	Cheque 003241	1,000.00		3,803.50C
17 Jan	Counter credit		120.00	3,923.50C
24 Jan	Cheque 003242	192.00		3,731.50C
24 Jan	Direct Debit – Cheltenham MBC – Rates	300.00		3,431.50C
25 Jan	Counter credit		200.00	3,631.50C
27 Jan	Counter credit		150.00	3,781.50C
28 Jan	Faster payment: Local Bank Ltd		480.00	4,261.50C
29 Jan	Cheque 003243	790.40		3,471.10C
30 Jan	Bank charges	12.40		3,458.70C
31 Jan	Bank interest	1.14		3,457.56C
31 Jan	Transfer	75.92		3,381.64C
	D = Debit C = Credit			

Task 13

Documentation of evidence

You are now required to generate the following documents to demonstrate your competence:

Document and reports	Save / upload as:
A document showing all transactions with each customer during January 20XX	File name = Evidence 1a – Name – AAT Number
A document showing the balance owed by each customer as at 31 January 20XX *The following information must be evidenced within these documents:* • Customer name • Account code • Payment terms	File name = Evidence 1b – Name – AAT Number Depending on your software you may need to save one or more documents.
A document showing all transactions with each supplier during January 20XX	File name = Evidence 2a – Name – AAT Number
A document showing the balance owed to each supplier as at 31 January 20XX *The following information must be evidenced within these documents:* • Supplier name • Account code • Payment terms	File name = Evidence 2b – Name – AAT Number Depending on your software you may need to save one or more documents.
Audit trail, showing full details of all transactions, including details of receipts/ payments allocated to items in customer/ supplier accounts and details in the bank account that have been reconciled.	File name = Evidence 3 – Name – AAT Number
Trial Balance as at 31 January 20XX	File name = Evidence 4 – Name – AAT Number
A screenshot of the recurring entry screen including all relevant input details.	File name = Evidence 5 – Name – AAT Number
A screenshot of the bank reconciliation screen showing the reconciled items.	File name = Evidence 6 – Name – AAT Number

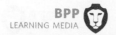

BPP PRACTICE ASSESSMENT 1
Using Accounting Software

ANSWERS

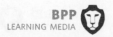

Using Accounting Software
BPP practice assessment 1

Some answers are given below. The answers we've provided are indicative of relevant content within the audit trail, the exact format of which will differ according to the computerised accounting package used.

Task	Transaction type	Account(s)	Date 20XX	Net Amount £	VAT £	Allocated against receipt/ payment ✓	Reconciled with bank statement ✓
1	Customer O/bal	ALW01	01 Jan	1,821.70		✓	
	Customer O/bal	LOC01	01 Jan	1,300.00			
	Customer O/bal	LAR01	01 Jan	800.80			
2	Supplier O/bal	BEL01	01 Jan	1,400.00			
	Supplier O/bal	DIS01	01 Jan	790.40		✓	
	Supplier O/bal	AND01	01 Jan	178.80			
3	Debit	Office equipment	01 Jan	3,567.00			
	Debit	Motor vehicles	01 Jan	12,750.00			
	Debit	Bank current account	01 Jan	3,101.80			✓
	Debit	Petty cash	01 Jan	200.00			
	Debit	Sales ledger control	01 Jan	3,922.50			
	Credit	Purchases ledger control	01 Jan	2,369.20			
	Credit	VAT on sales	01 Jan	1,540.60			
	Debit	VAT on purchases	01 Jan	1,080.20			
	Credit	Capital	01 Jan	20,000.00			
	Debit	Drawings	01 Jan	4,660.10			
	Credit	Sales – Desktops	01 Jan	8,780,00.00			
	Credit	Sales – Laptops	01 Jan	5,920.00			
	Credit	Sales – Computer repairs	01 Jan	620.80			
	Debit	Computers for re-sale – purchases	01 Jan	8,880.20			
	Debit	Rent and rates	01 Jan	810.00			
	Debit	Motor vehicle expenses	01 Jan	258.80			

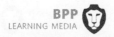

Task	Transaction type	Account(s)		Date 20XX	Net Amount £	VAT £	Allocated against receipt/ payment ✓	Reconciled with bank statement ✓
4	Purchases inv	BEL01	Computers for re-sale	03 Jan	2,100.00	420.00		
	Purchases inv	AND0	Motor vehicle expenses	09 Jan	160.00	32.00	✓	
	Purchases inv	DIS01	Computers for re-sale	21 Jan	2078.00	415.60		
	Purchases inv	BEL01	Computers for re-sale	28 Jan	500.00	100.00		
	Purchases Cr	BEL01	Computers for re-sale	23 Jan	400.00	80.00		
5	Sales inv	LOC01	Sales – Laptops	01 Jan	800.00	160.00	✓	
	Sales inv	LAR01	Sales – Desktops	15 Jan	2,520.50	504.10		
	Sales CN	LOC01		18 Jan	400.00	80.00	✓	
6a	Bank receipt (Other receipt in Sage One)	Bank	Sales – Computer repairs	07 Jan	50.00	10.00		✓
	Bank/Other receipt	Bank	Sales – Computer repairs	15 Jan	100.00	20.00		✓
	Bank/Other receipt	Bank	Sales – Laptops	23 Jan	166.67	33.33		✓
	Bank/Other receipt	Bank	Sales – Desktop	28 Jan	125.00	25.00		✓
6b	Bank payment	Bank	Drawings	12 Jan	180.00			✓
7	Customer receipt	ALW01	Bank	14 Jan	1,821.70			✓
	Customer receipt	LOC01	Bank	26 Jan	480.00			✓
8	Supplier payment on a/c	BEL01	Bank	11 Jan	1,000.00			✓
	Supplier payment	AND01	Bank	20 Jan	192.00			✓
	Supplier payment	DIS01	Bank	23 Jan	790.40			✓

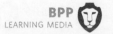

Task	Transaction type	Account(s)		Date 20XX	Net Amount £	VAT £	Allocated against receipt/ payment ✓	Reconciled with bank statement ✓
9	Bank payment	Bank	Rates – DD	24 Jan	300.00			✓
10	Cash payment	Petty cash	Travel	16 Jan	38.00			
	Cash payment	Petty cash	Stationery	20 Jan	31.60	6.32		
	Debit	Petty cash		31 Jan	75.92			
	Credit	Bank		31 Jan	75.92			✓
11	Journal debit	Drawings		15 Jan	85.00			
	Journal credit	Motor expenses		15 Jan	85.00			
	Journal debit	Sales – Desktops		30 Jan	400.00			
	Journal credit	Sales – Laptops		30 Jan	400.00			
12	Bank payment (Other payment in Sage One)	Bank	Bank charges and interest (Sage One) or Bank charges (Sage 50)	30 Jan	12.40			✓
	Bank / Other payment	Bank	Bank charges and interest (Sage One) or Bank interest paid (Sage 50)	31 Jan	1.14			✓

Additional guidance for individual tasks

If you struggled with the assessment, we suggest you read the guidance that follows and attempt the assessment again. Note that when we refer to 'Sage' in this section, this covers both Sage 50 and Sage One, unless otherwise stated.

Task 1 (guidance)

Make sure you set up all **customers** listed and be careful to set them up as customers, rather than suppliers. Enter the dates and opening balances carefully and check that all of your entries match the information you have been given.

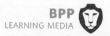

Note that if you are using Sage One, you need to enter the opening balance date as **31 December 20XW** as the program requires it to be one day before the accounts start date. Other programs, including Sage 50, may allow you to enter the opening balance date as 1 January 20XX.

Task 2 (guidance)

Make sure you set up all **suppliers** listed and be careful to set them up as suppliers, rather than customers. Enter the dates and opening balances carefully and check that all of your entries match the information you have been given.

Note that if you are using Sage One, you need to enter the opening balance date as **31 December 20XW** as the program requires it to be one day before the accounts start date. Other programs, including Sage 50, may allow you to enter the opening balance date as 1 January 20XX.

Task 3 (guidance)

Most of these accounts will already be on Sage, so you just need to enter the opening balances for these. However, for some accounts, you will need to either create new accounts or amend the names of existing accounts.

To help reduce the chance of error, be careful and methodical when entering the balances and selecting the appropriate nominal accounts. When finished, check you have not missed any accounts – you can do this by previewing a trial balance. Assuming you entered Task 1 and 2 data correctly, if you are using Sage, you will not need to enter opening balances for the sales ledger and purchase ledger control accounts.

Note that if you are using Sage One, you need to enter the opening balance date as **31 December 20XW** as the program requires it to be one day before the accounts start date. Other programs, including Sage 50, may allow you to enter the opening balance date as 1 January 20XX.

Task 4 (guidance)

When posting purchase invoices/credit notes, make sure you select the right supplier and an appropriate nominal account. VAT should be correctly accounted for and if you set the correct tax code in Sage 50 (VAT rate in Sage One), this will be calculated automatically – all you need to do then is check it matches the VAT shown on the invoice. Always check you have entered **all** of the transactions.

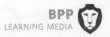

Task 5 (guidance)

Enter the invoices and the credit note carefully, ensuring you don't enter the credit note as an invoice or vice-versa. Remember that it is very important to select the correct income account in the nominal ledger. It is clear from the invoices which type of sale each invoice relates to. Always check you have entered **all** of the transactions.

Task 6a and 6b (guidance)

This task requires you to process payments and receipts that are not related to credit transactions with customers or suppliers. You should use the Other Payment/Other Receipt function in Sage One or the Bank Payment/Bank Receipt function in Sage 50.

Ensure you use the right way of accounting for VAT for cash sales. You are only given the gross amount. Therefore, in Sage One, you should enter the gross amount, and the program will automatically calculate and post the VAT. In Sage 50, although it may seem odd, firstly enter the gross amount in the Net field. Then press F9 and the program will automatically calculate the net amount.

As always, the choice of nominal account is important. Be careful not to omit any payments or receipts.

Tasks 7 and 8 (guidance)

When entering supplier payments or customer receipts using Sage, you should use the **Supplier Payment** or **Customer Receipt** functions (not the Bank Payment or Bank Receipt functions (Other Payment/Other Receipt functions in Sage One) as demonstrated earlier in this Text. You should find this makes it easy to allocate the payment/receipt to the correct supplier/ customer account. Don't miss out any transactions.

Task 9 (guidance)

Recurring payments are a bit tricky in Sage 50 – when you first enter the details, they do not impact on the nominal ledger. When you go back into Recurring items in Sage 50 to process the payment, remember **you only need to process the first payment.**

For Sage One however, the process is a bit different. You create and post the first payment using the **Other Payment** function. You then go back into the payment to set up the recurrence.

Details on how to do this were covered in Chapter 2/Chapter 4 of this Text.

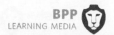
BPP
LEARNING MEDIA

Note that you are required to take a screen print in this task and you can do this by pressing **Print Screen** or **PrtScn (or PrtSc)**.

In Sage One, take a screenshot of both the 'Other Payment' screen with the details of the first payment, and the 'Make Recurring' screen with details of the recurrence.

In Sage 50 take a screenshot of the Add/Edit recurring entry screen with details of the first payment and recurrence.

Task 10 (guidance)

Remember to change the **nominal code** in Sage 50 to the **Petty Cash** ('Cash' in Sage One) nominal code when entering the payments in this task.

You can use the **Bank Transfer** function in Sage for the payment from the Bank account to the Petty cash account.

Task 11 (guidance)

Journals should be entered carefully to ensure you debit and credit the correct accounts. Don't get the debits and credits mixed up.

Task 12 (guidance)

Having entered the bank charges and bank interest (using the 'Other Payment' function in Sage One or the 'Bank Payment' function in Sage 50), you should reconcile the bank using the method covered in Chapter 2/Chapter 4.

In the answer provided, you can see which items you should have reconciled as they appear in the 'Matched transactions' section in the bottom half of the bank reconciliation screen in Sage 50. In Sage One, the reconciled items have a tick in 'Reconciled' column in the bank reconciliation screen.

Take a screenshot of the bank reconciliation screen just before you save the reconciliation (ie, before you click on Save button in Sage One, or the 'Reconcile' button in Sage 50).

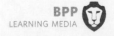

Task 13 (guidance)

This task tests your ability to generate the reports specified. You will get the marks available for this particular task by **generating the correct report**. You will receive these marks, even if some of the transactions within the report are incorrect, because you entered them incorrectly in earlier tasks.

There is a comprehensive section on generating reports in Chapter 2/Chapter 4 of this Text. You should look back at this if you were unable to generate and save as PDF files, any reports. **Make sure you check that you have saved all the reports.**

Specific guidance for each document/report is given below in **bold**.

Document and reports	Save / upload as:
Ensure you specify the correct date/date range for all reports:	**For the purpose of this practice assessment, save the documents to your desktop on your computer. In a real assessment you would also be required to upload these documents, but ignore the step of uploading for this practice assessment.**
A document showing all transactions with each customer during January 20XX **Run the 'Customer Activity' report. Run the 'Detailed' report in Sage 50. In Sage One, select all customers to obtain one report for all.**	File name = Evidence 1a – Name – AAT Number
A document showing the balance owed by each customer as at 31 January 20XX **Run the 'Aged Debtors Analysis – Detailed' report in Sage 50, or the 'Aged Debtors' report in Sage One and click the 'Detailed' button.**	File name = Evidence 1b – Name – AAT Number

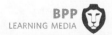

Document and reports	Save / upload as:
The following information must be evidenced within these documents: • Customer name • Account code • Payment terms **You need a separate document for payment terms – a screenshot of the Customer Record screen for each customer in Sage One. For Sage 50, you need the Credit Control screen within each Customer Record.**	Depending on your software you may need to save one or more documents. **Name these in the same way as above, continuing the sequence, eg, Evidence 1c...**
A document showing all transactions with each supplier during January 20XX **Run the 'Supplier Activity' report. Run the 'Detailed' report in Sage 50. In Sage One, select all suppliers to obtain one report for all.**	File name = **Evidence 2a – Name – AAT Number**
A document showing the balance owed to each supplier as at 31 January 20XX **Run the 'Aged Creditors Analysis – Detailed' report in Sage 50, or the 'Aged Creditors' report in Sage One and click the 'Detailed' button.**	File name = Evidence 2b – Name – AAT Number
The following information must be evidenced within these documents: • Supplier name • Account code • Payment terms You need a separate document for payment terms – a screenshot of the Supplier Record screen for each supplier in Sage One. For Sage 50, you need the Credit Control screen within each Supplier Record)	Depending on your software you may need to save one or more documents.

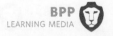

Document and reports	Save / upload as:
Audit trail, showing full details of all transactions, including details of receipts/payments allocated to items in customer/supplier accounts and details in the bank account that have been reconciled **Run the 'Audit Trail – Detailed' report.** **To show bank reconciled items:** *Sage 50 - reconciled items have an 'R' in the 'B' column of the report.* *Sage One - ensure the report is configured to include 'Bank Reconciled' column. Reconciled items have a tick in this column.* **To show receipts/payments allocated to items in customer/supplier accounts:** *Sage 50 - the report indicates the invoices that receipts/payments are allocated to, eg, '24.42 to PI 4' shows that a payment of 24.42 is allocated to purchase invoice no. 4.* *Sage One - use the Customer/Supplier Activity reports generated in 1a and 2a above. Allocated items are identified by having 0.00 in the 'Outstanding' column)*	File name = **Evidence 3 – Name – AAT Number**
Trial Balance as at 31 January 20XX **Run the 'Trial balance' report**	File name = **Evidence 4 – Name – AAT Number**

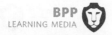

Document and reports	Save / upload as:
A screenshot of the recurring entry screen including all relevant input details. **From Task 9b** **In Sage One, take a screenshot of both the 'Other Payment' screen with the details of the first payment, and the 'Create Recurring Payment' screen with details of the recurrence.** **In Sage 50 take a screenshot of the Add/Edit recurring entry screen with details of the first payment and recurrence.**	File name = **Evidence 5 – Name – AAT Number**
A screenshot of the bank reconciliation screen showing the reconciled items. **From Task 12b** **Take a screenshot of the bank reconciliation screen just before you save the reconciliation (ie, before you click on Save button in Sage One and Reconcile button in Sage 50)**	File name = **Evidence 6 – Name – AAT Number**

BPP PRACTICE ASSESSMENT 2
Using Accounting Software

Time allowed: 2 hours

- You are now ready to attempt the BPP Practice assessment for Using Accounting Software.

- This assessment uses a standard rate of VAT of 20%.

- Answers are provided at the end of the assessment.

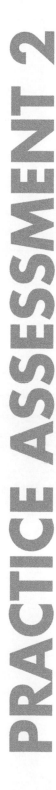

PRACTICE ASSESSMENT 2

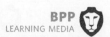

Using Accounting Software
BPP practice assessment 2

This is the old AQ2013 AAT sample assessment, adapted for the AQ2016 syllabus.

Assessment information (taken from AAT Sample Assessment)

The time allowed to complete this assessment is **2 hours.**

This assessment consists of **13 tasks** and it is important that you attempt them all.

- You will be asked to produce documents and reports to demonstrate your competence.

- You must then upload these documents so they can be marked by AAT.

All documents must be uploaded within the **total time** available. It is important that you upload **all** reports and documents specified in the tasks so your work can be assessed.

You will be able to attach and remove files throughout the duration of this assessment until you click on 'Finish', which will submit your assessment.

All uploaded documents should be saved and titled with the following information:

- Evidence number
- Your name
- Your AAT membership number

The evidence number to use for each document is stated in the table in Task 13.

Example

Your name is Simon White, and your AAT membership number is: 12345678

Evidence 1

A document showing all of the purchase invoices and credit notes (by purchase type) posted in May 20XX.

This document would be saved and uploaded as: Evidence 1 – Simon White – 12345678

If multiple documents are uploaded to show competency in an individual task, name these Evidence 1A and Evidence 1B and so on.

Unless the assessment asks for a specific format, you can choose the format which will best enable the marker to review and assess your work.

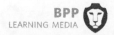
BPP
LEARNING MEDIA

During the assessment, you will only make entries to the nominal ledger accounts you created in Task 3. You will not be required to make any entries to any accounts other than those you have already created.

Information

This assessment is based on an existing business, **Campbell Kitchens**, an organisation that supplies kitchen furniture and equipment. The owner of the business is **Kitty Campbell** who operates as a sole trader. At the start of business, Kitty operated a manual bookkeeping system but has now decided that from **1 May 20XX** the accounting system will become computerised. You are employed as an accounting technician

Information relating to the business:

Business name:	Campbell Kitchens
Business address:	47 Landsway Road Stotton ST4 9TX
Business owner:	Kitty Campbell
Accounting period end:	30 April (each year)
VAT Number:	123456789 (standard scheme)
VAT rate:	Standard rate VAT of 20% charged on all sales

Sales

Kitty likes to keep a record of the different sales made by the business, by sales type:

- Kitchen furniture
- Kitchen equipment

You have been asked to carry out the bookkeeping tasks for May 20XX **only**, the first month that the business will be using computerised accounting software and the start of the new accounting period.

All documents have been checked for accuracy and have been authorised by Kitty Campbell.

Before you start the assessment you should:

- Set the system software date as **31 May of the current year**
- Set the financial year to start on **1 May of the current year**

Task 1

Refer to the customer listing below and set up customer records to open sales ledger accounts for each customer, entering opening balances at 1 May 20XX.

Customer Listing

CUSTOMER NAME AND ADDRESS	CUSTOMER ACCOUNT CODE	CUSTOMER ACCOUNT DETAILS AT 1 MAY 20XX
Fraser Designs 291 Tower Way Stotton ST7 4PQ	FRA001	Payment terms: 30 days Opening balance: £2,017.60
Fry and Partners 9 Carters Lane Brigtown BG1 3QT	FRY002	Payment terms: 30 days Opening balance: £1,597.60
SCL Interiors 14 Dingle Street Stotton ST4 2LY	SCL001	Payment terms: 30 days Opening balance: £1,906.50

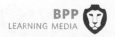

Task 2

Refer to the supplier listing below and set up supplier records to open purchases ledger accounts for each supplier, entering opening balances at 1 May 20XX.

Supplier Listing

SUPPLIER NAME AND ADDRESS	SUPPLIER ACCOUNT CODE	SUPPLIER ACCOUNT DETAILS AT 1 MAY 20XX
Hart Ltd 3 Lion Street Stotton ST8 2HX	HAR001	Payment terms: 30 days Opening balance: £1,012.75
Jackson Builders 75 Stevens Street Brigtown BG5 3PE	JAC001	Payment terms: 30 days Opening balance: £456.35
Vanstone plc 404 Larchway Estate Brigtown BG9 7HJ	VAN001	Payment terms: 30 days Opening balance: £2,097.40

Task 3

Refer to the list of **nominal ledger accounts** below:

Set up nominal ledger records for each account, entering opening balances (if applicable) at 1 May 20XX, ensuring you select, amend or create appropriate nominal ledger account codes.

Opening Trial Balance as at 01 May 20XX

ACCOUNT NAMES	Debit balance £	Credit balance £
Motor Vehicles	20,067.10	
Bank current account	4,916.26	
Petty Cash	68.24	
Sales tax control account		1,497.68
Purchase tax control account	909.23	
Capital		26,416.85
Drawings	350.00	
Sales – kitchen furniture		456.20
Sales – kitchen equipment		119.30
Goods for re-sale	224.00	
Sales ledger control* (see note below)	5,521.70	
Purchases ledger control* (see note below)		3,566.50
Bank interest received		NIL
Bank charges	NIL	
	32,056.53	**32,056.53**

* Note. As you have already entered opening balances for customers and suppliers, the software package you are using may not require you to enter these balances.

In the rest of the assessment, you will only make entries to the nominal ledger accounts you created in Task 3. You will not be required to make any entries to any accounts other than those you have already created.

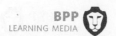

Task 4

Refer to the following summary of sales invoices and summary of sales credit notes and enter these transactions into the accounting software, ensuring you enter all the information below and select the correct sales account code.

Summary of sales invoices

Date 20XX	Customer name	Invoice number	Gross £	VAT £	Net £	Kitchen furniture £	Kitchen equipment £
7 May	Fry and Partners	523	2,011.68	335.28	1,676.40	1,676.40	
21 May	Fraser Designs	524	852.24	142.04	710.20		710.20
23 May	SCL Interiors	525	1,499.00	249.83	1,249.17	1,249.17	
27 May	Fry and Partners	526	535.40	89.23	446.17	446.17	
	Totals		4,898.32	816.38	4,081.94	3,371.74	710.20

Summary of sales credit notes

Date 20XX	Customer name	Credit note number	Gross £	VAT £	Net £	Kitchen furniture £	Kitchen equipment £
14 May	Fry and Partners	61*	500.16	83.36	416.80	416.80	
	Totals		500.16	83.36	416.80	416.80	0.00

* The credit note relates to some items that make up the opening balance of Fry and Partners at 1 May 20XX.

....

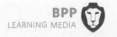

Task 5

Refer to the following purchase invoices and the purchases credit note and enter these transactions into the accounting software, ensuring you enter all the information below and select the correct purchases code.

Purchase invoices

<table>
<tr><td colspan="2" align="center">**Jackson Builders**
75 Steven Street, Brigtown, BG5 3PE
VAT Registration No 321 3726 89

INVOICE NO 5/219

Date: 12 May 20XX</td></tr>
<tr><td colspan="2">Campbell Kitchens
47 Landsway Road
Stotton
ST4 9TX</td></tr>
<tr><td></td><td align="right">£</td></tr>
<tr><td>Repairs to building</td><td align="right">909.25</td></tr>
<tr><td>VAT @ 20%</td><td align="right">181.85</td></tr>
<tr><td>Total for payment</td><td align="right">1,091.10</td></tr>
<tr><td colspan="2" align="center">**Terms: 30 days**</td></tr>
</table>

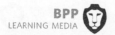

Vanstone plc
404 Larchway Estate, Brigtown, BG9 7HJ
VAT Registration No 119 0799 52

INVOICE NO 2017

Date: 18 May 20XX

Campbell Kitchens
47 Landsway Road
Stotton
ST4 9TX

	£
Supplying goods for re-sale	2,146.80
VAT @ 20%	429.36
Total for payment	2,576.16

Terms: 30 days

Purchase credit note

Vanstone plc
404 Larchway Estate, Brigtown, BG9 7HJ
VAT Registration No 119 0799 52

CREDIT NOTE NO 426

Linked to INVOICE NO 417

Date: 20 May 20XX

Campbell Kitchens
47 Landsway Road
Stotton
ST4 9TX

	£
Return of goods supplied for re-sale	612.75
VAT @ 20%	122.55
Total for payment	735.30

Terms: 30 days

Task 6a

Refer to the following cash sales listing and enter these into the accounting software.

Date	Payment method	Details	Amount
5 May 20XX	Cheque	A Davis – kitchen equipment	£375 including VAT
12 May 20XXX	Cash	P Kowalksi – kitchen furniture	£120 including VAT
17 May 20XX	Cash	M Ahmed - kitchen equipment	£74 including VAT
24 May 20XX	Cheque	JL Green – kitchen equipment	£474 including VAT

Task 6b

Refer to the following email from Kitty Campbell and enter this transaction into the accounting software.

Email
From: Kitty Campbell **To:** Accounting Technician **Date:** 10 May 20XX **Subject:** Premises insurance
Hello I have today paid our annual premises insurance of £819.40 by business debit card. Please record this transaction. VAT is not applicable. Thanks, Kitty

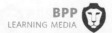

Task 7

Refer to the following BACS remittance advice notes received from customers and enter these transactions into the accounting software, ensuring you allocate all amounts as stated on each remittance advice note.

SCL Interiors
BACS Remittance Advice

To: Campbell Kitchens   15 May 20XX

An amount of £1,906.50 has been paid directly into your bank account in payment of the balance outstanding at 1 May.

Fry and Partners
BACS Remittance Advice

To: Campbell Kitchens   25 May 20XX

An amount of £1,097.44 has been paid directly into your bank account in payment of the balance outstanding at 1 May and including credit note 61.

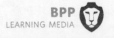

Task 8

Refer to the following summary of cheque payments made to suppliers. Enter these transactions into the accounting software, ensuring you allocate (where applicable) all amounts shown in the details column.

Cheques paid listing

Date 20XX	Cheque number	Supplier	£	Details
12 May	006723	Vanstone plc	1,200.00	Payment on account
24 May	006724	Hart Ltd	1,012.75	Payment of opening balance
31 May	006725	Jackson Builders	456.35	Payment of opening balance

Task 9

Refer to the following standing order schedule and:

(a) set up a recurring entry for rent standing order schedule below.

(b) save a screen shot of the screen, setting up the recurring entry prior to processing. You will be provided with required evidence number for this in Task 13.

(c) process the first payment.

Standing order schedule

Details	Amount	Frequency of payment	Total no. of payments	Payment start date 20XX	Payment finish date 20XX
Rent – VAT N/A	£750	One payment every 2 months	3	2 May	2 September

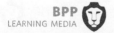

Task 10

(a) Refer to the following petty cash vouchers and enter these into the accounting software.

<table>
<tr><th colspan="2">Petty Cash Reimbursement
PCR No 29</th></tr>
<tr><td>Date: 1 May 20XX

Cash from the bank account to restore the petty cash account to £150.00.</td><td>£81.76</td></tr>
</table>

(b) Refer to the following petty cash vouchers and enter these transactions into the computer.

<table>
<tr><th colspan="2">Petty Cash Voucher</th></tr>
<tr><td>Date   7 May 20XX
PC212</td><td>**No**</td></tr>
<tr><td>Printer paper – including VAT

Receipt attached</td><td>£
45.60</td></tr>
</table>

<table>
<tr><th colspan="2">Petty Cash Voucher</th></tr>
<tr><td>Date   18 May 20XX
PC213</td><td>**No**</td></tr>
<tr><td>Rail fare

VAT not applicable

Receipt attached</td><td>£
37.90</td></tr>
</table>

Task 11

Refer to the following journal entries and enter them into the accounting software.

JOURNAL ENTRIES – 24 May 20XX	£	£
Premises insurance	10.00	
Bank		10.00
Being an error in the amount shown on Kitty Campbell's email of 10 May for premises insurance		

JOURNAL ENTRIES – 24 May 20XX	£	£
Drawings	600.00	
Bank		600.00
Being cash withdrawn from the bank by Kitty Campbell for personal use		

Task 12

Refer to the following bank statement. Using the accounting software and the transactions you have already posted:

(a) Enter any additional items on the bank statement that have yet to be recorded, into the accounting software (ignore VAT on any of these transactions).

(b) Reconcile the bank statement. If the bank statement does not reconcile, check your work and make the necessary corrections.

(c) Save a screenshot of the bank reconciliation screen. You will be provided with the required evidence number for this in Task 13.

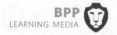

Rowley Bank plc
505 High Street
Stotton
ST1 9VG

Campbell Kitchens
47 Landsway Road
Stotton
ST4 9TX

Account number 62082176   31 May 20XX

STATEMENT OF ACCOUNT

Date 20XX	Details	Paid out £	Paid in £	Balance £
01 May	Opening balance			4,916.26C
01 May	Cash	81.76		4,834.50C
02 May	James Holdings Ltd – Rent	750.00		4,084.50C
05 May	Counter credit		375.00	4,459.50C
10 May	FH Insurance plc	829.40		3,630.10C
12 May	Cheque 006723	1,200.00		2,430.10C
12 May	Counter credit		120.00	2,550.10C
15 May	BACS – SCL Interiors		1,906.50	4,456.60C
17 May	Counter credit		74.00	4,530.60C
24 May	Cash withdrawn	600.00		3,930.60C
25 May	BACS – Fry and Partners		1,097.44	5,028.04C
28 May	Bank interest received		24.20	5,052.24C
30 May	Counter credit		474.00	5,526.24C
29 May	Bank charges	15.00		5,511.24C
	D = Debit C = Credit			

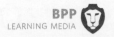

Task 13

Documentation of evidence

You are now required to generate the following documents to demonstrate your competence:

Document and reports	Save/upload as:
A document showing all customer invoices during May 20XX	File name = Evidence 1a – Name – AAT Number
A document showing the balance owed by each customer as at 31 May 20XX	File name = Evidence 1b – Name – AAT Number
The following information must be evidenced within these documents: • Customer name • Account code • Payment terms	Depending on your software you may need to save one or more documents.
A document showing all supplier invoices during May 20XX	File name = Evidence 2a – Name – AAT Number
A document showing the balance owed to each supplier as at 31 May 20XX	File name = Evidence 2b – Name – AAT Number
The following information must be evidenced within these documents: • Supplier name • Account code • Payment terms	Depending on your software you may need to save one or more documents.
Audit trail, showing full details of all transactions, including details of receipts/payments allocated to items in customer/supplier accounts and details in the bank account that have been reconciled .	File name = Evidence 3 – Name – AAT Number
Trial Balance as at 31 May 20XX	File name = Evidence 4 – Name – AAT Number

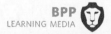

273

Document and reports	Save/upload as:
A screenshot of the recurring entry screen including all relevant input details.	File name = Evidence 5 – Name – AAT Number
A screenshot of the bank reconciliation screen showing the reconciled items.	File name = Evidence 6 – Name – AAT Number

BPP PRACTICE ASSESSMENT 2
Using Accounting Software

ANSWERS

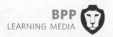

Using Accounting Software
BPP practice assessment 2

Some answers are given below, although these are not exhaustive. The answers provided are indicative of relevant content within the audit trail, the exact format of which will differ according to the computerised accounting package used.

Task	Transaction type	Account(s)	Date 20XX	Net Amount £	VAT £	Allocated against receipt/ payment ✓	Reconciled with bank statement ✓
1	Customer O/bal	FRA001	01 May	2,017.60			
	Customer O/bal	FRY002	01 May	1,597.60		✓	
	Customer O/bal	SCL001	01 May	1,906.50		✓	
2	Supplier O/bal	HAR001	01 May	1,012.75		✓	
	Supplier O/bal	JAC001	01 May	456.35			
	Supplier O/bal	VAN001	01 May	2,097.40			
3	Debit	Motor vehicles	01 May	20,067.10			
	Debit	Bank current account	01 May	4,916.26			✓
	Debit	Petty cash	01 May	68.24			
	Credit	VAT on sales	01 May	1,497.68			
	Debit	VAT on purchases	01 May	909.23			
	Credit	Capital	01 May	26,416.85			
	Debit	Drawings	01 May	350.00			
	Credit	Sales – kitchen furniture	01 May	456.20			
	Credit	Sales – kitchen equipment	01 May	119.30			
	Debit	Goods for re-sale	01 May	224.00			
	Debit	Sales ledger control*	01 May	5,521.70			
	Credit	Purchases ledger control*	01 May	3,566.50			
		*If appropriate					

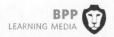

Task	Transaction type	Account(s)		Date 20XX	Net Amount £	VAT £	Allocated against receipt/ payment ✓	Reconciled with bank statement ✓
4	Sales inv	FRY002	Sales – Kitchen furniture	07 May	1,676.40	335.28		
	Sales inv	FRA001	Sales – Kitchen equip	21 May	710.20	142.04		
	Sales inv	SCL001	Sales – Kitchen furniture	23 May	1,249.17	249.83		
	Sales inv	FRY002	Sales – Kitchen furniture	27 May	446.17	89.23		
	Sales CN	FRY002	Sales – Kitchen furniture	14 May	416.80	83.36	✓	
5	Purchases inv	JAC001	Repairs	12 May	909.25	181.85		
	Purchases inv	VAN001	Goods	18 May	2,146.80	429.36		
	Purchases CN	VAN001	Goods	20 May	612.75	122.55		
6a	Bank receipt (Other receipt in Sage One)	Bank	Sales – Kitchen equip	5 May	312.50	62.50		✓
	Bank/Other receipt	Bank	Sales – Kitchen furniture	12 May	100.00	20.00		✓
	Bank/Other receipt	Bank	Sales – Kitchen equip	17 May	61.67	12.33		✓
	Bank/Other receipt	Bank	Sales – Kitchen equip	24 May	395.00	79.00		✓
6b	Bank payment	Bank	Premises insurance	10 May	819.40			✓
7	Customer receipt	SCL001	Bank	15 May	1906.50			✓
	Customer receipt	FRY002	Bank	25 May	1097.44			✓
8	Supplier payment on a/c	VAN001	Bank	12 May	1,200.00			✓
	Supplier payment	HAR001	Bank	24 May	1,012.75			
	Supplier payment	JAC001	Bank	27 May	456.35			
9	Bank payment	Bank	Rent – SO/DD	02 May	750.00			✓

Task	Transaction type	Account(s)		Date 20XX	Net Amount £	VAT £	Allocated against receipt/ payment ✓	Reconciled with bank statement ✓
10	Dr	Petty cash		01 May	81.76			
	Cr	Bank		01 May	81.76			✓
	Cash payment	Petty cash	Stationery	07 May	38.00	7.60		
	Cash payment	Petty cash	Travel	18 May	37.90			
11	Journal debit	Insurance		24 May	10.00			
	Journal credit	Bank		24 May	10.00			✓
	Journal debit	Drawings		24 May	600.00			
	Journal credit	Bank		24 May	600.00			✓
12	Bank/Other receipt	Bank	Bank interest received	28 May	24.20			✓
	Bank/Other payment	Bank	Bank charges	28 May	15.00			✓

Additional guidance for individual tasks

If you struggled with the assessment, we suggest you read the guidance below and attempt the assessment again. Note that when we refer to 'Sage' in this section, this covers both Sage 50 and Sage One, unless otherwise stated.

Task 1 (guidance)

All customers listed should be set up. Be careful to set them up as customers rather than suppliers. Enter the dates and opening balances carefully, as you will lose marks for inaccuracies. In Sage, when you enter the opening balances for customers, this creates a **debit to the sales ledger account** and a **credit to a suspense account**. When you enter either a debit or credit in each of Tasks 1 to 3 using the opening balance options within Sage, the opposite side of the entry will be posted to a suspense account. However, as the debits and credits you are given in the assessment are equal, the debits and credits to the suspense account will cancel each other off to a nil value, **if you have entered all opening balances correctly.** If you are left with a suspense account balance, then you will have made a mistake while entering the balances.

Note that if you are using Sage One, you need to enter the opening balance date as **30 April 20XX** as the program requires it to be one day before the accounts start date. Other programs, including Sage 50, may allow you to enter the opening balance date as 1 May 20XX.

▪▪

Task 2 (guidance)

It is important that you set up all **suppliers** listed and that you set them up as suppliers, rather than customers. Enter the dates and opening balances carefully and check that all of your entries match the information you have been given.

Note that if you are using Sage One, you need to enter the opening balance date as **30 April 20XX,** as the program requires it to be one day before the accounts start date. Other programs, including Sage 50, may allow you to enter the opening balance date as 1 May 20XX.

Task 3 (guidance)

Most of these accounts will already be on Sage, so you just need to enter the opening balances for these. However, for some accounts, you will need to either create new accounts or amend the names of existing accounts.

Be careful when entering the balances and selecting the appropriate nominal accounts to make entries to.

When you have finished entering the data, check you have not missed any accounts by previewing a trial balance. Remember – if you have a balance on the suspense account, then you have entered something incorrectly.

Note that if you are using Sage One, you need to enter the opening balance date as **30 April 20XX** as the program requires it to be one day before the accounts start date. Other programs, including Sage 50, may allow you to enter the opening balance date as 1 May 20XX.

Task 4 (guidance)

Both invoices and the credit note in the listings need to be entered carefully, ensuring you don't enter the credit note as an invoice, as you will be in the habit of posting invoices by the time you get to it. It is very important to select the correct nominal account if you want to score well in this task. Always check you have entered **all** of the transactions.

Task 5 (guidance)

When posting purchase invoices/credit notes, make sure you select the right supplier and an appropriate nominal account. Make sure you have accounted for the VAT properly too. Always check you have entered **all** of the transactions.

Task 6a and 6b (guidance)

This task requires you to process payments and receipts that are not related to credit transactions with customers or suppliers. You should use the Other Payment/Other Receipt function in Sage One or the Bank Payment/Bank Receipt function in Sage 50.

Ensure you use the right way of accounting for VAT for cash sales. You are only given the gross amount. Therefore, in Sage One, you should enter the gross amount, and the program will automatically calculate and post the VAT. In Sage 50, although it may seem odd, firstly enter the gross amount in the Net field. Then press F9 and the program will automatically calculate the net amount.

As always, the choice of nominal account is important. Be careful not to omit any payments or receipts.

Tasks 7 and 8 (guidance)

When entering supplier payments or customer receipts using Sage, you should use the **Supplier Payment** or **Customer Receipt** functions (not the Bank Payment or Bank Receipt functions (Other Payment/Other Receipt functions in Sage One) as demonstrated earlier in this Text. You should find this makes it easy to allocate the payment/receipt to the correct supplier/ customer account. Don't miss out any transactions.

Task 9 (guidance)

Recurring payments are a bit tricky in Sage 50 – when you first enter the details, they do not impact on the nominal ledger. When you go back into Recurring items in Sage 50 to process the payment, remember **you only need to process the first payment.**

For Sage One however, the process is a bit different. You create and post the first payment using the **Other Payment** function. You then go back into the payment to set up the recurrence.

Details on how to do this were covered in Chapter 2/Chapter 4 of this Text.

Note that you are required to take a screen print in this task and you can do this by pressing **Print Screen** or **PrtScn (or PrtSc)**.

In Sage One, take a screenshot of both the 'Other Payment' screen with the details of the first payment, and the 'Make Recurring' screen with details of the recurrence.

In Sage 50 take a screenshot of the Add/Edit recurring entry screen with details of the first payment and recurrence.

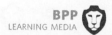

Task 10 (guidance)

You must remember to change the nominal code in Sage 50 to the Petty Cash (called 'Cash' in Sage One) nominal code when entering the payments in this task.

You can use the **Bank Transfer** button in Sage for the payment from the Bank current account to the Petty cash account.

Task 11 (guidance)

Enter journals carefully to ensure you debit and credit the correct accounts. Don't get the debits and credits mixed up.

Task 12 (guidance)

Having entered the bank charges and bank interest received, you should reconcile the bank using the method covered in Chapter 2/Chapter 4.

In the answer provided, you can see which items you should have reconciled as they appear in the 'Matched transactions' section in the bottom half of the bank reconciliation screen in Sage 50. In Sage One, the reconciled items have a tick in 'Reconciled' column in the bank reconciliation screen.

Take a screenshot of the bank reconciliation screen just before you save the reconciliation (ie, before you click on Save button in Sage One, or the 'Reconcile' button in Sage 50).

Task 13 (guidance)

This task tests your ability to generate the reports specified. You will get the marks available for this particular task by **generating the correct report**. You will receive these marks even if some of the transactions within the report are incorrect because you entered them incorrectly in earlier tasks.

There is a comprehensive section on generating reports in Chapter 2/Chapter 4 of this Text. You should look back at this if you were unable to generate and save as PDF files, any reports. **Make sure you check that you have saved all the reports**.

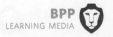

Specific guidance for each document/report is given below in **bold**.

Document and reports	Save / upload as:
Ensure you specify the correct date/date range for all reports:	**For the purpose of this practice assessment, save the documents to your desktop on your computer. In a real assessment you would also be required to upload these documents, but ignore the step of uploading for this practice assessment.**
A document showing all customer invoices during May 20XX	
Run the 'Day Books: Customer Invoices (Detailed)' report in Sage 50.	File name = Evidence 1a – Name – AAT Number
In Sage One, run the Sales Day Book report.	
A document showing the balance owed by each customer as at 31 May 20XX	
Run the 'Aged Debtors Analysis – Detailed' report in Sage 50, or the 'Aged Debtors' report in Sage One and click the 'Detailed' button.	File name = Evidence 1b – Name – AAT Number
The following information must be evidenced within these documents:	Depending on your software you may need to save one or more documents.
• Customer name • Account code • Payment terms	**Name these in the same way as above, continuing the sequence, eg, Evidence 1c...**
You need a separate document for payment terms – a screenshot of the Customer Record screen for each customer in Sage One. For Sage 50, you need the Credit Control screen within each Customer Record.	

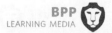

Document and reports	Save / upload as:
A document showing all supplier invoices during May 20XX **Run the 'Day Books: Supplier Invoices (Detailed)' report in Sage 50.** **In Sage One, run the 'Purchases Day Book' report.**	File name = **Evidence 2a – Name – AAT Number**
A document showing the balance owed to each supplier as at 31 May 20XX **Run the 'Aged Creditors Analysis – Detailed' report in Sage 50, or the 'Aged Creditors' report in Sage One and click the 'Detailed' button.** *The following information must be evidenced within these documents:* • Supplier name • Account code • Payment terms **You need a separate document for payment terms – a screenshot of the Supplier Record screen for each supplier in Sage One. For Sage 50, you need the Credit Control screen within each Supplier Record**	File name = **Evidence 2b – Name – AAT Number** Depending on your software you may need to save one or more documents.
Audit trail, showing full details of all transactions, including details of receipts/payments allocated to items in customer/supplier accounts and details in the bank account that have been reconciled **Run the 'Audit Trail – Detailed' report.** **To show bank reconciled items:**	File name = **Evidence 3 – Name – AAT Number**

Document and reports	Save / upload as:
Sage 50 - reconciled items have an 'R' in the 'B' column of the report. **Sage One - ensure the report is configured to include 'Bank Reconciled' column. Reconciled items have a tick in this column.** To show receipts/payments allocated to items in customer/supplier accounts: **Sage 50 - the report indicates the invoices that receipts/payments are allocated to, eg, '24.42 to PI 4' shows that a payment of 24.42 is allocated to purchase invoice no. 4.** **Sage One - use the Customer/Supplier Activity reports generated in 1a and 2a above. Allocated items are identified by having 0.00 in the 'Outstanding' column)**	
Trial Balance as at 31 May 20XX **Run the 'Trial balance' report**	File name = **Evidence 4 – Name – AAT Number**
A screenshot of the recurring entry screen including all relevant input details. **From Task 9b** **In Sage One, take a screenshot of both the 'Other Payment' screen with the details of the first payment, and the 'Create Recurring Payment' screen with details of the recurrence.** **In Sage 50 take a screenshot of the Add/Edit recurring entry screen with details of the first payment and recurrence.**	File name = **Evidence 5 – Name – AAT Number**

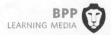

Document and reports	Save / upload as:
A screenshot of the bank reconciliation screen showing the reconciled items . **From Task 12b** **Take a screenshot of the bank reconciliation screen just before you save the reconciliation (ie, before you click on Save button in Sage One and Reconcile button in Sage 50)**	File name = **Evidence 6 – Name – AAT Number**

Index

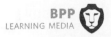

P

Payments, 50, 51, 59, 138, 139, 147
PDF, 4, 94
Petty cash, 64, 154
Print screen, 5, 94
Program date, 35, 46, 134
Purchase invoices, 36, 121
Purchases and Purchases Returns Day Books, 77

R

Receipts, 50, 51, 57, 58, 70, 138, 147
Recurring payments, 61, 151
Reports, 72, 77, 80, 159
Restore files, 10

S

Sales and Sales Returns Day Books, 77
Sales invoices, 41, 42, 127

Screenshots, 5, 94
Standing orders, 61, 151
Statements, 75, 164
Supplier, 25, 88, 111, 175
Supplier account, 26, 112
Supplier codes, 25, 111
Supplier invoices, 36, 121
Supplier payments, 51, 139
Supplier record, 88, 175
Supplier report, 74, 175

T

Tax codes, 20, 21, 46, 108, 110
Trade creditors ledger, 25, 88, 122, 175
Trade debtors ledger, 88, 111, 123, 175
Trial balance, 78, 81, 170

V

VAT, 14, 20, 21, 46, 108, 110, 134